T0210856

"This is a rare and compelling text. With captivating ease, clarity, and insight, this book inspires interest in understanding language, society and the media. Marcel Danesi is not only one of the great minds of our time, he is a wonderfully effective teacher."

Elliott Gaines, *Wright State University, USA*

"This is a welcome addition to discussion of the interlocking roles of language and the media through which it works. Students and researchers alike will be delighted to receive Marcel Danesi's thinking on the digital and web contexts that are driving, at what seems a dizzying rate, a qualitative and quantitative change in language use."

Nick Regan, *University of Bath, UK*

"Marcel Danesi provides the reader with an up-to-date and accessible account of the most recent research in sociolinguistics, linguistic anthropology, and the new media through the use of clear and comprehensible prose together with useful graphics (charts, tables, figures) that reinforce the textual material to ensure that the student has a clear grasp of the content. Exercises and discussion questions provide the user with a mechanism to demonstrate a functional and practical knowledge of the content of each section. The discussion of important new concepts such as multimodality, artificial intelligence, and language acquisition in immigrant settings address the most current research in these fields."

Frank Nuessel, *University of Louisville, USA*

"Danesi provides a compelling and informative survey of mediated language use featuring an admirable blend of inner (cognitive-psychological) and outer (socio-cultural) dynamics. The text brings ideas and methods from cognitive science, cultural studies and metaphor studies into conversation with foundational concepts in sociolinguistics and linguistic anthropology through lively prose and an abundance of vivid examples. Through the discussion of case studies and practical exercises, students and practitioners learn to be mindful of language use in historical, contemporary and cross-cultural contexts."

Jamin Pelkey, *Ryerson University, Canada*

"The third edition of this book provides a comprehensive, thorough and up-to-date discussion of language dynamics, functioning and uses. In a clear, detailed and engaging way, and from an interdisciplinary perspective, the volume offers parameters and frameworks for tracing and understanding the relationship between language, culture, communicative contexts and media."

Michele Sala, *University of Bergamo, Italy*

"One of the best texts available on the dynamics of language use and social change!"

Fletcher Ziwoya, *University of Nebraska-Kearney, USA*

"Engaging throughout, Danesi's book brings together so many topics that students might choose to neglect were it not for the writing's ability to incorporate them in a constantly appealing synthesis."

Paul Cobley, *Middlesex University, UK*

Language, Society and New Media

This book presents an interdisciplinary approach to the scientific study of the relation between language and society, language and culture, language and mind. It integrates frameworks from sociolinguistics and linguistic anthropology and emerging strands of research on language and new media, in order to demonstrate how language undergirds human thought and social behaviors. It is designed as an introductory textbook aimed at students with little to no background in linguistics. Each chapter covers the main aspects of a particular topic or area of study, while also presenting future avenues of study. This edition includes discussions on:

- social media and the creation of identity;
- gestural communication;
- emoji writing;
- multimodality;
- human–computer interaction.

Discussions are supported by a wealth of pedagogical features, including boxes, as well as activities, assignments, and a glossary at the back. The overall aim is to demonstrate the dynamic connections between language, society, thought, and culture, and how they continue to evolve in today's rapidly changing digital world. It is ideal for students in introductory courses in sociolinguistics, language and culture, and linguistic anthropology.

Marcel Danesi is Full Professor of Linguistic Anthropology and Director of the Program in Semiotics and Communication Theory at the University of Toronto, Canada. He has authored numerous books and articles on language in use and on applications of sign theory to language and culture.

Language, Society and New Media

Sociolinguistics Today

Third edition

Marcel Danesi

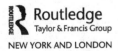
Routledge
Taylor & Francis Group

NEW YORK AND LONDON

Third edition published 2020
by Routledge
52 Vanderbilt Avenue, New York, NY 10017

and by Routledge
2 Park Square, Milton Park, Abingdon, Oxon OX14 4RN

Routledge is an imprint of the Taylor & Francis Group, an informa business

© 2020 Taylor & Francis

First edition published by Routledge 2015

Second edition published by Routledge 2017

Library of Congress Cataloging-in-Publication Data
Names: Danesi, Marcel, 1946- author.
Title: Language, society and new media : sociolinguistics today / Marcel Danesi.
Description: Third edition. | New York, NY : Routledge, 2020. | Includes bibliographical references and index. |
Identifiers: LCCN 2019054050 |
Subjects: LCSH: Mass media and language. | Socialization. | Language and culture. | Sociolinguistics.
Classification: LCC P40.5.S57 D36 2020 | DDC 302.2301/4--dc23
LC record available at https://lccn.loc.gov/2019054050

ISBN: 978-0-367-45629-0 (hbk)
ISBN: 978-0-367-46514-8 (pbk)
ISBN: 978-1-003-02942-7 (ebk)

Typeset in Sabon
by Taylor & Francis Books

Contents

Figures

Tables

Boxes

Preface

Language is a fascinating and enigmatic phenomenon. Why did it come about in the human species? What is it? What does it allow humans to do that other species cannot? The discipline that aims to investigate questions such as these is known as *linguistics*. Within this science, the particular focus on the relation between language, society, thought, and culture is known with various designations—sociolinguistics, linguistic anthropology, cultural linguistics, the sociology of language, and a few others. The purpose of this book is to introduce the formal study of this relation—a study that has become increasingly more complex in an age, designated the "global village" by the late communication theorist Marshall McLuhan, where languages, societies, and cultures are in constant contact and flux. Traditionally, sociolinguistics has aimed to document and examine the use of languages in specific societies or by particular communities and groups, focusing on how they bind people together in specific ways. Linguistic anthropology has focused instead on how languages correlate with cultural symbols, rituals, rites, and belief systems. This book will amalgamate these two main approaches, although it remains essentially an introductory text in sociolinguistics. The underlying premise that has guided the presentation of the topics and themes in each of its nine chapters is the idea that language varies according to individuals, situations, and media of communication.

This third edition has been designed to respond to the various comments made to me by both instructors and students who have used previous editions. Based on these, it retains the features of previous editions that have been found to be the most useful. The chapters have also undergone streamlining and reorganization. And some have been augmented to include topics such as meme communication and human-machine interaction.

Overall, I have attempted to make this edition more responsive to user needs. I sincerely hope that it will be a useful introduction to the fascinating and ever-broadening field of sociolinguistics. I feel privileged to have had so many students over the years who have inspired me to bring all my experiences together and to write a book that I hope will be worth reading.

Marcel Danesi
University of Toronto, 2019

Features of the Book

This textbook covers the main aspects of sociolinguistic analysis and research in an introductory fashion; it also blends themes covered more specifically in linguistic anthropology, such as the relation between language, concepts, and culture. It is intended primarily for undergraduate courses.

Each chapter contains:

1 a non-technical presentation of the main aspects of a specific topic;
2 practical examples and illustrations;
3 boxes providing further information or else explaining technical terms;
4 a reference section at the end.

The back of the book contains:

1 exercises and questions for discussion that can be done as assignments or as suggestions for further investigations;
2 appendices that provide information on technical matters such as phonetic transcription and basic statistics;
3 a glossary of technical terms.

Rapid Overview

General linguistics focuses on language as a system of internal structures (sounds, grammar, vocabulary, and so on); sociolinguistics focuses on language as a social tool, revealing how humans use it to think, act, and behave in groups. This book will introduce basic notions and describe key findings in this fascinating branch of linguistics.

Language is a highly adaptive and context-sensitive instrument that is shaped by its everyday usage—that is, its internal structures are susceptible to the subtle influences that communication has on them. Language is also a variable instrument that fluctuates across geographical and social spaces. The variants that emerge from this fluctuation are known as *dialects* and *sociolects*. Dialects arise over time as a consequence of the separation of groups from a speech community; sociolects arise instead as a result of divisions within a society, based on gender, economic class, education, and the like.

In his study of American aboriginal languages, Franz Boas discovered features that suggested to him that words served people as mental tools for coming to grips with their particular environments and social realities. This can be seen in the fact that the vocabulary of a language serves the specific classificatory and communicative needs of its speakers. For example, speakers of English have very few words for *seals* at their disposal, whereas those who live in regions such as the Arctic have developed a sophisticated vocabulary to refer to them in their native languages. English-speaking societies have instead developed an elaborate vocabulary of color terms, probably because of the social role that fashion plays within them. Boas' approach is very relevant today where new communities are cropping up online. Because of communication in the new online media, language and its uses are undergoing changes literally at the speed of light. Sociolinguistics and linguistic anthropology today are becoming evermore important in understanding how language is evolving and what the future of human communications may be like.

1 Sociolinguistics

From the dawn of history, humans have used a unique ability—*language*—to think, to classify the world, to communicate with one another beyond the instinctual use of body signals, to encode and transmit knowledge to subsequent generations, and to carry out an infinite array of intellectually sophisticated activities. Civilization is built on language. Each word is, at once, an instantiation of time-specific knowledge, an act of human consciousness, a memory capsule, and an implicit principle of cultural organization and social structure. Cumulatively, the repository of words of the world's languages constitutes humanity's collective knowledge system. The Greek philosophers saw language as a manifestation of *lógos*, which meant both "word" and "mind." Jumping forward a couple of millennia to the nineteenth century, a discipline called *linguistics* emerged to study *lógos* scientifically. Subsequently, in the twentieth century, linguists developed theoretical models, precise methods of research, and various branches of their discipline in order to answer the overall question of what language is and what it allows humans to accomplish. One of the branches is *sociolinguistics*, the investigation of the relation of language to social systems, ideas, and behaviors; another one is *linguistic anthropology* (originally called *anthropological linguistics*), the study of how language, mind, and culture interact to produce people's beliefs and worldviews. These two branches are typically considered to be separate today, even though they share a considerable domain of research interests. So, while sociolinguistics proper is the primary focus of this textbook, many aspects of linguistic anthropology will be incorporated into its overall presentation.

Humans have always been curious about language. Already in the 400s BCE, an Indian scholar named Pāṇini described the Sanskrit language he spoke with a set of about 4,000 rules. His work, called the *Ashtadhayayi*, is considered to be one of the first grammars of any language on Earth. Pāṇini showed that many words could be decomposed into smaller meaning-bearing units. In English, for example, the word *incompletely* is made up of three such units: *in* + *complete* + *ly*. Two of these (/in-/ and /-ly/) recur in the formation of other words and are thus structural units of English grammar; *complete* is, instead, a non-decomposable unit, part of a collection of units called a *lexicon*. Pāṇini also described with precision how Sanskrit words were pronounced, looking forward to the modern-day study of sound systems. Moreover, he argued that Sanskrit grammar and vocabulary provided an indirect historical record of how a particular society emerged, developed, and shaped the beliefs of its speakers.

This chapter will provide an introductory overview of what the systematic study of language, culture, and society is fundamentally about. The contemporary sociolinguist focuses on how language units such as those described by Pāṇini underlie and reveal details of social and cultural systems. The ideas presented here are discussed in a schematic way. Many of these will be developed and illustrated in subsequent chapters.

1.1 Language

Defining language is an exercise in circular reasoning, because we need words to do so, and language is, in a reductive sense, a collection of words. The English term *language* comes ultimately from the Latin word *lingua*, meaning "tongue." So, a working definition of this phenomenon is the use of the tongue and other organs to create words. But the more appropriate term for this definition is *speech*—the physical means that are (or can be) used to deliver or express language. *Language* is a faculty of the brain that is expressed as physical speech in some way.

From the dawn of history, the lengths to which some have gone to throw light on the origin of language are quite extraordinary. It is reported by the Greek historian Herodotus (c. 484–425 BCE) that in the seventh century BCE the Egyptian king Psamtik devised an "experiment" to determine the original language of humanity. The story goes that he gave two new-born babies of ordinary people to a shepherd to nurture among his flocks. The shepherd was commanded not to utter any speech before them. The children were to live by themselves in a solitary habitation. At the due hours the shepherd was instructed to bring food to them to eat, to give them their fill of milk, and to carry out all the necessary tasks to ensure their survival. After two years, the shepherd brought the babies raised in the prescribed manner before Psamtik. The first word uttered by the two sounded like *becos*—the ancient Phrygian word for "bread." The ecstatic Psamtik immediately declared Phrygian to be the mother tongue of humanity. It is unlikely that Psamtik's "experiment" ever took place. But even if it had, it certainly would not have proved anything. The babbling sounds made by the children—in probable imitation of something they had heard—were interpreted, or more accurately misinterpreted, as sounding like the word *becos* by Psamtik.

Language allows humans to refer to, and think about, objects, states, ideas, feelings, and events that are felt to be important by a particular society at a point in time. A certain kind of plant thus becomes a *tree* or a *flower*, if the given society makes these distinctions; otherwise it remains an unnamed generic plant. When we come across something for which we have no name, but which we want to identify and encode into our language in some way, then we employ several ingenious strategies—we can make up a new word, we can use paraphrases (other words) to describe it, or we can borrow a word from another language that seems to fill in the gap that exists in our own language. Language is an adaptive tool that we employ to name the world around (and within) us so that we can carry it around in our minds, so to speak, in the form of words and other structures.

Wherever there are humans living in groups, there are languages. Animals communicate with their innate signaling systems. Humans also use signals (body language and facial expressions). But verbal language is a unique evolutionary endowment. Unlike signaling systems, which tend to be stable and largely uniform across time and space, language varies and fluctuates according to where it is used and to the time period of its usage. Different languages emerge in accordance to the specific experiences and needs of the people who speak them. There is no better or worse language. All languages serve human needs equally well, no matter if the language is spoken by millions of people (like Mandarin Chinese) or a small handful (like some indigenous languages of America); and no matter if it is the main language of a nation-state or used by a small community of people. Each language allows people to solve common problems of knowledge, understanding, and social organization.

There are between 6,000 and 7,000 languages spoken in the world today. There are a little more than 200 languages with a million or more speakers. Of these, around 20 have 50 million or more. More than half of the languages spoken today are expected to disappear in the next century—a tragedy that parallels the corresponding loss of natural species and resources on earth. Diversity (biological, intellectual, linguistic, cultural) is a principle of life. If we lose linguistic-cultural diversity, we are at serious risk of losing diversity of thought, which is a critical resource for human knowledge making. Languages in danger of extinction include the indigenous ones of America (North and South), Australia, and Siberia. Preserving endangered languages is an objective of many sociolinguists and anthropologists today. Language loss (known technically as *language attrition*) is a worldwide problem.

1.1.1 Language Classification

Languages are classified in two main ways (Campbell and Poser 2008; Song 2011). One is in terms of *families*, that is, groups of languages that have split off from a common ancestor language. For example, Latin, Greek, and Sanskrit are all part of the language family called *Indo-European*, established by the fact that they share phonetic, grammatical, and vocabulary patterns that are traceable to that ancestral source. Over time, each of these produced "linguistic offspring" of its own. As a concrete example, consider the presence of certain Latin *cognates* in Italian, French, and Spanish, the linguistic offspring of Latin—cognates are words having the same linguistic root or origin (see Table 1.1).

A close examination of the cognates makes it evident that a specific pattern of phonetic correspondences exists among them. The *tt* in the Italian words corresponds to *it* in the French words and to the *ch* in Spanish words

Table 1.1 The Development of Latin Words into Italian, French, and Spanish

Latin source	Italian	French	Spanish
nocte(m)(night)	*notte*	*nuit*	*noche*
tectu(m)(roof)	*tetto*	*toit*	*techo*
lacte(m)(milk)	*latte*	*lait*	*leche*
factum(m)(fact)	*fatto*	*fait*	*hecho*

(pronounced more or less like English *ch* in the word *church*). Clearly, these correspondences are phonetic derivatives of the original Latin consonant cluster *ct* = /kt/. Many other patterns, phonetic, grammatical, and lexical, can be established among these languages. As such, they are said to belong to the same language family, known as the Romance languages. The use of cognates to determine membership in a language family is known technically as *genetic classification*. There are around 15 major language families that have been identified by using this method.

Another method is called *typological*; it involves classifying languages according to how they construct their words. *Agglutinative* or *synthetic* languages typically use so-called bound morphemes, or elements that are combined to make up words; *isolating* languages, in contrast, tend to form each word with a single morpheme. An example of a language classified as agglutinative is Turkish: the word *evlerinizden*, which means "of/from your houses" consists of four morphemes: *ev + ler + iniz + den* = "house + plural + your + from." Mandarin Chinese is classified instead as an isolating language. Its version of the same phrase, "from your houses," consists of four distinct words: *Cóng nǐ de fángzi* (从你的房子). Needless to say, there is no such thing as an exclusively agglutinative or isolating language. It is a matter of degree—of more or less.

Edward Sapir (1921) developed one of the first typological systems for classifying languages. He took into consideration both the number of morphemes used in word formation and the degree of synthesis in the formation process. For example, the English words *goodness* and *depth* are similar in that they are composed of a root morpheme (*good* and *deep*) and a suffix (*-ness* and *-th*). The word *depth*, however, shows a greater degree of synthesis, since it has evolved from a complete fusion of the root and suffix morphemes, while in the case of *goodness* the suffix is added to the root without the same type of fusion. The American linguist Joseph Greenberg (1966) further elaborated Sapir's technique, introducing the concept of "morphological index" as a means to establish the degree of synthesis mathematically. The index is calculated by taking large, representative samples of the words in a language, and then dividing the number of morphemes (M) by the number of words (W):

$$I = M \div W$$

In a perfectly isolating language, the index is equal to 1, because there would be a perfect match between number of words (W) and number of morphemes (M), or M = W. In agglutinating languages, M is greater than W. The greater it is, the higher the index, and thus the higher the degree of agglutination. The highest index Greenberg discovered with his method was 3.72 for a Native American language. He suggested that:

- languages in the 1.0–2.2 range should be classified as *analytic*
- languages in the 2.2–3.0 range should be classified as *synthetic (agglutinative)*
- languages in the 3.0 and above range should be classified as *polysynthetic*.

The main weakness in classifying languages in this way lies in the lack of a definitive criterion for determining what constitutes a word in one language or another. The typological classification of languages has, nevertheless, gained wide acceptance because of the central role of words in language structure. Generally, linguists use a combination of both genetic and typological methods to classify languages today. Although the two methods often coincide in classifying certain languages consistently, they also produce results that contrast with each other. The use of computers and algorithms to compile and organize relevant data has greatly enhanced classification efforts today.

1.1.2 Features of All Languages

All languages share a basic set features. The main ones are as follows:

1. Languages have a finite set of distinctive sound units and a finite set of grammatical units (such as /in-/ and /-ly/, seen earlier in the word *incompletely*) for constructing words; the former are called *phonemes* and the latter *morphemes*.
2. Languages have a set of rules for combining morphemes to form larger units of meaning (phrases, sentences, and texts) systematically and cohesively. These rules constitute the *syntax* of a language.
3. Languages have a set of meaning-bearing units (actual words, phrases, etc.), called a *lexicon*, that allow people to carry out intellectual, expressive, and communicative activities.
4. Languages have writing symbols (pictographs, alphabet characters) for representing words or ideas in some physical medium.
5. Languages provide the resources to coin words for referring to new objects, ideas, and events whenever they are needed. This means that languages are constantly changing and evolving along with other human expressive systems (music, drawing, art, etc.).
6. Languages allow humans to communicate with each other in specific contexts and for various personal, social, and intellectual purposes.

7   Languages permit people to encode and preserve knowledge, and thus to transmit it across generations and across geographical spaces.
8   Languages make purposeful social interaction possible, including the carrying out of rituals, interpersonal relations, and the like.
9   Languages are highly variable across time and space, splitting into variants known as dialects.

It is remarkable to note that with a small set of phonemes, a language allows people to make and use as many words, sentences, and texts as they need ad infinitum. This feature is called *double articulation*, a term introduced by the French linguist André Martinet (1955). The English word *cat*, for example, is composed of the sounds *c* = /k/, *a* = /æ/, and *t* = /t/, in that order, which are meaningless as separate sounds in themselves; they bear meaning through the specific way in which they are combined: *cat* = /kæt/. Now, the same sounds can be used in various other combinations, and with other sounds, to create different words with other meanings. For instance, the /k/ sound is found in words such as *cup, ache, act, tarmac*; /æ/ in *bat, mail, train, sane*; and /t/ in *tip, lot, tail, abstain* (see Box 1.1 for an explanation). Without the principle of double articulation, it would require a huge inventory of phonemes to create distinct words and an enormous mental effort just to remember them. In sum, the property of double articulation allows for the creation of a potentially infinite number of messages with a small repertory of phonetic resources. This is in line with an inherent "principle of least effort" in language, which can be characterized informally as "doing a lot with a little." (See Appendix A for a chart of phonetic symbols used by linguists, known as the International Phonetic Alphabet.)

Box 1.1   Phonetic and Phonemic Transcription

In linguistics, the symbols between square brackets represent speech sounds as they are actually pronounced. This is called *phonetic* transcription. Whereas spelling symbols may vary in representing the same sound, phonetic transcription does not:

[k] = in *cat, kind, quick, ache* ...
[æ] = in *bat, tail, aesthetic* ...
[t] = in *top, caught, attire* ...

Now, let's take any two sounds, such as [k] and [b], putting them in word pairs such as *cat* = [kæt] and *bat* = [bæt]. As this shows, the two sounds allow us to distinguish one word from the other. Because of this, they are called *phonemes*, and identified with slant lines: /k/ and /b/. The phoneme is defined technically as a minimal unit of sound that can distinguish one word from another in a language. This implies that /k/ can replace other consonants, such as /w/, /p/, etc. to make English words: *kin—win—pin*—etc. If we wish to refer to the actual physical pronunciation features of a phoneme, we use phonetic transcription (within square brackets). See Appendix A for a more detailed explanation.

As mentioned, language is a faculty of the brain, and speech the physical ability to produce and use language. Speech can be vocal, produced with the vocal organs (tongue, teeth, lungs, etc.), or nonvocal, as in writing, gesturing, and sign languages. The two are intrinsically intertwined, as will become obvious throughout this book.

1.1.3 Acquiring Language

Children acquire the language to which they are exposed in their everyday lives spontaneously, without any need for training. They do so by listening to samples of speech and imitating them as best they can; in a short time they start making up verbal messages on their own. By the age of 5 or 6, children demonstrate a sophisticated control of the language in which they have been reared. Remarkably, if they have been exposed to more than one language, they will acquire both to varying degrees, becoming *bilingual* speakers—a situation that is more common than one might expect, as will be discussed subsequently. The spontaneous childhood acquisition of two languages is called *primary bilingualism*. When people add another language to their linguistic repertoire, either by necessity (as in situations of immigration) or by choice (as in the learning of another language at school), it is called *secondary bilingualism*.

Vocal speech is made possible because of the lowered larynx (the muscle and cartilage at the upper end of the throat containing the vocal cords)—a feature that is unique to the human species (see Figure 1.1). At birth, the larynx is located high in the neck. Because of this, during their first months of life, infants breathe, swallow, and emit sounds in ways that are similar to other primates. At some point around the third month of life, the larynx starts to descend, gradually altering how the child will breathe and swallow. This entails a few risks—food can easily become lodged in the entrance to the larynx; and drinking and breathing simultaneously can lead to choking. In compensation, the lowered larynx permits vocal speech to emerge by leaving a chamber above the vocal cords that can modify sound. At that point, children start emitting sounds that are imitative of the words to which they are exposed.

Intrigued by the naturalness with which infants acquire language, the Greek philosopher Plato asked the following question: How it is that children, whose contacts with the world are brief and limited, are able to speak with no effort by simply being exposed to random and poor (imperfect)

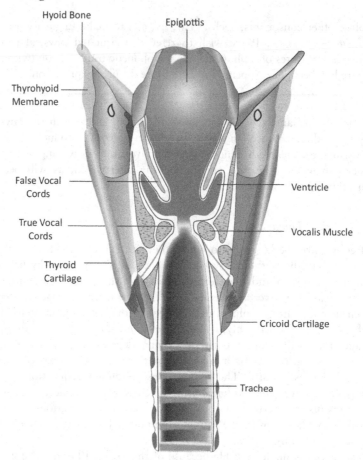

Figure 1.1 The Human Larynx

samples of a language? This is known as the *poverty of the stimulus* con-undrum, or the puzzle of why infants, who are not exposed to rich enough speech input within their environments to figure out the features of their language, still do so with little or no effort. So, Plato concluded that lan-guage is innate and thus will develop naturally as do other innate human traits. However, this does not capture the importance of the interplay between the environment in which children are reared, the creative impulses in infants, and the connection of language to other faculties. Needless to say, if nurturing is not present, then language does not emerge, as the study of "feral children"—children who have survived without normal rearing con-ditions—has dramatically shown (Curtiss 1977).

The linguist who has been influential in promoting Plato's view from a modern-day perspective is the American linguist Noam Chomsky (1975, 2000,

2002). Chomsky posits the presence of a universal grammar (UG) in the human brain. The UG, he maintains, is the blueprint from which all specific languages are built, constituting the set of rule-making principles that are available to all human infants and from which they can construct their specific grammars. When children learn one fact about the language to which they are exposed, they can easily infer other facts without having to learn them one by one. Differences in languages are thus explainable as differences in rule types within the UG, known as *parameters*. Linguist Stephen Pinker (2007) refers to the UG as a "language of thought" that endows children to infer the appropriate rules they need to produce their own particular "language of speech." Pinker suggests that the UG may be present in our genes. Seemingly in support of the possibility that language is transmitted through the genetic channel is the discovery of a gene, called FOXP2, that some believe passes on language impairments to one's offspring. But the evidence for this is not strong. Moreover, as Burling (2005: 148–149) points out, FOXP2 may not even be a specifically marked language gene:

> FOXP2 should not be considered a language gene, however. Several thousand other genes are believed to contribute to building the human brain, and a large portion of these could contribute, in one way or another, to our ability to use language. Any one of these might interfere with language if it were to mutate in a destructive way. Nor is the influence of FOXP2 confined to language or even the brain, for it is known to play a role in the embryological development of lung, heart, and intestinal issues.

Critiques like this one notwithstanding, one the main theoretical premises of UG theory is a plausible one, namely that language is part of human nature, and this is why languages are not invented *tabula rasa* with new generations of speakers (see, for example, Roberts 2017). However, creativity in this paradigm is a restricted notion—it is seen as the ability to create words and sentences in childhood by a specific utilization of the UG in particular circumstances. But this paradigm seems to ignore a different kind of creativity that involves making comparisons, associations, and analogies. For instance, if a child does not know the word for "moon" but knows the word for "ball," the child might refer to the moon as a ball. In so doing, the child has used a creative form of analogy that connects the moon to a ball via resemblance in shape. Only later, as the child learns that these two objects are labeled in different ways, does that same child start to differentiate between the moon and other round objects with distinct words. As the Russian psychologist Lev S. Vygotsky (1962) pointed out in his studies of language development, children are essentially "little poets," making analogies and inferences about the world that are similar to the verbal creations of poets. The brain is more likely to be a creative poetic organ, rather than a strictly parameter-setting one, allowing children to grasp the meaning of things through inferences, hunches, and comparisons, and then converting them into verbal structures according to the specific language forms to which they are exposed.

1.2 Field of Study

Children realize that the words they are acquiring in their environments are more than convenient labels for naming things. By later childhood, they start understanding that they can use them to bring about some action or to express needs, as well as to interact in a socially appropriate way with others. If they are reared in English-speaking cultures, they learn soon enough that if the person to whom they are talking is a superior or someone in a position of authority or of importance (such as a family physician or a school teacher) then they should address the person differently (and deferentially), perhaps using a title ("Mrs. Jones," "Mr. Smith," "Dr. Brown," and so on). In contrast, they know that it would be bizarre to address friends or close family members with titles, unless they wanted to be humorous. Children learn, in effect, that language is not only a naming device, but also a social one. The study of language as a primary means for carrying out social actions is a central goal of socio-linguistics. The first scientific studies that are recognizable as sociolinguistic in focus—apart from research on dialects and bilingualism that can be traced as far back as the early nineteenth century—emerged in the middle part of the twentieth century (Shuy 1997; Tagliamonte 2016). The American scholar Thomas Callan Hodson is sometimes identified as the first to use the term *sociolinguistics* in a 1939 article titled "Sociolinguistics in India," signaling that a new mode of inquiry was taking shape within linguistics.

Sociolinguistics can be defined as the discipline studying the social functions of language and how the units and structures of a language bear socially sensitive meanings. In Koasati (an indigenous language spoken in Louisiana), for instance, men are expected traditionally to use the word *lawawhol* to refer to the action of "lifting," whereas women are expected to use *lakawhos* (Haas 1944). Arguably, the Koasati people perceive the lifting abilities of the two genders as different and thus have historically seen a need to convey this dissimilarity through lexical differentiation. The men are probably expected to be the "heavy lifters," the women are not. Such vocabulary differences are keys to understanding how specific communities perceive gender roles and abilities (Taylor 1977; Eckert and McConnell-Ginet 2013). But there is always a doubling-back of language on the worldview of its users. Gender-based lexical dichotomies shape thought and affect behavior in subtle (and not so subtle) ways in subsequent generations of speakers, often leading to differential treatments of males and females. The same is true of racially-based, age-based, and class-based lexical forms. In sum, language both encodes social differences, wherever and whenever they are required, and in so doing shapes how these are understood. This is a basic principle of sociolinguistic theory.

1.2.1 The Birth of Linguistics

In the sixteenth and seventeenth centuries, the first systematic surveys of the known languages were attempted, in order to determine which facts (phonetic, grammatical, lexical) were universal and which were specific to each language. In the eighteenth century, the surveys became increasingly more precise, culminating in the assertion by the scholar Sir William Jones (1746–1794) that Sanskrit, Greek, and Latin developed from a common source. Shortly thereafter, the German philologist Jacob Grimm (1785–1863) and the Danish philologist Rasmus Christian Rask (1787–1832) started comparing languages systematically, noticing that in some languages the sounds in related words corresponded in regular ways. For example, they found that the initial /p/ sound of Latin *pater* ("father") and *pede(m)* ("foot") corresponded consistently to the initial /f/ sound in the English cognates *father* and *foot*. They concluded that there must be a historical link between Latin and English, traced back to Indo-European. The method of making such linkages came to be called *comparative grammar*—a term coined initially in 1808 by the German scholar Friedrich Schlegel (1772–1829). Towards the end of the nineteenth century, a group of scholars started to study how languages were constructed, developing a set of principles and analytical tools for investigating them. The Swiss philologist Ferdinand de Saussure (1857–1913) put the finishing touches to the emerging blueprint for this science by making a distinction between the study of how languages change over time, which he called *diachronic*, and the systematic study of languages at a specific point in time, which he called *synchronic*. He also proposed that the new science should focus on *langue* ("language"), the faculty of language itself (the ability shared by all humans), rather than on *parole* ("word"), or the specific use of a language in conversations, writing, and other expressive ways.

Saussure's approach came to be known as *structuralism*, a term used also in psychology and anthropology, disciplines that were coming into being at about the same time as linguistics. In Europe, structuralism was adopted and elaborated by a group of linguists who congregated in the Czech city of Prague; the group eventually came to be known as the Prague Circle in the 1920s. One of the techniques that the Circle established as basic to linguistic science was the *minimal pair*—a technique that is used to this very day. The words *cat* and *bat* constitute a minimal pair (as discussed previously); that is, they are composed of the same sequential combination of sounds except for the one in initial position. This allows the linguist to flesh out the differential sound cue, known as the phoneme (as we saw), that keeps these words distinct. In general, by analyzing minimal pairs, it is possible to identify all the phonemes in a language.

1.2.2 Sociolinguistics

Sociolinguistics is now a major branch of linguistics. As mentioned, its overarching goal is to study the relation between a language and the society (or societies) that employs it. In a reductive sense, theoretical linguistics deals with the Saussurean notion of *langue* and sociolinguistics with *parole* The range of phenomena that sociolinguists deal with today is a broad one indeed. It includes the investigation of *bilingualism* (the acquisition and use of two languages) and the related phenomenon of *code switching* (the admixture of languages in the speech of bilinguals); the study of *communicative competence* (the ability to use language to communicate purposefully), known technically as *pragmatics*, which focuses on the nature and function of *conversations* (verbal interactions of all kinds) and *discourses* (specific modes of speech to signal group membership); the investigation of *dialects* and *sociolects* (respectively the geographical and social variants of a language), as well as *diglossia* (the assignment of social prestige to linguistic variants); the study of how language encodes and, in turn, shapes social perceptions of gender, age, class, identity, ethnicity, and race.

Other areas of interest to sociolinguists include *language aesthetics* (the social functions of expressive or creative forms of language, such as poetry), *language planning* (the role of legislation and governmental policies in regulating language use), *registers* (the levels of language use that denote social distinctions), *slang* and *jargon* (forms of language that are used for group solidarity or emerge in specific kinds of speech contexts), *style* (the use of language to fit in with certain social roles or models), and *literacy* (writing traditions and their impact on a society).

The foregoing list is a partial one, although it covers the main areas of research. In general, it can be said that sociolinguistics encompasses the study of how language varies according to social context. A number of its research areas overlap with linguistic anthropology. For this reason, the two disciplines are sometimes combined into a general line of inquiry, as will be done in this textbook.

1.2.3 Linguistic Anthropology

The Prague Circle structuralists were among the first to examine the relation between internal linguistic structures (such as phonemes) and external (social) ones. A similar approach to the study of the indigenous languages of America was adopted by the anthropologist Franz Boas (1858–1942) at Columbia University, starting in the 1920s. Boas saw the objective of linguistics as understanding how groups of people developed their native languages for their particular needs and purposes. For example, in the traditional Nuer society, a herding people of eastern Africa, a sophisticated vocabulary is used for referring to the colors and markings of cattle; by the same token, the Nuer people have very few words to describe the colors of clothes. This indicates that cattle play a much more important role in traditional Nuer society than does fashion (Evans-Pritchard 1940). Modern urbanized societies, by way of contrast, have many words for clothes, because fashion has more salience than livestock does. Languages, therefore, are windows into a society's main concerns, emphases, and interpretations of the world. Boas' approach laid the foundations for *linguistic anthropology*, a branch of linguistics that is thriving today. Linguistic anthropology and sociolinguistics share many research methods and intellectual traditions, as will be illustrated throughout this book (Gumperz and Cook-Gumperz 2008).

A central tenet of linguistic anthropology is that language, mind, and culture are intrinsically intertwined—one depends synergistically on the others. This principle was explored systematically by Boas and his student Edward Sapir (1921), and then by Sapir's own student Benjamin Lee Whorf (1956). Whorf translated the tenet into an hypothesis, known alternatively as the *Linguistic Relativity Hypothesis* or the *Whorfian Hypothesis* (WH)—the view that different societies encode into their languages those concepts they feel are important and necessary to them; but these, in turn, influence how they come to perceive reality, called the doubling-back effect referred to earlier (Miller 1968; Mathiot 1979; Niyaz 2017). This does not, however, block mutual understanding among speakers of different languages, because analogies, metaphors, paraphrases, and other strategies can always be used to explain the specific perceptions encoded by a society's lexicon or grammar.

The WH will be discussed in more detail in subsequent chapters, since it is somewhat controversial (McWhorter 2016). Suffice it to say here that in its generic form it posits that languages predispose speakers to attend to certain concepts as being necessary, even though it may not necessarily shape perception per se. This means that we encode into language whatever we need to make sense of the world in which we live and that this doubles back on us, shaping how we habitually see that world. For example, before the advent of cellphones and mobile phones, no word existed for taking self-portrait photographs, although this was nonetheless carried out in various ways such as with the use of tripods. When self-portraiture became easy to do with the new devices, a word for it was coined—the *selfie*, which is often ascribed to an Australian man named Nathan Hope, when he shared a photo of his busted lip in 2002 on his forum post, having taken the picture by himself. The word gained global usage and was named the Word of the Year in 2013 by the *Oxford Dictionary*. Hope has claimed that he did not really coin the word; it was around in urban slang. Whatever the case, *selfie* fit in perfectly with a new reality, where the meanings of *self* and *selfie* may have merged cognitively, leading to the designation of *selfie culture*, whose impact on society has been acknowledged by various sources, including *the Guardian*, which produced a film series titled *Thinkfluencer* in 2013 that explored the implications of this culture. There was even a short-lived sitcom in 2014 on ABC, titled *Selfie*, which revolved around a woman who was obsessed with gaining fame through the selfies she posted on Instagram. She ended up discovering, in true cautionary tale tradition, that this whole new trend was meaningless and alienating.

When we name something, we are not simply identifying it as something important or useful to us; we are also connecting it to social trends and social evolutionary tendencies. What we name is not only a record of its existence, but also of its effects on us.

1.3 Methodology

Each science has its particular procedures, techniques, and research methods for gathering relevant information and data. Sociolinguistics does as well, and like other sciences, it is constantly revising and revamping them to meet new conditions. Both sociolinguistics and linguistic anthropology utilize the method of *ethnography*, or the systematic observation and annotation of how people use language in specific contexts. Sociolinguistics also utilizes quantitatively based techniques such as interviews and case studies—both of which are common methods in other social sciences. In a phrase, the methodology of sociolinguistics is eclectic and wide ranging.

American linguist William Labov is regarded as the founder of contemporary sociolinguistics, with his classic studies on the social implications of pronunciation differences that started in the 1960s (Labov 1963, 1967, 1972). Labov made audio recordings of conversations of New York City residents of different ethnic and social backgrounds. One of the features that stood out in the collected data was the perceptions people had with regard to the pronunciation of /r/ after vowels in words such as *bird, tired, beer*, and *car*. An "/r/-less" pronunciation was felt to be prestigious in the past, modeled after British English. However, after World War I the prestige declined, quickly becoming an old-fashioned way of pronouncing words. Labov's study confirmed this, recording the highest occurrence of the pronunciation of /r/ in young people, aged 8 to 19.

He also discovered that people aspiring to move from a lower class status to a higher one attached great prestige to the way in which the /r/ was pronounced. He chose as his subjects employees working at three stores in New York City in order of prestige at the time: Saks Fifth Avenue, Macy's, and S. Klein. He found that the rates of pronunciation of /r/ were highest in Saks, less in Macy's, and lowest in S. Klein. Labov concluded that workers in these stores identified with the prestige of their employers and customers and that this identification influenced their pronunciation habits. In other words, he established that the phonemic system of a language is hardly an abstract one; it correlates directly with social perceptions and aspirations of social mobility.

1.3.1 *Interviews*

To collect the data he required, Labov conducted interviews and then analyzed the data with statistics. The fusion of statistical and interview techniques is common in sociolinguistic methodology (Milroy and Gordon 2003; Tagliamonte 2006; Chambers 2010). Labov's research was preceded by the fascinating work of John Fischer in 1958, who used an interactive conversational technique to gather data. Fischer would talk with a group of elementary schoolchildren, finding that they often alternated between two verb suffixes, formal /-ing/ versus informal /-in/ (as in *reading* versus *readin'*). The choice, Fischer realized, was not random; it varied initially according to the gender, social class, personality, and mood of the speakers. If they were girls, if they came from families with an above average income, if they had dominating or assertive personalities, or if they were tense, the children tended to use the more formal /-ing/ ending. As the interviews progressed, however, the children became more relaxed and were more likely to use the informal /-in/ suffix, no matter their gender, social class, or family income. In other words, Fischer's study brought out the fact that speakers of a language are sensitive both to the context in which it is used and to the perceptions associated with such use (conscious or unconscious).

Research projects like the ones carried out by Fischer and Labov continue to characterize sociolinguistics generally. In order to assay how a specific linguistic form is used and what it tells us about its relation to some social behavior the researcher chooses subjects (informants) that are part of a specific target group. The basic idea is to craft questions that are designed to produce the information required in an unobtrusive manner (Briggs 1986). The interview may be done person-to-person, by telephone, emails, or via social media.

In order to collect authentic speech data, the sociolinguist must get subjects to talk spontaneously, given that interviews might engender stress in people, causing their speech to become more guarded and cautious than it would otherwise be in natural conversations. This was called the "observer's paradox" by Labov. The main way around the paradox is to create questions and a style of interviewing that simulates casual or relaxed conversations. Elicitation tasks should also be constructed to be straightforward and congenial: "What would you call this in your language?" "How would you pronounce this word?"

The specific set of questions will depend on the researcher and the project, but, typically, it would involve comparing a social variable (age, gender, race, class, region) with a specific aspect of language (a phoneme, morpheme, phrase) or communication strategy (honorifics, politeness). The interview sessions are recorded and are afterwards analyzed in various ways, such as counting the frequency of a feature and then assessing it statistically. Today, there are apps and appropriate software that can do this kind of analysis rapidly. Moreover, interviewing has also migrated to cyberspace, so that today online interviews are common and used in tandem with, or separately from, face-to-face interviews. Overall, the sociolinguistic interview, which is typically structured in a loose way, is guided by a few general principles that are worth paraphrasing here:

1   The one-to-one interview should be as casual, conversational, and informal as possible; Labov called this the *vernacular principle*, a technique aiming both to make the subject feel at ease and to deflect the subject's conscious attention away from the speech samples that the interview is designed to elicit.

2   The interview questions should focus on the relevant topics, which should be inserted spontaneously into the flow of the conversation as it unfolds.

3   The subjects should always be encouraged to talk as long as they desire on any of the topics that particularly interests them, even if they digress somewhat from the main topic.

4   The interview should include a series of tasks that bring the topic at hand into sharp focus, such as a reading passage, a relevant word list, or a list of minimal pairs. In the above study on the pronunciation of /r/, Labov used minimal pairs such as *sauce—source* in order to identify the pronunciation features of his subjects, simply asking them how they would pronounce each item in the pair.

5   Researchers should always strive to make the subject feel in control, rather than the other way around. So, the reading tasks used should be consistent with what is known about the interests of the subject.

6   If need be, peer pairs or groups, rather than individual subjects, should be used to attenuate any sense of discomfort individuals might have.

7   Sometimes self-recordings, rather than formal interview sessions, might be required, allowing subjects to make relevant commentaries as they go about their daily routines in a variety of settings.

8   A combination of the one-to-one with other types of interviewing formats may be required for a specific research project.

1.3.2 Fieldwork

Fieldwork is conducted in a natural social environment or in a specific context, rather than in an artificial way such as, for example, in a laboratory or other formal setting. Labov conducted his fieldwork by going to the three stores, as mentioned, and interviewing workers in those stores in a conversational style. Fieldwork allows for relevant information to be gathered through observation, interviews, and conversations with subjects. It may also involve participating in a variety of social functions and activities with the subjects during the period of study. This allows a linguist to observe linguistic features as they relate to various social functions. These are then collected in a report called a *case study*. This helps the linguist deconstruct the complex verbal patterns and activities observed and recorded during the fieldwork stage.

The first to establish fieldwork as the main procedure in linguistic research was Boas (mentioned earlier). But even before Boas, dialectologists (linguists who specialize in the study of dialects) used surveys to collect speech data in order to create dialect atlases, collections of maps that display the linguistic features used in specific regions. The first survey was carried out in 1876 in Germany by a linguist named Georg Wenker (1852–1911). Wenker sent a list of sentences written in Standard German to schoolteachers in northern Germany, asking them to return the list with each word transcribed phonetically into their local dialects. By the end of the project, he had compiled over 45,000 questionnaires. Wenker then produced two sets of maps, with each one highlighting a single feature. The maps were bound together under the title *Sprachatlas des Deutschen Reichs*.

The method used by Wenker remains a point-of-reference for conducting dialect surveys to this day, although the fieldwork procedure for gathering the data has, of course, changed. Dialectologists now send trained observers into the designated region(s) to conduct and record interviews or else they use online and social media to carry out surveys.

1.3.3 Ethnography

Ethnography also started with Boas (1920). Since then, it has become a fundamental method of research in both linguistic anthropology and sociolinguistics. Ethnographers gather the relevant information by living among a group of people, observing their communication habits, questioning them when appropriate, and then annotating their observations through diary entries, occasional jottings, and daily logs. Afterwards, they collate these into formal field notes. Ethnography requires sensitivity to others and this entails, above all else, treating them as individuals, not as mere "subjects." Actually, *ethnology* is the term used more specifically to refer to the method of data gathering itself, and *ethnography* to the technique of writing down one's observations. In practice, however, only the latter term is used to refer to both (Hymes 1964) (see Box 1.2).

Three classic anthropological ethnographies are Bronislaw Malinowski's *Argonauts of the Western Pacific* (1922), E. E. Evans-Pritchard's *The Nuer* (1940), and Boas' book on the Kwakiutl (1940), a native society on the northwestern coast of North America. Through ethnography, Boas was able to observe firsthand how the grammar and vocabulary of the Kwakiutl language served the specific needs of its speakers, providing them with the resources for talking about their particular world in culturally relevant ways, making social interaction fluid and meaningful. The language also revealed the particular worldview that the Kwakiutl espoused, which was based on a sense of connection to the land and to each other as equal beings. Norman K. Denzin (1996) provides a list of useful principles and procedures that define ethnographic research, including the following four:

1   All behaviors and practices should be considered equal and recorded unselectively.
2   Symbolic and ritualistic practices should be tied to patterns of interaction and communication.
3   The viewpoints of the people should be prioritized, although a distinction between these and the ethnographer's technical annotations should be maintained.
4   Casual explanations (and personal judgments) should be avoided.

Box 1.2 Ethnography and Ethnology

Ethnology is the method of living among groups of people and interacting with them spontaneously, so as to gain insights about them as collectivities.

Ethnography refers more specifically to the annotation of such insights as a set of observations. However, this term is used more generally to include ethnology as well.

The ethnographer's main goal is to observe and describe language in its everyday social contexts and to elicit people's explanations for how words, symbols, and rituals overlap. By looking at the world through the eyes of the "Other," the ethnographer aims to enrich and deepen our understanding of human nature, without any bias or prejudicial perspective. Grasping the worldview of the "Other" with reverence is the ultimate goal of ethnography.

1.3.4 Data Collection

To gather data on language use today, especially in online venues, techniques such as data mining are becoming common. These will be discussed in more detail in Chapter 9. Suffice it to say here that there are commonly available softwares that allow for data collection, data processing, information searching, data classification, etc., making it possible to quantify information and use it for various purposes, such as pinpointing preferences on websites by users. The relevant techniques include the automatic grouping of documents or files, categorizing them into rubrics that are relevant to the research objective, and analyzing patterns and interrelationships within them.

One particular type of AI software, called an expert system, enables a computer to ask questions and respond to information the answers provide, thus allowing the analyst to assess the information required in a pre-organized way. The computer can narrow the field of inquiry until a potential solution or viable theory is reached. However, if the rules and data available to the system are incomplete, the computer will not yield the best possible solution.

1.3.5 Statistics

In the mid-1700s, the word *Statistik* came to be used in German universities to describe a systematic mathematical comparison of data about different nations. Given the demonstrated efficacy of the technique, statistics was quickly adopted by the emerging psychological and social sciences in the subsequent century and has since become a primary analytical tool of these sciences. The first task in statistical analysis is to organize the information gathered from interviews or fieldwork, according to frequency or recurrence.

Sociolinguistic research projects are often guided initially by principles of statistical design. As difficult as these may seem to those entering into this field, the basic concepts of statistics are actually straightforward and, nowadays, can be easily applied to a case study with the use of appropriate software. Nonetheless, some basic understanding of these principles is useful, because the two main aspects of sociolinguistic research—ethnography and interviewing—must inform one another in the overall design of a project, otherwise one ends up gathering tidbits of information that may be interesting in themselves but are otherwise of little overall theoretical or scientific value. Basic relevant statistical notions and ideas are found in Appendix B. A good detailed and comprehensive treatment can be found in Tagliamonte (2006).

1.4 Merging Sociolinguistics and Linguistic Anthropology

As mentioned several times, sociolinguistics and linguistic anthropology share much common ground, theoretically and methodologically. The two branches are considered to constitute a singular paradigm in this book—the former provides the analytical tools for describing social phenomena as they manifest themselves through specific language structures and uses, while the latter allows us to hone in on how these structures reveal worldview and cultural emphases. Neither treats the various subsystems of language (phonemic, grammatical, lexical, etc.) as autonomous phenomena, to be studied in and of themselves, but in relation to cognition, culture, and the social systems that they undergird. Through his in-depth study of the Hopi language of the southwestern US, Whorf posited, in essence, that the categories of one's particular language are much more than simple mediators of thought. He saw them as the "shapers" of the very thought patterns they embodied, constituting both social strategies and cultural filters of perception: "The world is presented in a kaleidoscopic flux of impressions which has to be organized by our minds—and this means largely by the linguistic systems in our minds" (Whorf 1956: 153).

1.4.1 Sociolinguistic Research

Some areas of sociolinguistic research (see 1.2.1) have a long tradition of study, such as dialect analysis; others have a more recent history, such as the study of language use in social media. It is worthwhile taking an initial glimpse here into some of the issues that motivate sociolinguistic research. Sociolinguistics is an applied science, in the sense that it applies linguistic theories, techniques, and ideas to the study of the language–society link. This does not mean that sociolinguistics has had no impact on theories of language. Research findings in sociolinguistics suggest that studying language separately from its uses is somewhat artificial, because language use itself tends to have a direct impact on how the language will evolve.

Already in the 1930s, Russian psychologist Lev Vygotsky (1962, 1978) showed that the use of language for intellectual and social purposes surfaces early on in life as children come to think reflectively about the world through the words they have acquired. When children speak to themselves as they play, they are engaging in an internal dialogue, testing out the meanings and concepts imprinted in the words that they have acquired from everyday usage. A broad distinction is thus made in linguistics generally between *linguistic competence* and *linguistic performance* or, to use Saussure's terms again, *langue* and *parole*—that is, between the system of language itself and the ability to use it for some purpose. The study of *parole* was initially relegated to subsidiary status within linguistics proper, because it was felt that it had no implications for the study of language per se, and thus fell outside the proper domain of linguistic science. But this stance came to be viewed as an artificial one early on, because ethnographic research on languages consistently revealed that a language served communicative needs, and when the latter changed, so too did the language (Andersch, Staats, and Bostrom 1969). After Vygotsky, linguists became keenly aware that a systematic study of verbal communication produced relevant insights into language itself. The study came to be designated *pragmatics*. Work in pragmatics has shown that the ways in which people talk not only taps into a system of implicit social rules and rituals, but also shapes and changes a society itself as speech patterns change in subsequent generations. The American linguist Dell Hymes called the ability to utilize language meaningfully *communicative competence* in 1971. With this term, he wanted to suggest that the ability to use language is as systematic as knowing the rules of grammar (Saville-Troike 1989).

Canadian sociologist Erving Goffman (1959, 1978) saw language use as a key to understanding how we present ourselves to others and how we perceive each other. Conversations thus play a crucial role in imparting a sense of identity as well as a sense of bonding with like-minded people. As Robin Lakoff (1975) found, speakers will even refrain from saying what they really mean in some situations in the service of the higher goal of preserving group solidarity.

Another important offshoot of work in pragmatics is the notion of *discourse*. This refers to the unconscious use of a specific type of *parole* that is designed to bind people or groups together in terms of shared values, worldviews, beliefs, ideologies, and intentions. Discourse is typically characterized by keywords that appear frequently in conversations (Stubbs 2008) and by other interlinking strategies such as allusions to ideas shared by the group (Searle 1969; Tannen 1989, 1993a, 1993b, 1994; Fairclough 1995; Van Dijk 1997; Scollon and Wong Scollon 2001). Schools, corporations, universities, politicians, the media, and other collectivities all develop discourse styles that determine how members speak to one another and thus understand the world. As the Russian scholar Mikhail Bakhtin (1981) argued, discourse is shaped by values and presuppositions that interlocutors endorse and reinforce through communication. Formal rites, rallies, political debates, academic lectures, among others, are anchored in particular types of discourse, either unconsciously or specifically intended for the occasion. Discourse allows speakers to maintain or indicate allegiance to a group and its views and causes, implicitly or explicitly. For this reason, it can be dangerous, because it can spread stereotypes and biases (Foucault 1971).

Varying patterns of *parole* also correlate with social rituals and norms. In most societies, it would be considered rude or adversarial to address a superior at work with an informal mode of speech, unless the superior permits it ("Hey, Jack, what's up?"); contrariwise, it would be felt as aberrant or strange to carry out a conversation with a close friend using formal speech ("Hello, my dear friend, I would like to inquire how you are"). In other words, social relations and rituals are encoded in linguistic cues that sociolinguists call *registers*. In the traditional Javanese society of Indonesia, different social classes were once expected to utilize specific registers according to situation (Errington 1998). At the top of the traditional social hierarchy were the aristocrats; in the middle, the townsfolk; and at the bottom, the peasants. The most formal register was used by aristocrats who did not know one another very well, but also by townsfolk if they happened to be addressing a high government official. The mid-formal register was used by townsfolk who were strangers, and by peasants when addressing their social superiors. The low register was used by peasants among themselves, or by an aristocrat or town official talking to a peasant, and among friends on any social level. It was also the register used to speak to children of any class. Today, the speech registers have changed somewhat, as the traditional society has evolved, but these have residues in various linguistic protocols and in politeness strategies.

A fascinating study by James Pennebaker (2011) has illustrated another dimension of the relation between *langue* and *parole*—the link between language and personality. Pennebaker examined the speeches of several American presidents and found, for example, that President Barack Obama was the "lowest I-word user" of any of the modern-day presidents. Pennebaker argued that when presidents used the pronoun "I" abundantly in their speeches their intent was to personalize their message, conveying to audiences that they were committed personally to specific causes. Obama's apparent disdain for the first-person singular pronoun "I" did not mean, however, that he was humble, insecure, or uncommitted; on the contrary, it showed confidence, self-assurance, and a high degree of commitment, because, by omitting the pronoun, Obama's assurance and commitment to political change was implicit and thus more suggestive and powerful. The gist of Pennebaker's study is that a simple pronoun reveals more about personality than do content words (nouns, adjectives, verbs) or any psychological profile. Pronouns have an "under-the-radar" meaning to them, constituting traces to character.

Pennebaker started his research project by looking at thousands of diary entries written by subjects suffering through traumas and depressions of various kinds. He discovered that pronouns were indicators of mental health, claiming that recovery from a trauma or a depression entailed a form of "perspective switching" that pronouns facilitated. Pennebaker also found that younger people and those from lower classes used "I" more frequently than others, indicating a socially and psychologically based perception of selfhood. His work has received significant attention both on the part of sociolinguists and medical practitioners, who use what Pennebaker calls "expressive writing" for therapeutic reasons. This line of research reveals, in terms of the present purposes, that we all have a "personal language style," which linguists call *idiolect*. This is an individual's particular manner of speaking that identifies a person instantly, including pronunciation, tone of voice, choice of vocabulary, types of sentence used, and so on. Research on pronouns has actually shown that they constitute what Paul Bouissac (2019: 4) calls "a sensitive zone at the seams of social fabric."

1.4.2 Variation

A main focus of sociolinguistics is variation—that is, how language varies in social and regional situations and environments. Regional or ethnic varieties of a language are called *dialects*; variants that vary according to social contexts are called *social dialects* or *sociolects*. The traditional study of dialects comes under the rubric of *dialectology*, which consists of three main techniques:

1   the comparison of specific forms and structures between dialects
2   a plausible explanation for the differences identified (usually based on an historical analysis of the dialects)
3   a comparison of dialect speech against a "norm" or "standard."

Determining whether two dialects are related, or whether they have changed enough to be considered distinct languages, has often proved to be a difficult task. Dialectologists rely on what they call, loosely, *mutual intelligibility* as a criterion for making such a determination. If two speech codes can be understood mutually by the speakers of both, at the same time that the speakers are able to perceive differences between them as being minor, then they are likely to be dialects of a common language. If they are not intelligible, then they are different languages (or dialects of different languages). There are problems with this criterion, because many levels of mutual intelligibility exist (even among unrelated languages), and dialectologists must decide at what level speech codes should no longer be considered mutually intelligible. This has turned out to be rather difficult to establish. For one thing, if a speaker of one variety wants to understand a speaker of another, then intelligibility is more likely to ensue than if this were not the case. In addition, one can never downplay the role of cultural and sociopolitical factors in shaping the perception of what constitutes a dialect and what constitutes a separate language.

The study of dialect variation within a broader sociolinguistic framework involves such research questions as the following:

1   Are migrations away from tight-knit dialect-speaking communities changing the way the dialects are used and thus obliterating some of their traditional functions?

2 Are social media and online communications generally generating new dialectal forms? If so, what are they and how do they function?
3 How do we determine today which dialect in a multilingual society is perceived as more useful than others and why?
4 Do dialectal differences reflect broader social tendencies, including political or ideological ones?
5 Which specific dialectal traits indicate allegiance to a group or groups?

1.4.3 Markedness

A primary focus of sociolinguistic research is on how language and social perceptions affect each other. As a corollary, sociolinguistics looks for changes in language as reflexes of changes in society. The decline in usage of the masculine grammatical gender in words to indicate people in general, which started towards the middle part of the twentieth century, mirrored the movement towards gender equality. In the not-too-distant past, terms like *chairman* and *spokesman* revealed how English grammar predisposed its users to view certain social roles as "typical" for the men. The grammar and lexicon reflected that the men were at the center of the society. This is why in the past (and somewhat even today) it was said that a woman married into a man's family, and why at wedding ceremonies expressions such as "I pronounce you man and wife" were used. Today, such gendered phraseology is on the wane, as the language catches up to changes in society. The point is that gender roles and language forms are intertwined. Investigating gender in the Iroquois language, Alpher (1987) found, contrary to English, that the feminine gender was the default one grammatically, with masculine terms being marked by a special prefix. In other words, Alpher found the reverse of pairs such as *waiter—waitress* or *actor—actress,* in which the special suffix /-ess/ is used to identify the person as female, whereas the /-er/ suffix is used for the general category. Alpher related this to the fact that Iroquois society is matrilineal. The women hold the land, pass it on to their heirs in the female line, are responsible for agricultural production, control the wealth, arrange marriages, and so on. Iroquois grammar thus reflects the fact that women play a more central organizational role than do the men in society.

Traditionally, the word *man* has been used to refer not only to adult males but also to human beings in general, regardless of their sex. In Old English, the principal sense of this word was "human being," whereas the words *wer* and *wif* referred respectively to "male person" and "female person" (Miller and Swift 1971, 1988). Subsequently, *wer* was replaced by *man* as the normal word for a male, but the older sense of a human being also remained in its meaning range. It thus encoded two referents—males and humans. The result of this semantic blending virtually rendered females invisible. Studies investigating the mental images that are elicited when *man* is used as a generic form of reference have confirmed this (Doyle 1985). The image that comes to mind typically is that of a male, not a genderless one.

Changes made to the English language since the 1960s have attempted to correct this biased perception with terms such as *chairperson* or simply *chair* (instead of *chairman*) and *humanity* (rather than *mankind*).

The mechanism that links the grammar and the lexicon to social perception is known generally as *markedness*. Initially, the theory of markedness was applied simply to identify certain forms in a language as more common or neutral and others as more distinctive or "marked." In English, the article form, *a*, occurs before another word beginning with a consonant (*a boy, a girl*); and its complementary form, *an*, is used instead before a word beginning with a vowel (*an apple, an egg*). Linguists refer to the *a*-form as *unmarked* and the *an*-form as *marked*, because the former is more typical or representative (non-specific) of a class or system (in this case, the indefinite article system); the latter is the conditioned or exceptional member—it occurs in a specific phonetic location. Soon, linguists found that markedness characterizes all levels of language and reference. In Italian, for example, the masculine plural form of nouns referring to people is the unmarked one, referring (nonspecifically) to any person, male or female; whereas the feminine plural form is marked, referring only to females (see Table 1.2),

This markedness pattern in Italian is a residue of the fact that, traditionally, the males in that society were likely to be the political leaders, the writers, the artists, and so on, even though many women were also prominent in these roles. The situation has changed, of course; neither was it always this clear-cut; so, the grammatical gender of certain nouns is more a memento of the past today. As King (1991: 2) aptly puts it, in societies where the masculine is the unmarked system in grammar, "men have traditionally been the political leaders, the most acclaimed writers, the grammarians, and the dictionary makers, and it is their world view that is encoded in language." In societies (or communities) where the feminine is the unmarked system, the reverse seems to be true, as various studies have indicated (such as the one by Alpher, already discussed). The close relation between markedness in language and social structure can be seen when change takes place, because it occurs simultaneously in both. Consider job designations as a case-in-point. In the 1920s, the women who entered into traditionally male-based occupations had their job titles marked linguistically by the /-ess/ suffix. This produced doublets: *waiter—waitress, actor—actress*. Things have since changed. Although the word *actress*

Table 1.2 Italian Masculine and Feminine Forms

Masculine plural forms (= unmarked)	Feminine plural forms (= marked)
i turisti = all tourists, males and females	*le turiste* = female tourists only
gli amici = all friends, males and females	*le amiche* = female friends only
i bambini = all children, males and females	*le bambine* = female children only
gli studenti = all students, males and females	*le studentesse* = female students only

is still around, it is no longer marked socially; that is, by and large, people use the /-ess/ suffix when they want to refer to the actor's sex, not her social gender; otherwise the general term for the job category today is *actor*, and it includes men and women.

As another case-in-point, consider feminine titles in English. *Mrs.* is a marked form, indicating a woman's marital status. So too is *Miss*, which implies that the woman is not married. The term *Ms.* was introduced in the 1970s to rectify this representation of women according to marital status. The new title was designed to provide a parallel term to *Mr.*, thereby eliminating marital status from the semantics of female titles. This shows that we no longer necessarily identify women by their relationship to men and that women's traditional titles no longer properly represent their current realities (King 1991: 48). Today, markedness studies in areas such as transgendered identification and racist speech are among the most important ones being undertaken by sociolinguists. As an applied science, sociolinguistics attempts to deconstruct the linguistic features that encode sexist and racist values that are destructive of social harmony (Alim, Rickford, and Ball 2016). In a phrase, racist or racializing language is constantly at work in reproducing prejudicial ideas about races and assigns certain people to them.

1.4.4 Research in Linguistic Anthropology

The study of how worldview is built into a language is a central focus of linguistic anthropology. Ethnography is the principal method by which the anthropological linguist attempts to collect relevant speech data. A fieldworker who does not know the meaning of a particular word may look for clues in the data collected, relating the word to other information or material by comparison or contrast. The linguist might also turn to nonverbal clues for insights. Of these, hand gestures or spontaneous gesticulations are the most important (as will be discussed). Obviously, the larger "meaning-making picture" is critical in refining the overall ethnographic analysis of linguistic meaning and its relation to cognition and culture.

One way to examine features that are culturally relevant is to classify words together into what are known as *lexical fields*. For example, one such field is that of color terms, which all share the feature of chromaticism. Now, distinguishing between individual color terms will depend on what a specific term denotes and what it tells us about the role of color in a culture. The topic of color terminology will be discussed in more detail subsequently. Lexical fields are useful because they allow for further differentiation to be carried out and what this tells us about the culture. For example, the group of words that refer to "objects on which to sit," such as *chair*, *sofa*, *stool*, and *bench*, among others, belong to the same lexical field. Within the field they can be distinguished from one another according to how many people are accommodated and whether a back support is included. The complexity and conceptual sophistication of this lexical field in English suggests that English culture has a long tradition of manufacturing objects to sit on, which, in turn, implies an emphasis on sitting patterns and their meanings in different social contexts.

1.4.5 Internet Linguistics

The theoretical and methodological tools of sociolinguistics and linguistic anthropology are especially powerful today for studying language use in the new digital media and, thus, for discerning commonalities and differences between computer-mediated communication (CMC) and face-to-face (F2F) communication. Has communicative competence changed radically, or has it simply adapted to new media of interaction? How are registers determined and negotiated in cyberspace (see Box 1.3)? How does CMC reflect the usual sociolinguistic variables of gender, race, class, and ethnicity? Have the conversational functions changed? Does language use change according to the medium or digital device involved (Papacharissi 2011; Farman 2012)? These and other questions have expanded sociolinguistic research broadly. This whole area is now called *Internet linguistics* (Crystal 2011, McCulloch 2019).

Box 1.3 Cyberspace

Cyberspace is the term coined by American novelist William Gibson in his 1984 novel *Neuromancer*, and Gibson's description of cyberspace is worth repeating here (Gibson 1984: 67):

> Cyberspace. A consensual hallucination experienced daily by millions of legitimate operators. A graphic representation of data abstracted from the banks of every computer in the human system. Unthinkable complexity. Lines of Light ranged in the nonspace of the mind, clusters of constellations of data. Like city lights, receding.

Cyberspace now has its own speech communities and its own set of sociolinguistic conventions for communicating and interacting.

Mass communications technologies have always affected how people interact and even think. Already in 1922, the American journalist Walter Lippmann feared that the mass media of his era (print, radio, and cinema) had a direct negative effect on people's minds. The scholar Harold Lasswell echoed Lippmann's worry in 1927, arguing that the mass media adversely influenced people's worldviews and beliefs. If these critics are correct, then the study of the new digital media is truly a pivotal one for understanding how societies and languages are evolving—for better or worse. One of the more influential theorists on the mass media is the late Marshall McLuhan

(1911–1980) (see McLuhan 1962, 1964). A change in mass communications media, he claimed, brings about an intensification and acceleration of social change. Moreover, he foresaw the kind of routine interconnected world that electronic technologies now make possible, calling it an electronic "global village," where the "medium is the message."

Digital media have enhanced the delivery of *parole*. They have made *multimodality*—the use of more than one mode of communication (visual, audio, etc.)—a simple matter of clicking or touching parts of a screen. Studying CMC involves assessing the role of two different modes of communication: *synchronous* and *asynchronous*. Asynchronous CMC occurs when the intended receiver is not necessarily aware that a message has occurred—this characterizes emails, bulletin boards, blogs, and chatrooms. Synchronous CMC occurs, instead, when the interlocutors are aware of the communication as an ongoing one, as in text messaging and Skype interactions. Sociolinguistic research is revealing some differences between F2F communication and both synchronous and asynchronous CMC. The research on politeness speech, for example, has traditionally sought to determine the role of styles and registers for conveying respect during communication (Brown and Levinson 1987; Wierzbicka 1991). But in CMC one may ask whether the same rules of politeness still apply. Are social media platforms changing politeness protocols?

Digital messages can be subdivided into *informational* and *conversational*. The former are messages, such as those on sites such as Wikipedia, that simply provide information. These have few implications for sociolinguistic inquiry. However, the language used on social media sites, such as Facebook, Instagram, Snapchat, and Twitter, is of primary relevance to sociolinguistics. The notion of speech community has always been an important one in F2F contexts. In his classic textbook on linguistics, Leonard Bloomfield (1933: 42) defined a speech community as "a group of people who interact by means of speech." Bloomfield pointed out that the members also were aware of what kind of speech was proper and what kind was improper. Dell Hymes (1964: 51) elaborated Bloomfield's definition as follows: "A speech community is defined as a community sharing knowledge of rules for the conduct and interpretation of speech. Such sharing comprises knowledge of at least one form of speech, and also knowledge of its patterns of use." Because such definitions are rather generic, Lesley and James Milroy (1978) introduced the term *speech network*, adding frequency of interaction and the strength of the contact to Bloomfield's definition. People in "dense networks" have frequent (daily) contact with each other, and are thus likely to be linked by more than one type of bond than do those with infrequent contact, forming "weak networks."

The idea of dense network is particularly applicable to social media research, because people now have the technological ability to keep in contact more than in physical space. As Milroy and Milroy realized, dense networks put pressure on people to conform because their values can be more readily revealed. This is particularly true in cyberspace. Twitter, for example, can form the basis of interlinked personal networks—and even of a new sense of community—even though Twitter was not designed to support the development of online communities. Studying Twitter is thus important for understanding how people use specific networks to form social connections and preserve existing ones.

Another major goal of Internet linguistics is how the new media are affecting writing practices (Baron 2000). For example, the second person singular pronoun in English, *you*, is written typically as *u* in informal media texts (such as text messages); many other commonly used abbreviated forms have emerged, arguably, to allow for a message to be written more rapidly. But these bear more information than economy of form for efficiency of delivery. The spelling *u* is a common one in text messages and other digital texts; but when the completely spelled form *you* is used instead to the same interlocutor, such as a paramour, it may convey irony, anger, or some other emotion. As Coleman (2010) has written, CMC is clearly leading to new forms of pragmatic competence, as will be discussed throughout this textbook.

References and Further Reading

Alim, S., Rickford, J. and Ball, A. F. (eds.) (2016). *Raciolinguistics: How Language Shapes Our Ideas about Race*. Oxford: Oxford University Press.

Alpher, B. (1987). Feminine as the Unmarked Grammatical Gender: Buffalo Girls Are No Fools. *Australian Journal of Linguistics* 7: 169–187.

Andersch, E. G., Staats, L. C., and Bostrom, R. C. (1969). *Communication in Everyday Use*. New York: Holt, Rinehart & Winston.

Bakhtin, M. M. (1981). *The Dialogic Imagination*. Trans. C. Emerson and M. Holquist. Austin, TX: University of Texas Press.

Baron, N. S. (2000). *Alphabet to Email: How Written English Evolved and Where It's Heading*. London: Routledge.

Bloomfield, L. (1933). *Language*. New York: Holt.

Boas, F. (1920). The Methods of Ethnography. *American Anthropologist* 22: 311–322.

Boas, F. (1940). *Race, Language, and Culture*. New York: Free Press.

Bouissac, P. (ed.) (2019). *The Social Dynamics of Pronominal Systems*. Amsterdam: John Benjamins Publishing Company.

Briggs, C. L. (1986). *Learning How to Ask: A Sociolinguistic Appraisal of the Role of the Interview in Social Science Research*. Cambridge: Cambridge University Press.

Brown, P. and Levinson, S. C. (1978/1987). *Politeness: Some Universals in Language Usage*. Cambridge: Cambridge University Press.

Burling, R. (2005). *The Talking Ape: How Language Evolved*. Oxford: Oxford University Press.

Campbell, L. and Poser, W. J. (2018). *Language Classification: History and Method*. Cambridge: Cambridge University Press.

Chambers, J. (2010). *Sociolinguistic Theory: Linguistic Variation and Its Social Significance*. Malden, MA: Wiley-Blackwell.

Chomsky, N. (1975). *Reflections on Language*. New York: Pantheon.

Chomsky, N. (2000). *New Horizons in the Study of Language and Mind*. Cambridge: Cambridge University Press.

Chomsky, N. (2002). *On Nature and Language*. Cambridge: Cambridge University Press.

Coleman, E. C. (2010). Ethnographic Approaches to Digital Media. *Annual Review of Anthropology* 39: 487–505.

Crystal, D. (2011). *Internet Linguistics: A Student Guide*. New York: Routledge

Curtiss, S. (1977). *Genie: A Psycholinguistic Study of a Modern-Day Wild Child*. New York: Academic.

Denzin, N. K. (1996). *Interpretive Ethnography*. London: Sage.

Doyle, J. A. (1985). *Sex and Gender: The Human Experience*. Dubuque, IA: Wm. C. Brown Publishers.

Eckert, P. and McConnell-Ginet, S. (2013). *Language and Gender*. Cambridge: Cambridge University Press.

Errington, J. J. (1998). *Shifting Languages: Interaction and Identity in Javanese Indonesia*. Cambridge: Cambridge University Press.

Evans-Pritchard, E. E. (1940). *The Nuer*. Oxford: Oxford University Press.

Fairclough, N. (1995). *Media Discourse*. London: Arnold.

Farman, J. (2012). *Mobile Interface Theory: Embodied Space and Locative Media*. London: Routledge.

Fischer, J. L. (1958). Social Influences in the Choice of a Linguistic Variant. *Word* 14: 47–57.

Foucault, M. (1971). *The Archeology of Knowledge*. Trans. A. M. Sheridan Smith. New York: Pantheon.

Gibson, W. (1984). *Neuromancer*. London: Grafton.

Goffman, E. (1959). *The Presentation of Self in Everyday Life*. Garden City, KS: Doubleday.

Goffman, E. (1978). Response Cries. *Language* 54: 787–815.

Greenberg, J. H. (1966). *Language Universals*. The Hague: Mouton.

Gumperz, J. J. and Cook-Gumperz, J. (2008). Studying Language, Culture, and Society: Sociolinguistics or Linguistic Anthropology? *Journal of Sociolinguistics* 12: 532–545.

Haas, M. (1944). Men's and Women's Speech in Koasati. *Language* 20: 142–149.

Hodson, T. C. (1939). Sociolinguistics in India. *Man in India* 19: 23–49.

Hymes, D. (1964). *Foundation of Sociolinguistics: An Ethnographic Approach*. Philadelphia, PA: University of Pennsylvania Press.

Hymes, D. (1971). *On Communicative Competence*. Philadelphia, PA: University of Pennsylvania Press.

Kardos, G. and Smith, C. O. (1979). On Writing Engineering Cases. Proceedings of ASEE National Conference on Engineering Case Studies. www.civeng. carleton.ca.

King, R. (1991). *Talking Gender: A Nonsexist Guide to Communication*. Toronto: Copp Clark Pitman Ltd.

Labov, W. (1963). The Social Motivation of a Sound Change. *Word* 19: 273–309.

Labov, W. (1967). The Effect of Social Mobility on a Linguistic Variable. In: S. Lieberson (ed.), *Explorations in Sociolinguistics*, pp. 23–45. Bloomington, IN: Indiana University Research Center in Anthropology, Linguistics and Folklore.

Labov, W. (1972). *Language in the Inner City*. Philadelphia, PA: University of Pennsylvania Press.

Labov, W. (2001). *Principles of Linguistic Changes: Social Factors*. Malden: Wiley-Blackwell.

Labov, W. (2008). Quantitative Reasoning in Linguistics. www.ling.upenn.edu/~wlabov/Papers/QRL.pdf.

Lakoff, R. (1975). *Language and Woman's Place*. New York: Harper & Row.

Lasswell, H. D. (1927). *Propaganda Techniques in World War I*. Cambridge, MA: MIT Press.

Lippmann, W. (1922). *Public Opinion*. New York: Palgrave Macmillan.

Malinowski, B. (1922). *Argonauts of the Western Pacific*. New York: Dutton.

Martinet, A. (1955). *Économie des changements phonétiques*. Paris: Maisonneuve & Larose.

Mathiot, M. (ed.) (1979). *Ethnolinguistics: Boas, Sapir and Whorf Revisited*. The Hague: Mouton.

McCulloch, G. (2019). *Because Internet: Understanding the New Rules of Language*. London: Penguin.

McLuhan, M. (1962). *The Gutenberg Galaxy: The Making of Typographic Man*. Toronto: University of Toronto Press.

McLuhan, M. (1964). *Understanding Media: The Extensions of Man*. London: Routledge.

McWhorter, J. H. (2016). *The Language Hoax*. Oxford: Oxford University Press,

Miller, C. and Swift, K. (1971). *Words and Women*. New York: Harper & Row.

Miller, C. and Swift, K. (1988). *The Handbook of Nonsexist Writing*. New York: Harper & Row.

Milroy, L. and Gordon, M. (2003). *Sociolinguistics: Method and Interpretation*. London: Wiley-Blackwell.

Milroy, L. and Milroy, J. (1978). Belfast: Change and Variation in an Urban Vernacular. In: P. Trudgill (ed.), *Sociolinguistic Patterns in British English*, pp. 19–36. London: Edward Arnold.

Miller, R. L. (1968). *The Linguistic Relativity Principle and Humboldtian Ethnolinguistics: A History and Appraisal*. The Hague: Mouton.

Niyaz, N. (2017). *Metaphorical Framing, the Sapir-Whorf-Hypothesis and How Language Shapes Our Thoughts*. Grin Verlag.

Papacharissi, Z. (2011). *A Networked Self: Identity, Community and Culture on Social Network Sites*. London: Routledge.

Pennebaker, J. W. (2011). *The Secret Life of Pronouns*. London: Bloomsbury Press.

Pinker, S. (2007). *The Stuff of Thought: Language as a Window into Human Nature*. New York: Viking.

Roberts, I. (ed.). (2017). *The Oxford Handbook of Universal Grammar*. Oxford: Oxford University Press.

Sapir, E. (1921). *Language*. New York: Harcourt, Brace, & World.

Saussure, F. de. (1916). *Cours de linguistique générale*. Paris: Payot.

Saville-Troike, M. (1989). *The Ethnography of Communication: An Introduction*, 2nd ed. Oxford: Wiley-Blackwell.

Scollon, R. and Wong Scollon, S. (2001). *Intercultural Communication*, 2nd ed. Oxford: Wiley-Blackwell.

Searle, J. R. (1969). *Speech Acts: An Essay in the Philosophy of Language*. Cambridge: Cambridge University Press.

Shuy, R. (1997). A Brief History of American Sociolinguistics: 1949–1989. In: C. B. Paulston and G. R. Tucke (eds.), *The Early Days of Sociolinguistics: Memories and Reflections*, pp. 11–32. Dallas, TX: Summer Institute of Linguistics.

Song, J. J. (ed.) (2011). *The Oxford Handbook of Linguistic Typology*. Oxford: Oxford University Press.

Stubbs, M. (2008). Three Concepts of Keywords. Paper presented to the conference on Keyness in Text, University of Siena.

Tagliamonte, S. (2006). *Analysing Sociolinguistic Variation*. Cambridge: Cambridge University Press.

Tagliamonte, S. (2016). *Making Waves: The Story of Variationist Sociolinguistics*. Chichester: John Wiley & Sons.

Tannen, D. (1989). *Talking Voices*. Cambridge: Cambridge University Press.

Tannen, D. (1993a). *The Social Constructions of Sex, Gender, and Sexuality*. Englewood Cliffs, NJ: Prentice Hall.

Tannen, D. (1993b). *Framing in Discourse*. Oxford: Oxford University Press.

Tannen, D. (1994). *Gender and Discourse*. Oxford: Oxford University Press.

Taylor, D. M. (1977). *Languages of the West Indies*. Baltimore, MD: Johns Hopkins.

Van Dijk, T. (ed.) (1997). *Discourse as Social Interaction*. London: Sage.

Vygotsky, L. S. (1962). *Thought and Language*. Cambridge, MA: MIT Press.

Vygotsky, L. S. (1978). *Mind in Society*. Cambridge: Cambridge University Press.

Whorf, B. L. (1956). *Language, Thought, and Reality*, J. B. Carroll (ed.). Cambridge, MA: MIT Press.

Wierzbicka, A. (1991). *Cross-Cultural Pragmatics: The Semantics of Human Interaction*. Berlin: Mouton de Gruyter.

2 Language and Society

As mentioned briefly in the previous chapter, the ancient Indian scholar Pāṇini was among the first to carry out a systematic study of the grammatical structure of words and phrases, and how the meanings imprinted in them reflected the thoughts, experiences, and beliefs of Sanskrit society. Some little time later, the Greek philosopher Aristotle (384–322 BCE) analyzed sentences as being constructed with "parts of speech," such as *subject* and *predicate*, each one with a specific purpose. For example, the *subject* is a statement about something (a referent), and the *predicate* is what is affirmed or denied about the referent. Two centuries later, Greek scholar Dionysius Thrax (170–190 BCE) subdivided the parts of speech into eight main categories: *nouns, verbs, articles, pronouns, prepositions, conjunctions, adverbs*, and *participles*—categories adopted by the Roman scholar Priscian, in the sixth century CE, forming the basis for writing the grammars of emerging vernacular (non-Latin) languages in Europe. These are used to this day in linguistics and grammar study generally.

In antiquity, the notion of "good grammar" also emerged, referring to a use of language that mirrored social elegance and skill in elocution. It was a metric of social status, and still is. It was in the sixteenth and seventeenth centuries that a different view of grammar emerged, separating it from its social implications. A group of French scholars, called collectively the Port-Royal Circle, started examining grammar not as part of social manners and etiquette, but as a mental faculty, aiming to determine which aspects were universal and which were specific to various languages. They prefigured Chomsky's notion of universal grammar (introduced in Chapter 1), by claiming that all languages possessed the same set of rule-making principles that were applied to the construction of specific grammars. Chomsky (1966) acknowledged his debt to the Port-Royal grammarians, indicating that their view of language was similar to his own.

A century later, the German scholar Wilhelm von Humboldt (1767–1835) took a different approach, foreshadowing the Whorfian Hypothesis (WH), also discussed briefly in Chapter 1. Rather than focusing on a set of universal principles of grammatical structure, Humboldt argued that the grammar and vocabulary of each language reflected the historically significant experiences of the people who used it. Each language revealed an *innere Sprachform* (internal speech form) that shaped how its speakers came to view reality. He put it as follows (Humboldt 1836 [1988]: 43):

> The central fact of language is that speakers can make infinite use of the finite resources provided by their language. Though the capacity for language is universal, the individuality of each language is a property of the people who speak it. Every language has its *innere Sprachform*, or internal structure, which determines its outer form and which is a reflection of its speakers' minds. The language and the thought of a people are thus inseparable.

The topic of the relation between language and mind will be discussed in Chapter 8. This chapter will look, more specifically, at the relation of the *innere Sprachform*—the vocabulary, grammar, and sound system of a language—to the social constructs (gender, race, class, and so on) that it reflects. This topic is a fundamental one in sociolinguistics, because it brings out conspicuously how language, speech, and society are intrinsically intertwined. The chapter constitutes an overview of central notions and methods for studying the language–society interface, as well as the language-new media one that is constantly evolving in cyberspace. A discussion of *sociolects*, which is a more focused one with regards to this interface, is found in Chapter 5.

2.1 Vocabulary and the Lexicon

When we hear a word such as *spaghetti* we might think of Italians, *Wiener Schnitzel* of Germans, and *fried chicken* of southern Americans. Clearly, a word is more than an arbitrary name for something; it also encodes social and ethnic connotations. To study this type of phenomenon, linguistics makes use of a dual terminology—*vocabulary* refers to the actual set of words and phrases in a language; *lexicon* is preferred instead to indicate the abstract knowledge of words, known more technically as *lexemes* (see Box 2.1). The lexicon is part of *langue* (to use Saussure's apt term) and *vocabulary* is part of *parole* (the use of the lexicon to make messages). In practice, however, these two terms are used synonymously, unless there is a specific technical reason to use them differentially.

Box 2.1 The Lexicon and Vocabulary

In linguistics, the term *lexicon* refers to the set of *lexemes*, the words or phrases, real and potential, that are part of linguistic competence (*langue*). *Vocabulary* refers instead to the actual use of words and phrases for communicative purposes (*parole*). The lexicon is the abstract knowledge of the kind of words that belong to a language; vocabulary is the specific use of that knowledge in social interactions.

People have two kinds of vocabulary—*active* and *passive*. The former refers to the lexemes they use typically in speaking or writing; the latter consists of lexemes that people understand when listening or reading, but which they do not use with regularity. Generally, people have a passive vocabulary several times larger than their active one. For the average speaker of a language, the active vocabulary is estimated to be around 10,000 lexemes, while the passive vocabulary is around 30,000 to 40,000. The range of a person's vocabulary is often studied as part of the person's education, experiences, preferences, or interests.

2.1.1 Core Vocabularies

Some aspects of the lexicon might be universal or display universal properties; this feature is called the *core vocabulary*, a minimal set of lexemes referring to things and concepts that people across the world have tended to encode linguistically, because they refer to experiences and concepts that play a central role in human life—words for *mother, father, sun, moon,* and so on. Early work on core vocabularies can be traced to the philologists of the nineteenth century who examined cognates to determine if languages were related. As mentioned in Chapter 1, these are words that are derived from the same linguistic source or root. For example, *domicile* ("residence," "home") in English and *domicilio* ("residence") in Italian derive from the same Latin root word *domicilium* ("dwelling"), a fact that is used, with other facts, to link the two languages through the evolutionary-historical channel. The American linguist Morris Swadesh (1951, 1959, 1971) saw core vocabularies as a means to reconstruct early societies by determining which words united them and which words set them apart. Table 2.1 gives an example of a core vocabulary of 11 lexemes in eight different Bantu languages, spoken in parts of Africa, some of which are facing extinction due to the encroachment of modernity into these parts.

Several interesting observations can be made by inspecting this list in a cursory fashion. For instance, the lack of a word for *wand* in some Bantu languages suggests several possibilities—the languages may have other ways of conveying the same referent (such as through metaphor or paraphrase); the speakers of those languages may not use wands for social practices; and so on. In other words, although it is included in this particular set of core lexemes for a language family, it turns out to be culture specific rather than a universal lexical item. The word *umuntu* in Zulu, translated as "human," reveals a social value of Zulu culture; it actually means that a human being becomes a true person through other people (a meaning that is not identified as such in the list). This implies the importance of Otherness in the Zulu worldview that is imprinted in the meaning of the word. In effect, core vocabularies partially reflect universal naming tendencies, but may also be used to identify culture-specific experiences. The role of the latter can never be underestimated.

Table 2.1 Core Vocabulary Items in the Bantu Family

Concept	Zulu	Chwana	Herero	Nyanja	Swahili	Ganda	Giau	Kongo
human	umuntu	motho	omundu	muntu	mtu	omuntu	umundu	muntu
humans	abantu	vatho	ovandu	antu	watu	abantu	babandu	antu
tree	umuti	more	omuti	mtengo	mti	omuti	—	—
trees	imiti	mere	omiti	mitengo	miti	emiti	—	—
tooth	ilizinyo	leino	eyo	dzino	jino	erinyo	lisino	dinu
teeth	amazinyo	maino	omayo	mano	meno	amanyo	kamasino	menu
chest	isifuba	sehuba	—	chifua	kifua	ekifuba	—	—
chests	izifuba	lihuba	—	zifua	vifua	ebifuba	—	—
elephant	indhlovu	tlou	ondyou	njobvu	ndovu	enjovu	itsofu	nzau
elephants	izindhlovu	litlou	ozondyou	njonvu	ndovu	enjovu	tsitsofu	nzau
wand	uluti	lore	oruti	—	uti	—	—	—

Source: Werner 1919

The linguist Morris Swadesh (1971) was among the first to put forth several principles for the construction of core vocabularies:

1   A core vocabulary should contain words for concepts that probably exist in all languages ("skin," "blood," "bone," "drink," "eat," and so on).
2   Culturally biased words, such as the names of specific kinds of plants or animals, are to be included in the core vocabulary only if relevant to the analysis at hand.
3   Variation in lexical reference, as for example Russian *ruká*, which covers the same referential domain as two English words, *arm* + *hand*, should be considered in the overall construction. This means that the same core concept will be encoded differentially in a lexicon.

Research on core vocabularies has been extensive, and need not concern us here. Such lists have been used by historical linguists to estimate the relative length of time that might have elapsed—known as *time depth*—since two languages in a family began to diverge into independent ones. The method of calculating time depth is known as *glottochronology*. It starts by counting the number of cognates among the languages being compared. The lower the number, the longer the languages are deemed to have separated. Two languages that can be shown to share 60 percent cognates are said to have diverged before two that have, instead, 80 percent in common (Lees 1953; see also Dyen 1975; Gray and Atkinson 2003).

2.1.2 Vocabulary and Social Systems

An underlying objective of the core vocabulary concept is to allow for a reconstruction of a previous society via its core lexemes, since this will show what cultural emphases are at play in its foundation. It constitutes a kind of "archeological sociolinguistics," which gives us a glimpse into past societies via their vocabularies. In effect, the notion of core vocabularies brings out the fact that there has always been an intrinsic interconnection between language and society. So, in order to establish links between specific parts of the lexicon and social systems, the linguist must at times delve into the history and evolution of core vocabularies in order to understand why they have undergone changes in meaning. Consider how the two Latin root words *domu(s)* and *casa(m)* changed their meanings after they evolved into Italian lexemes—as mentioned in Chapter 1, Latin is the source language of Italian (see Table 2.2).

This table allows us to deduce an implicit sociolinguistic principle—the words used by people to designate certain things reflect social conditions. Most speakers of early vernacular Italian clearly lived in homes that were "shacks." Thus, the fact that the word for "shack" (*casa*), and not the Latin word for "house" (*domus*) and its Italian derivative *duomo* (used for churches), became the source for "house in general" reflects the social class of most of the first speakers of vernacular Italian.

Table 2.2 Changes in Meaning in Italian Words

Latin source	Original meaning	Italian form	New meaning
domu(s)	house	*duomo*	dome
casa(m)	shack	*casa*	house

In effect, the lexicon constitutes a culture-specific strategy for understanding the world. In a relevant study, William Labov (1973) showed how this manifested itself in simple naming tasks. He presented drawings of cups, and cuplike containers, asking subjects to name the items with words such as *cup, mug, bowl, dish,* and *pitcher.* The subjects were then asked to imagine a series of objects containing coffee, mashed potatoes, or flowers. The subjects were most likely to label untypical objects as *cups* if they contained coffee and least likely to do so if they held flowers. It seems that speakers cannot get away from the established meanings of words and what they typically refer to.

Recall the theory of markedness from the previous chapter. In the area of vocabulary it implies that certain lexemes are marked for gender, class, ethnicity, or some other social variable. For instance, in the case of the relation between lexemes and gender categories three main findings have emerged from the relevant sociolinguistic research (Coates 1986; Eckert and McConnell-Ginet 2003):

1 In some societies, the adult male vocabulary is perceived as the standard or unmarked one, and women's speech as a deviation from the male benchmark; the opposite situation is rarer, but also occurs in some societies, such as the Iroquois one (as discussed in Chapter 1).
2 In some societies, gendered differences in vocabulary allow individuals to refer to their specific situations meaningfully, as discussed with regard to Koasati in Chapter 1.
3 A gender-neutral lexicon is used mainly in societies where equality between the sexes is stressed.

With the expansion of the meaning of gender identity, there now exist lexical gaps in languages to make reference to this expansion. In English, this gap is being filled with the pronoun *they/them* as the unmarked or gender-neutral pronoun, which now includes transgendered individuals. Inclusiveness involves a lexical response.

A key notion in the study of vocabulary is that of *speech community,* defined as a group of people connected to each other by means of a common *code* (Chapter 1). Basil Bernstein (1971), an early founder of sociolinguistics, was the one who used this notion to tackle the question of how linguistic distinctions unfold in speech communities according to class. The higher classes typically used an *elaborated code* (the standard or official language) and the lower classes a *restricted code* (a dialect or regional variant). Of specific interest to the theme of the present chapter is that the vocabulary used in one code or the other varies markedly, allowing people in their particular communities to bond and to make social differentiations that are crucial to them. In Britain, for example, Bernstein found that restricted codes emphasized groupthink, whereas elaborated codes emphasized individualism. This dichotomy had an effect on broader social outcomes. He discovered that children with a restricted code struggled at school where the elaborated code is the main language. The reason for this was not lack of intelligence, but the fact that the children had to learn how to distinguish between the social and educational functions of the two codes. Bernstein also found that in working-class neighborhoods, using the elaborated code was perceived as a sign of pretentiousness. The restricted code was, instead, felt to be "natural" and a means to maintain group solidarity.

2.1.3 Group- and Community-Based Vocabularies

Vocabularies are also fashioned to define groups. For instance, *argots* and *cants*, both of which refer to the type of slang used by criminals, are intended to prevent outsiders from understanding conversations among group members and to reinforce group solidarity. *Argot* designates more specifically the type of code that develops among street gangs and *cant* of organized criminal groups. Thus, argot is likely to be more comprehensible to outsiders, because deviation from the norm is not as drastic as it is in cant speech, which is marked by a highly specialized, secret vocabulary.

The first dictionary of criminal cant was published in 1819. It was compiled by an English nobleman, James Hardy Vaux, who had spent his early life in London and Liverpool and who had become a thief to support his addiction to gambling (Nicaso and Danesi 2013). Vaux recorded the cant spoken by common thieves and wrote the dictionary probably to gain a pardon, which he did in fact receive in 1820. Historical documents show that English criminal cants were spoken centuries prior to Vaux's book, many going back to the medieval period. Members of organized criminal groups are expected to develop fluency in their particular cant, because it is crucial for keeping their operations secret and in conveying unity through the "insider savvy" imprinted in the lexemes. A classic example is the cant used by the Russian Mafia (Lunde 2004), which is a trace to the gang's social structure, activities, and mindset. For example, *akademiya* (literally, "academy") refers to the prison where the gangster (*vory v zakone*) learns his trade; *dan* stands for extortion money; *Panama* is the descriptive English name given to the dummy company set up to launder extortion money; and *khoda* refers to a gang meeting. Likewise, the Italian Mafia, the Japanese yakuza, and the Chinese triads have developed cants that allow members to communicate in specific group-based ways.

Vocabularies also emerge for political and sociocultural reasons. These are called community-based vocabularies. A case-in-point is African American Vernacular English (AAVE), whose vocabulary has traditionally been replete with lexemes that convey nuances that are of relevance and importance to

African American history and culture. As Janice Rahn (2002) suggests, AAVE is a means for many African Americans to take control of their own lives through the empowerment that it encourages. AAVE, as Geneva Smitherman (2000: 34) also points out, connotes attitudes of "rebelliousness against societal constraints" and the "fierce determination to live on one's own terms." Phrases such as *boyz in blue* (police) and *government cheese* (welfare) are defiant descriptors of the discriminatory environment in which many African Americans live. This makes AAVE vocabulary an anti-hegemonic code, standing in defiance of the traditions of Standard American English.

Samy Alim (2004) characterizes AAVE as "Hip-Hop Nation Language," promoting a "subtle, yet powerful, rejection of racial discriminatory practices." It is a kind of linguistic antidote to inherent racism. Alim's research has also shown that social mobility among African Americans involves a form of bilingualism, whereby a socially mobile young African American might use AAVE in a contextualized fashion—among peers for in-group identification purposes—and SAE (Standard American English) for broader social functions (see also Thomas 2007; Reeves 2008; Alim and Smitherman 2012; Alim, Rickford, and Ball 2016). Racism is a menace to the integrity of American society, and AAVE is, in an indirect way, a means to understand how African Americans interpret it. Sociolinguistic research on racism and prejudice today has become of great significance, given the social destructiveness that it brings about.

2.1.4 Semantics

The study of the meanings of lexemes and their use in larger structures (sentences, utterances, etc.) comes under the rubric of *semantics* (see Box 2.2). In sociolinguistics, the relevant aspect of semantic analysis is the investigation of how meaning reflects social systems. The most common technique for identifying semantically coded social differences is to collect lexical data that allows the researcher to extract the relevant connotations from it. This can be done through the usual forms of sociolinguistic research—surveys, interviews, ethnography (Chapter 1).

Box 2.2 Semantics

Semantics is the study of the meaning of words, phrases, sentences, and utterances. It is subdivided into several branches, including:

- formal semantics, which studies the logical structure of meaning
- lexical semantics, which studies word meanings and word relations
- cognitive semantics, which studies how linguistic meaning reflects the structure of concepts.

The technical term for what a lexeme encodes is *referent* (as already indicated). So, for example, the referent of the word *cat* is an animal with certain features (a tail, body hair, whiskers, retractile claws, and so on). This meaning is called *literal* or *denotative*. If cats play specific roles in a given society, the word will accumulate additional meanings, called *senses* or *connotations*. For example, in some societies, a cat is perceived to be a household companion, whereas in others, it is considered to be a sacred animal. These are connotations that go beyond the denotative meaning of the word. Connotations are of particular relevance to sociolinguists, because they indicate the value of certain referents in social terms. If a specific word for *cat* does not exist in a language, the implication is that this kind of mammal either does not exist in the territory where the language is spoken or that it has few, if any, social connotations.

Consider color lexemes as a case-in-point. In English, terms such as *red, blue, green, yellow, brown, white*, and *black* are used commonly to cover a broad range of denotative meanings. Further semantic distinctions can be made with terms such as *crimson, navy blue, pea green*, and so on. The topic of color is actually one that has generated much debate in sociolinguistics and linguistic anthropology. It is worth discussing briefly here, since it reveals both the relation of language to perception and social emphases. As discussed briefly in Chapter 1, languages that have a sophisticated color vocabulary put great value on fashion, visual aesthetic traditions, and other areas that require such a vocabulary. At a denotative level, color terms refer to gradations of hue. Languages might segment and organize the gradations on the color spectrum in denotatively different ways. A simple example is the word *blue* in English. The hue designated by *blue* is covered by three different terms in Italian—*azzurro, celeste*, and *blu* (see Table 2.3). These are not just shades of *blue*; they are separate lexemes for different color hues, even though they seem to fall, more or less, into the same perceptual category as English *blue*.

Psychologists estimate that we can distinguish perhaps as many as 10 million hues. Obviously, then, our limited number of color terms is far too inexact to describe all the colors we are potentially capable of discerning. So, each term designates a culture-based category of color, rather than referring to a specific frequency of light. This is the reason why people often have difficulty trying to describe a specific color in some detail. To fill in the lexical gaps within the *red* category, for example, we might use metaphors such as *crimson, ruby, rusty*, and so on.

Table 2.3 "Blue" in Italian

English	Italian	Equivalents
blue	*azzurro*	basic blue
blue	*celeste*	light blue
blue	*blu*	dark blue

Consider what speakers of English would "see" if they were to put a finger at any point on the color spectrum. They would perceive only a negligible difference in the hues adjacent to the finger at either side. Depending on where it is put, however, one might name the difference in a specific way. This is because speakers have become accustomed to "seeing" the spectrum in terms of their particular color terms. But there is nothing inherently natural about the lexical system used in English. So, when an English speaker refers to something as *blue*, an Italian speaker might refer to it as either *azzurro* or *celeste*. This in no way implies that culture-specific color terminology blocks people from perceiving color gradations. All languages have the lexical resources available to them to indicate a specific gradation if required; and specific color terms in no way preclude the ability to perceive how other cultures recognize and name color. This is what foreign language learners do when they are acquiring a different language, and thus a different lexicon.

This whole line of analysis raises a fundamental question: Are there any universals in color terminology? In 1969, the linguists Berlin and Kay examined this very question. Using the judgments of the native speakers of 20 widely divergent languages, they came to the conclusion that there were "focal" points in basic (single-term) color systems that clustered in certain predictable ways. They identified 11 such points, which corresponded to the English words *red, pink, orange, yellow, brown, green, blue, purple, black, white*, and *gray*. Not all the languages they investigated had separate terms for each of these points, but they detected a pattern in naming practices. If a language had two focal colors, then these were equivalents of English *black* and *white*. If it had three, then the third one corresponded to *red*. A four-term system added either *yellow* or *green*; whereas a five-term system had both of these. A six-term system included *blue*; a seven-term one had *brown*. Finally, terms for *purple, pink, orange*, and *gray* were found to occur in any combination in languages that had the previous focal colors. Berlin and Kay thus discovered, remarkably, that languages with, say, a four-term system consisting of *black, white, red*, and *brown* did not exist.

Examples of languages possessing from 2 to 11 focal terms can be seen in Table 2.4.

In 1975, Kay revised the sequence to account for the fact that certain languages—such as Japanese—lexicalized a color that can be paraphrased in English as "green-blue." He gave it the name GRUE and placed it next to *yellow* in the original sequence. Since then it has been found that further differentiation is required because Russian and Italian (as we have seen) do not have a single focal color term for *blue*, but rather distinguish "light blue" and "dark blue" as focal colors. Other factors have also been found to interrupt the sequence, which need not concern us here.

Suffice it to say that the main implication of Berlin and Kay's study is that color vocabularies are organized according to a sequence, implying that some hues are likely to be perceived as more fundamental across the world than others. These constitute core vocabularies for color referents. When

Table 2.4 Focal Color Terms

Number	Terms (English equivalents)	Example of language
2	*white, black*	Jale (New Guinea), Ngombe (Africa)
3	*white, black, red*	Arawak (Caribbean), Swahili (eastern Africa)
4	*white, black, red, yellow/green*	Ibo (Nigeria), Tongan (Polynesia)
5	*white, black, red, yellow, green*	Tarascan (Mexico), !Kung (southern Africa)
6	*white, black, red, yellow, green, blue*	Tamil (India, Sri Lanka), Mandarin (China)
7	*white, black, red, yellow, green, blue, brown*	Nez Percé (Montana), Javanese
8–11	*white, black, red, yellow, green, blue, brown, purple/pink/orange/ gray*	English, Zuñi (New Mexico), Dinka (Sudan), Tagalog (Philippines)

words do not exist for a color, then metaphor or borrowing is used to fill in the gaps. For example, Swahili has a three-color-term system, but its vocabulary is bolstered by metaphorical constructions (for example, yellow = *manjano* "turmeric") and by borrowing (blue = *buluu*). Metaphor may even be the source for the origin of the focal terms themselves (Wescott 1980). In Hittite, the earliest documented Indo-European language, the words for colors were metaphors designating plant and tree names corresponding to English *poplar, elm, cherry, oak,* and so on.

2.2 Cognitive Semantics

The approach to the study of language as a system of concepts grounded in figurative language is known as *cognitive semantics*. Boas, Sapir, and Whorf (see Chapter 1 for references), among other early anthropological linguists, would have actually been called cognitive semanticists today, because they too saw figurative language as a basic feature in semantics and communication. Interestingly, the source of interest in the formal study of such language may have come from early AI research in the 1940s and the work of mathematician Warren Weaver and scientist Andrew D. Booth in the 1950s (see Booth 1955; Weaver 1955). Given the low power of computers of the era, various problems emerged that nonetheless became of great interest to linguists. For example, at Georgetown University in 1954, from a widely publicized experiment in machine translation of Russian sentences into English, it was clear that the algorithms in the experiment lacked the kind of conceptual sophistication that humans have when it comes to tapping into the figurative nuances of utterances. A classic example from the experiment was the automatic translation of the Russian version of "The spirit is willing, but the flesh is weak" as "The vodka is strong, but the meat is rotten." It was obvious that the problem of figurative language and of context (the situation in which language is used) were important ones in semantics.

Linguist Yehoshua Bar-Hillel (1960) argued, shortly thereafter, that humans use contextual information to make sense of messages. Various studies soon led to the analysis of contextual inferences in discourse, leading to the growth of pragmatics and discourse analysis as major emphases in sociolinguistics. It also led, a few decades later, to the first scientific studies that laid the foundations for the rise of the cognitive semantic movement.

2.2.1 Context

The meanings of words are constrained by the context in which they are used (Duranti and Goodwin 1992; Kay 1997). Consider a sentence such as "The pig is ready to eat." Denotatively, the word *pig* refers to a type of mammal. But when the sentence is uttered in different contexts, its meaning will vary. If it is spoken by a farmer during feeding time, then *pig* retains its denotative meaning: "There is an animal called a *pig* that is ready to eat its food." If the same sentence is uttered by a cook who is announcing the fact that a cooked *pig* has become available for consumption, then the word has a different meaning: "The (cooked) *pig* is ready for people to eat." If the sentence is meant to be sarcastic, describing a person who appears voracious while waiting for food to be served, then *pig* has ironic meaning: "The *pig* (slob) is ready to eat."

The anthropologist Bronislaw Malinowski (1884–1932) argued that word meanings are adaptive, allowing speakers to make sense of situations (Malinowski 1923). Even the words we use to make social contact carry with them connotations, rather than literal referential meanings—a phenomenon that Malinowski called *phatic*. If we meet someone we know well, invariably we will make contact with an expression such as "Hi, how are you?" With this expression, we are not inquiring about the person's health or state of mind. We are simply acknowledging the person's presence and the implicit social relationship we have with the person. It has phatic, rather than literal, meaning. The literal meaning of the expression is constrained to a situation whereby the interlocutor is a medical doctor or else if it is known that the person has a medical condition. The branch that studies the role of context on speech is called, as mentioned in Chapter 1, *pragmatics*, a term coined by the American philosopher Charles S. Peirce (1931) and adopted in the 1930s by psychologist Charles Morris (1938). Pragmatics will be discussed in Chapter 6.

The sociologist Erving Goffman (1922–1982) put forth the idea that the context will shape how people talk about themselves (Goffman 1959). Goffman insisted that everyday life shaped people's consciousness, introducing the method of *frame analysis* into sociolinguistics—the technique of dividing human interaction into separate frames of behavior that can then be analyzed in terms of constituent units of self-portrayal. Goffman's term "presentation of

Self" has become a widely used one in the social and psychological sciences, as a way of characterizing human consciousness and behavior in social contexts, such as how people talk in specific situations.

2.2.2 Metaphor

Research on figurative language has become widespread, constituting a central area of interest within cognitive semantics. We hardly realize how prevalent figurative language is in everyday conversations. When asked how we feel about something, we might say that we are "*cool* about it," or that we are "*lukewarm* about it." These expressions reveal that we perceive feeling in terms of the sensations we experience in response to physical conditions that we have named *cool* and *lukewarm*. They are not exceptional or idiomatic; they are systematic and thus revelatory of an unconscious conceptual system guiding linguistic choices in ordinary contexts of communication, not exceptional ones (such as in the use of poetry or rhetorical oratory).

The term *metaphor* designates a figure of speech that connects referents so that we can understand each one in terms of the other. So, when we say something like "That linguist is a snake" the probable reason for correlating the two referents—*linguist* and *snake*—is an unconscious sense that human character and perceived animal features are interconnected existentially. In this case, the connotative features associated with snakes (treachery, deceit) come from a longstanding cultural tradition of perceiving snakes as dangerous. The meaning of *snake* in the metaphor thus refers to a treacherous or deceitful person.

Scientific interest in metaphor started with the pivotal work of certain psychologists in the latter half of the nineteenth century and the early part of the twentieth. They were the first to conduct experiments to determine how people processed figurative language (Wundt 1901). The linguist Karl Bühler (1908/1951) collected some truly intriguing data on how subjects paraphrased and recalled proverbs, which are frozen metaphorical expressions. He found that the recall of a given proverb by subjects was excellent if it was linked to another proverb; otherwise it was easily forgotten. So, an expression such as "You're playing with fire" would be better recalled if followed by a metaphorically connected one such as "You're throwing caution to the wind." Bühler concluded that metaphorical-connective thinking produced an effective retrieval form of memory and was, therefore, something to be investigated further by linguists and psychologists.

A few decades later, the literary critic I. A. Richards (1936), argued that the meaning of an expression such as "The linguist is a snake" can never be completely captured by literal paraphrases such as "The linguist is sneaky," "The linguist is deceptive," and so on. A metaphorical concept is larger than its literal paraphrases—a principle that has remained intrinsic to cognitive semantics. The philosopher Max Black (1962) expanded Richards' theory by suggesting that a specific metaphorical utterance was a particular token of a broader and unconscious mode of thinking. So, utterances such as "The linguist is a snake" and "The linguist is a tiger" are tokens of the same concept—*people are animals*. In 1977, a study by psychologists Pollio et al. found that such expressions are hardly simple rhetorical strategies, but rather they pervade everyday speech in a systematic way. Speakers of English utter, on average, an astounding 3,000 metaphors and 7,000 idioms per week. Figurative language could no longer be construed as a mere ornamental accessory to literal language. This became even more evident after the publication of several collections of studies (Ortony 1979; Honeck and Hoffman 1980) and a pivotal 1980 book by George Lakoff and Mark Johnson, *Metaphors We Live By*. These set the stage for cognitive semantics to crystallize and spread broadly.

Lakoff (1979) expanded Black's distinction by differentiating between a specific, or *linguistic*, metaphor and the broader unconscious concept from which it is derived, which he called a *conceptual metaphor*. So, linguistic metaphors such as "The linguist is a snake" or "My friend is a butterfly" are not disconnected from one another, but are manifestations of the same conceptual metaphor, *people are animals*. *People* is called the *target domain* and *animals* the *source domain*. Research has found that common discourse is not only replete with conceptual metaphors, but also guided by them (Lakoff and Johnson 1980, 1999; Johnson 1987, 2007; Danesi 2017). As target domains are associated with various kinds of source domains, the conceptual metaphors become increasingly more unconscious and intertwined, leading to what Lakoff and Johnson called *idealized cognitive models* (ICMs). To see what this means, consider the target domain of *ideas*. The following source domains, among others, shape how we talk about this concept:

sight

(1) I can't *see* the point of your idea.
(2) *Seeing* is believing.

geometry

(3) Her ideas are *parallel* to ours.
(4) His idea is *diametrically* opposite to ours.

plants

(5) That idea has deep *roots* in Cartesian philosophy.
(6) Hers is a *budding* new idea about atomic structure.

buildings

(7) Quantum ideas today are *constructed* on mathematical notions.
(8) The *cornerstone* of that idea goes back considerably in time.

food

(9) It is difficult to *digest* those ideas easily.
(10) That is an *appetizing* idea.

fashion

(11) Those ideas went *out of style* years ago.
(12) That idea is in *fashion* nowadays.

commodities

(13) I don't *buy* your ideas.
(14) She must *package* her ideas differently.

The constant use of such source domains to convey the target concept of *ideas* produces, cumulatively, an ICM. This is the network of source domains that allows us to navigate a conversation meaningfully. If the target of a conversation is *ideas* then the following statements would make sense:

> *Speaker A:* I just couldn't *digest* what he said.
> *Speaker B:* Yeah, I didn't *buy* it either. I don't *see* his point.

Speaker A utilized the *ideas are food* conceptual metaphor, and Speaker B employed the *ideas are commodities* and *ideas are sight* conceptual metaphors together. The fact that we can understand these utterances is evidence that ICMs are part of how we encode and decipher utterances, not exceptions to it. Before cognitive semantics, the study of metaphor fell within the discipline of rhetoric, where it was viewed as one of various *tropes* (figures of speech). But since the early 1980s the practice has been to consider various tropes as revealing particular kinds of conceptual metaphor. Thus, *personification* ("My cat speaks Italian") would be classified as a conceptual metaphor in which the target domain is an *animal* or *inanimate object* and the source domain a set of lexemes that are normally associated with human beings. Two tropes, however, are considered to be conceptually different—metonymy and irony. *Metonymy* entails the use of an entity within a domain to represent the entire domain:

1   She loves *South Park* (= the sitcom with that name).
2   There are too many new *faces* around here (= people).
3   They bought a *FIAT* (= car called a FIAT).
4   The *buses* are on strike (= bus drivers).
5   The *Church* does not condone that act (= theologians, priests).
6   The *White House* made another announcement today (= the president, the American government).

Irony is defined as a strategy whereby words are used to convey a meaning that seems to be contradictory or paradoxical—for example, "I love being tortured" uttered by someone in excruciating pain. Clearly, context is crucial in gleaning ironic meaning. If the sentence is uttered by a masochist, then it would hardly have ironic meaning (Winner 1988). Comedic uses of irony have always functioned to make people think about the world in which they lived. So too today, comedy and satire help us cope with societal events that confront us and challenge us on a daily basis.

2.2.3 Metaphor and Society

In the language spoken by the Batammaliba people who live in the border region between the West African states of Togo and the Benin Republic, the parts of the house are named with body terms (Tilley 1999: 41–49). Known as *anthropomorphism*, this common naming strategy suggests that we project our bodies metaphorically onto the referents that make up our lives in order to, perhaps, connect conceptually and existentially with them.

Anthropomorphism is common across cultures. As a concrete example, take the Western Apache language of east-central Arizona, which names the parts of the automobile in terms of body parts because they resemble each other in an imaginary way (Basso 1990: 15–24) (see Table 2.5).

Basso (1990) explains the use of such metaphors in two ways. First, there is the fact that cars came forward initially to replace horses in Apache life and, thus, the terms used to describe equine anatomy have been projected onto the names of car parts. Second, because vehicles can generate and sustain locomotion, they are perceived as metaphorical extensions of the anatomical constituents of equine or human movement.

Take, as another example of the link between metaphor and social naming practices, the verb system of Navajo. In that language, the categorization of motion is a major conceptual focus of that system (Young 2000). Many verbs designate specific aspects of motion and of objects affected by motion. For this reason, Navajo uses metaphors of motion, which manifest a specific kind of understanding and experience of the world that contrasts with English, as the examples in Table 2.6 show.

The gist of the foregoing discussion is that metaphor is the basis for understanding many essential aspects of social life. It is also connected to symbolic and ritualistic practices. Take, for instance, the *love is a sweet taste* conceptual metaphor in English, which manifests itself in such common linguistic metaphors as "She's my *sweetheart*," "They went on a *honeymoon*," and the like. The same concept also undergirds the practice of giving sweets to a romantic partner on St. Valentine's day, consuming a piece of wedding cake as symbolic of matrimonial love, sweetening the breath with candy before kissing a paramour, and so on. Incidentally, in Chagga, a Bantu language of Tanzania, similar practices exist. It is thus no coincidence that the language possesses the same conceptual metaphor. In Chagga, the man is

Table 2.5 Metaphorical Terms for Car Parts in Apache

English equivalent of Apache term	Auto part
fat	grease
chin and jaw	front bumper
shoulder	front fender
hand and arm	front wheel
thigh and buttock	rear fender
mouth	gas pipe opening
foot	rear wheel
back	bed of truck
eye	headlight
face	area from top of windshield to bumper
nose	hood
forehead	top, front of cab
entrails	machinery under hood
vein	electrical wiring
liver	battery
stomach	gas tank
intestine	radiator hose
heart	distributor
lung	radiator

Table 2.6 Navajo Concepts

English concept	Navajo concept translated literally
one dresses	one moves into clothing
one lives	one moves about here and there
one is young	one moves about newly
to sing	to move words out of an enclosed space
to greet someone	to move a round solid object to meet someone

perceived to be the *eater* and the woman his *sweet food*, as can be detected in expressions that mean, in translated form, "Does she taste sweet?" "She tastes sweet as sugar honey" (Emantian 1995: 168). Ongoing research on the relation between metaphor and social practices is showing that material, symbolic, and ritualistic culture is mirrored in, and even built from, conceptual metaphors.

Metaphor is also a trace to the unconscious knowledge and folk wisdom of a society. A proverb such as "He has fallen from *grace*" refers in its origin to a Biblical narrative. Today, we continue to use it with only a dim awareness (if any) of its origins. Conceptual metaphors that portray life as a journey—"I'm still a *long way* from my goal," "There is no *end* in sight"—are similarly rooted in Biblical narrative. As the Canadian literary critic Northrop Frye (1981) pointed out, one cannot grasp the meaning of such expressions without having been exposed, directly or indirectly, to the original stories. These are the unconscious source domains for many of the words and proverbs we use for judging human actions and offering advice, bestowing on everyday life an unconscious metaphysical meaning and value. When we say "An eye for an eye and a tooth for a tooth" we are invoking imagery that reverberates with implicit Biblical meaning. Every culture has similar proverbs, aphorisms, and sayings. They constitute a remarkable code of practical knowledge and ethics that anthropologists call "folk wisdom." Indeed, the very concept of wisdom implies the ability to apply proverbial language insightfully to a situation.

2.3 Grammar and Phonology

In addition to vocabulary, the grammar and phonology of a language also play crucial roles in encoding and cuing social realities. The word *grammar* has assumed many meanings since antiquity, as pointed out at the start of this chapter. In linguistics, it has a technical designation—knowledge of how lexemes are constructed and combined according to rules that allow speakers to produce and understand utterances. The study of grammar is divided traditionally into two main areas—*morphology* and *syntax*. The former is the analysis of how words are formed or put together from smaller units (morphemes), and the latter of how these are organized into phrases, sentences, and texts. Sociolinguistics does not focus on grammar per se, but on what it tells us about social phenomena. Recall that in Italian the masculine gender is the unmarked category in the domain of gender reference (Chapter 1). This aspect of Italian grammar once mirrored (and still does somewhat) differentiated perceptions of gender roles in Italian society. In other words, a specific aspect of Italian morphology was once marked for social gender roles.

Recall also how William Labov was able to link the pronunciation of a phoneme, /r/, to social identity and upward social mobility. His study brought out the fact that phonology matters to people, who are sensitive to its many socially based nuances. In effect, phonemes are suggestive structures. The way certain words are pronounced, as studies in pragmatics have shown, bear social value, conveying meaning in specific contexts. For example, Clopper and Pisoni (2004) found that the perception of phonological differences between regional dialects of American English by naïve listeners involved classifying the speakers. In one experiment, they used acoustic techniques to identify sentences that revealed different dialectal features. Then, recordings of the sentences were played back to listeners who were asked to categorize speakers into one of six geographical dialect regions and to the potential social class to which they belonged. The results showed that listeners were able to categorize speakers using three broad dialect clusters (New England, south, north/west), but that they had more difficulty categorizing speakers into six smaller regions. Taken together, the results confirmed that listeners have unconscious knowledge of phonological differences between dialects and social status, and use this knowledge unconsciously to categorize talkers by region and class.

2.3.1 Morphology

As discussed several times, the units that make up words are called morphemes. The word *cats*, for instance, consists of two morphemes: *cat* (phonemically /kæt/), whose meaning can be rendered broadly as "feline animal," and /-s/, whose meaning is "more than one." If the meaning of the morpheme is lexical (*cat*), then it is called a root morpheme or lexeme; if it recurs systematically in the formation of other words (such as /-s/ as a plural marker in *cats, pots, tips, pucks*), it is called a grammatical morpheme, or simply morpheme. The technique for identifying morphemes is known as *segmentation*. This entails breaking up a word into meaningful segments (morphemes) that cannot be split any further. The word *unfriendly* can be broken down into three segments: /un-/, /friend/, and /-ly/. Of these, /friend/ is the lexeme, whereas /un-/ and /-ly/ are grammatical morphemes: /un-/ is added as a prefix to adjectives, participles, and their derivatives to indicate the absence of a quality or state (*unbearable, unending*, and so on); and /-ly/ is added as a suffix to transform adjectives into adverbs, chiefly denoting manner or degree (*happily, easily*, and so on).

Morphological structure can encode differences in gender roles (Adler 1978). As briefly mentioned in Chapter 1, in the quasi-extinct Koasati language of Louisiana, verb endings identify the sex of the speaker (Haas 1944). Table 2.7 contains a few Koasati verbs in English-spelling transcription (for Koasati pronunciation see Appendix C).

As these examples show, the addition of /-s/ indicates a male speaker. In terms of markedness theory, this suggests that the masculine gender in Koasati is the marked one, and the feminine the unmarked one, which, in turn, suggests that the society is matrilineal. And this turns out to be the case. Koasati was part of a native civilization called *Muskogee*, in which clan structure is matrilineal and authority over the clan is ascribed to the women (mainly elderly).

Table 2.7 Gendered Differences in Koasati Verbs

English gloss	Women say ...	Men say ...
lift it	*lakawohl*	*lakawohs*
he is saying	*ka*	*kas*
don't sing	*taalawan*	*taalawas*
he is building a fire	*ot*	*os*

Thus, the distinction in the morphology of Koasati verbs is a reflection of a distinction in social structure based on matrilineage. In Kurukh, a Dravidian language spoken in northern India, the verb suffixes are similarly gender coded (Ekka 1972), but with a reverse markedness system—one set for the men speaking to women and another for the women speaking to women. When men and women interact, the masculine suffixes are the unmarked forms.

2.3.2 Syntax

Investigating the ways in which morphemes and lexemes are organized to produce phrases, sentences, and texts is called *syntactic analysis*. If the words in (1) "Alex teased Sarah" are reversed to (2) "Sarah teased Alex," the meanings are also reversed. The collocation of words in English sentences mirrors an actor-action-receiver relationship. The actor is converted into the grammatical subject of an active English sentence, the action into a verb, and the receiver into its aim (or object). In (1), *Alex* is the actor whereas in (2) it is *Sarah*. In (1) *Sarah* is the receiver of the *teasing* action, whereas in (2) the receiver is *Alex*. This is why the meanings are also reversed. Edward Sapir (1921) was among the first to argue that a change in the order of words in a sentence, or omitting any words from it, reflects different concepts. As he put it (Sapir 1921: 87): "The sentence is the outgrowth of historical and of unreasoning psychological forces rather than of a logical synthesis of elements that have been clearly grasped in their individuality." As Sapir went on to suggest, syntax is not an arbitrary system of sentence formation; it is a guide to how thoughts are formed (Crawford 1995; Hall and Bucholtz 1996).

Psychologist Cheris Kramer noted in 1974 that the speech of American men and women was differentiated by a distinctive blend of marked characteristics, such as tone, profanities, and the use of tag questions ("Don't you think?" "Isn't it?"). Kramer presented captions of cartoons taken from a number of magazines to a group of college students (25 men, 25 women), asking them to guess the sex of the speakers in the cartoons. The subjects classified the captions according to male and female speech characteristics, as instructed, with no hesitation. In other words, Kramer was able to show that we tend perceive some syntactic structures as gendered. Her work was carried out in the 1970s. Since then, syntactically marked categories in English have become largely neutralized, although some persist (Holmes 1984; Cameron, McAlinden, and O'Leary 1988; Macaulay 2009).

Gender is not the only social code that is mirrored in syntax. In 1969, Jacqueline Lindenfeld found a correlation between syntactic complexity, degree of formality of conversations, and class membership. Using notions such as sentence length and embedded clauses (clauses starting with *that*, *which*, or *who*), she discovered that the greater the length and degree of embedding in certain contexts, the more the utterance was associated with educated and higher class speech, regardless of gender. Similar findings have been reported across the world, including in Belgium (Van den Broek 1977) and Turkey (Huls 1989). Overall, as Jenny Chesire (2009) has cogently argued, the sociolinguistic studies on syntax show that specific syntactic structures correlate with social variables, such as a speaker's social class or gender.

2.3.3 Phonology

In a classic sociolinguistic study, Peter Trudgill (1974), was able to connect phonological features to differentiated speech in a community in Norwich, England. He found, predictably, that the higher the level of education attained by people in the community, the more they aspired to use standard forms of pronunciation. But, more significantly, he discovered that in casual speech situations it was the women, regardless of educational background, who used standard pronunciation the most—for example, they were more inclined to completely pronounce the /-ing/ verb ending instead of the informal /-in/ one in lexical pairs such as *walking* versus *walkin'*. Even in the lowest class, the women were the ones who were more inclined to use standard pronunciation than were the men. Trudgill's study suggested that, in some societies or speech communities, women tend to be more sensitive to the social value of phonemic cues, whereas men prefer to speak in a manner that binds them socially to their male peers. He called this "covert prestige." For the women in Norwich, the covert prestige is towards the norm, for the men it is away from it.

Gender-based differentiations in pronunciation abound across languages. For example, in Atsina, an Algonquin language once spoken in Montana (Goddard 2001), women used palatalized velar stops (/ky/ rather than /k/) and men palatalized dental stops (/dy/ rather than /d/). So, for example, the word for "bread" was pronounced as *kjatsa* = /kyatsa/ by the women and as *djatsa* = /dyatsa/ by the men. In 1922, Bogaras documented similar doublets in the Chukchee language of Siberia, where the consonants /č/ (pronounced like the *ch* in *change*) and /r/ in male speech are replaced with /s/ or /š/ (pronounced like *sh* in *shore*) in female speech. So, the lexeme for the phrase "by a buck" would be pronounced as /čumñata/ by the men and as /šumñata/ by the women, and "people" as /ramkičin/ by the men and as /šamkiššin/ by the women. In another relevant study, Levine and Crockett (1967) found that white women speakers in North Carolina tended to use standard pronunciation more than men if the situation required formal speech. Wolfram (1969) discovered that in AAVE-speaking communities in Detroit, the women tended to use the more prestigious /-r/ in words such as *far* and *car* more than the men when the occasion called for the use of the standard language.

Research has also shown that specific vowel phonemes often correlate with class variables. In a northern Indian village called Khalapur, pronunciation differences in the local Hindi dialect called Khari Boli signal caste differences (Gumperz 1971). The lower castes use the single vowels /a/, /u/, /o/ before consonants, whereas the higher castes use the more standard Hindi diphthongs /ai/, /ui/, /oi/. So, the word for "ear of corn" would be pronounced as /bal/ by the lower castes and as /bail/ or just /bai/ by the higher ones. Contrasts of this type characterize the phonemic vowel system of the dialect. Differentiated vowel pronunciations also allow people to signal their distinctive identities. The inhabitants of Martha's Vineyard, in Massachusetts, have adopted particular vowel phonemes to keep themselves apart from people vacationing on the island (Labov 1963).

2.4 Language and Social Media

The overall objective of this chapter has been to discuss the language–society nexus, that is, to show how the units and structures of a language (lexical, grammatical, and phonological) encode social variables, reveal social emphases, define speech communities, and how sociolinguistics has traditionally studied these phenomena. The discussion and exemplification was based on research in real-world situations. However, the world has changed since the advent of the Internet, and sociolinguistics is being applied increasingly to examine how the language–society nexus has changed in online culture and communications.

As we saw in the previous chapter, the linguistic investigation of online speech falls generally, but not exclusively, under the rubric of Internet Linguistics. One general finding concerns the style of writing that has emerged, named *netlingo* by British linguist David Crystal (2006, 2008). This is a style that is characterized by compactness, allowing interlocutors to increase the speed at which their messages can be inputted and sent. For this reason, a series of common abbreviations, acronyms, and other reduced forms have become conventionalized in what is essentially a "digital dialect." These are easy to explain from a purely structural perspective: for example, removing vowels in frequently used words and expressions does not impact comprehension in any obstructive way, and using single letters for entire words also requires little effort to decode messages: *I have g2g* ("I have got to go"), *How r u?* ("How are you?"), etc.

Research has shown that register (level of formality) is determined by whether abbreviations are used (or not) in online communications. In formal email messaging, words tend to be spelled out completely and traditional grammar and punctuation are used. In informal text messaging, tweets, and other routine social media-based communications, however, the reverse is often true. If a word is spelled out completely it is either because the software used by the device is a corrective one or because semantic nuances are intended: *How are you?* versus *How r u?* The latter is the normally expected one among friends; the former is not, and thus might be interpreted in nuanced ways, such as conveying subtle anger or irony (Danesi 2013). It is relevant to note that no less an authority on language trends than the Oxford English Dictionary has listed items from netlingo into its dictionary (*lol*, 24/7, g2g, and many more). It also chose an emoji for its "Word of the

Year" in 2015—an event that will be discussed in Chapter 7. In this final section of this chapter, a few general findings and commentaries on the language of social media will be put forth. More detailed aspects will be discussed in due course.

2.4.1 Social Media

As Nazir (2012) has shown in her research, the use of social media has not drastically changed the patterns in the language–society nexus discussed in this chapter. She found, for instance, that the same system of marked gendered speech in English conversation is still evident on Facebook. Similar findings have been documented across languages (Lewis and Fabos 2005; Zappavigna 2012, 2018; Schwartz et al. 2013; Vandergriff 2013). However, several changes have been documented. One is the notion of speech community. In the social media universe, it is typically *virtual* or *imaginary*, rather than based on real-world historical traditions. Social media systems have allowed anyone to interact with anyone else in the world, regardless of social or ethnic backgrounds. A virtual community has the following features:

1   A common language, such as Twitterspeak or netlingo, based on a set of linguistic conventions constructed by the participants, including the use of hashtags to identify topics. The hashtag is part of a "folksonomy," a user-created naming system, which is quite distinct from a taxonomy, a centrally created naming system.
2   A dual-faceted community structure, which is both collective and personal. It is collective because social media users belong to a worldwide group who understand the common language and its norms. Moreover, almost all messages are searchable, except for a small number of partially locked private pages. Virtual communities are also personal because members imagine they are following and talking to other members, as in F2F conversations.
3   There is a belief that personal tweets have the ability to influence people in the network through replies and retweeting.
4   In such communities, there is regular communication around a shared purpose or interest.
5   Social and linguistic identities are negotiated within the virtual community.

The promise of social media has been to allow human needs to be expressed individualistically, even though most users soon start to realize that its true force lies in the compulsive attachment it instills in them. In the past, social relations, enduring cultural traditions, and stable patterns of work, life, and leisure assured people that stable patterns of meaning and experience united them in real space. The Internet has shattered this assurance, impelling individuals to develop new strategies to manage the shocks of everyday life. Social media have also engendered addictive behaviors, such as *FOMO* (fear of missing out), which is the irrational fear that others, such as friends on Facebook, may be experiencing enjoyment or excitement, which stimulates a desire to stay continually connected to what others are doing via social media. Another is *FONK* (fear of not knowing), or the belief that if we only knew more, we would be able to do much more, including enjoy ourselves more.

One particularly interesting new form of speech is called "searchable talk" (Zappavigna 2018), which is connected to hashtag culture. Hashtags have a "commentary" function. A hashtag referencing the target of evaluation in a tweet, not only renders the content searchable, but also constitutes a means to affiliate with values expressed in the tweet. The subtext is "Search for me and affiliate with my values." Hashtags can become ideologically and politically subtle codes.

2.4.2 Multimodality

A major technological difference between F2F and CMC communication involves multimodality. Simply put, this is the use of a combination of *modes* of communication—writing, audio, images, animation, etc.—that allows for a message to be delivered and processed in a complementary way.

The American philosopher Susanne Langer (1948) referred to the linear-sequential process of encoding and decoding verbal (written) texts as a *discursive* one; whereas, texts such as paintings or musical works are processed holistically, rather than linearly; she called this type of modality *presentational*. Discursiveness has the salient feature of detachment, which means that the constituent parts of a text can be considered separately—for example, one can focus on a specific word, detaching it from its location in the text, without impairing the overall understanding of the text. Presentational texts cannot be similarly deconstructed. For example, we experience a work of art not as an isolated event, but in its entirety as a unitary structure. Trying to understand what it means forces us, however, to analyze why the art work so moved us. However, no matter how many times we try to explain the experience, it somehow remains beyond analysis. One can analyze the opening movement of Beethoven's *Moonlight Sonata* as a series of harmonic progressions and melodic figures based on the key of C# minor. However, the elements of melody and harmony come into focus as components of the work only during a discursive analysis of the sonata's structure. When one hears it played as an artistic performance, however, one hardly focuses on these constituent elements. One experiences the music holistically.

In making multimodality routine, CMC is both discursive and presentational. For example, an emoji added to a written text will add a visually based presentational component that complements the alphabetically constructed text. We do not read an emoji or an animated video as composed of individual bits and pieces, but presentationally, as a totality which encloses and reveals its meaning holistically, connecting it to the verbal text. The multimodality feature of CMC implies a more flexible form of sociolinguistic research that must be used in tandem with the traditional ethnographic methods of observation, interviewing, and discourse analysis in order to understand the language–society nexus that has evolved in cyberspace (see, for example, Norris 2004; Bolander and Locher 2014; Yang 2019).

2.4.3 Memes

A feature of online communications that is grabbing the attention of linguists more and more is the phenomenon of *memes*, a term coined by sociobiologist Richard Dawkins in *The Selfish Gene* (1976), which he defines as replicating patterns of information (ideas, fashions, artworks, etc.) and of behavior that people inherit directly from their cultural environments. An Internet meme, more specifically, may be an image (for example a photo of a cat), a video (such as the dance craze), a hyperlink, a hashtag, a website, or even just a word or phrase. Memes spread virally via social media networks, blogs, and email, constituting a new form of discourse that is based on the ephemerality of everyday events. As Mark Deuze (2010) observes, the technologies associated with online culture, especially the mobile ones, make content a personalized transportable form, and thus embedded in the variability and randomness of everybody's life. Studies have shown that memes can, in fact, be studied as units analogous to the usual structural units of a language (lexemes, morphemes, etc.) (Blackmore et al. 2000).

Lestari (2019) carried out an extensive analysis of memes on Instagram, showing how memetic communication has become a powerful one, transcending physical and national boundaries. Memes allow for a larger community, independent of national language, to form and coalesce around similar topics of interest. Three relevant features of memes are the following:

- Memes are highly reproducible and thus can spread virally.
- As they traverse social media, memes can be altered and thus mutate, whereby the original meme is tweaked to conform to the specific interests of particular virtual communities. This suggests that there are "dialect memes" that speak directly to certain communities.
- Hashtag memes are often used as incentives for social change.

Memetic theory is itself in a state of flux, and thus any sociolinguistic approach to the study of memetic communication must be tempered accordingly (see, for example, Deacon 2004). Such communication depends on the nature of technology—as this changes so too will memetic communication. The usual questions in this regard apply here as well, such as the following: Are memes intertwined with social variables (that is, are memes gendered, group based, etc.)? Are they part of a new multimodal lexicon, and if so, what semantic structures underlie it? Are they connected to conceptual metaphors? Do they display semantic ambiguity as do linguistic forms? And so on.

References and Further Reading

Adler, M. K. (1978). *Sex Differences in Human Speech: A Sociolinguistic Study.* Hamburg: Helmut Buske.

Alim, S. (2004). Hip-Hop Nation Language. In: E. Finegan and J. Rickford (eds.), *Language in the USA.* New York: Cambridge University Press.

Alim, S. and Smitherman, G. (2012). *Articulate While Black: Barack Obama, Language, and Race in the U.S.* Oxford: Oxford University Press.

Alim, S., Rickford, J., and Ball, A. F. (eds.) (2016). *Raciolinguistics: How Language Shapes Our Ideas about Race.* Oxford: Oxford University Press.

Bar-Hillel, Y. (1960). The Present Status of Automatic Translation of Languages. *Advances in Computers* 1: 91–163.

Basso, K. H. (1990). *Western Apache Language and Culture: Essays in Linguistic Anthropology.* Tucson, AZ: University of Arizona Press.

Berlin, B. and Kay, P. (1969). *Basic Color Terms.* Berkeley, CA: University of California Press.

Bernstein, B. (1971). *Class, Codes and Control: Theoretical Studies Towards a Sociology of Language.* London: Routledge.

Black, M. (1962). *Models and Metaphors.* Ithaca, NY: Cornell University Press.

Blackmore, S., Dugatkin, L. A., Boyd, R., Richerson, P. J., and Plotkin, H. (2000). The Power of Memes. *Scientific American* 283(4): 64–73.

Bogaras, W. (1922). Chukchee. In: *Handbook of American Indian Languages,* pp. 631–903. Washington, DC: Bureau of American Ethnology.

Bolander, B. and Locher, M. A. (2014). Doing Sociolinguistic Research on Computer-Mediated Data: A Review of Four Methodological Issues. *Discourse, Context, and Media* 3: 14–26.

Booth, A. D. (1955). Use of a Computing Machine as a Mechanical Dictionary. *Nature* 176: 565.

Bühler, K. (1908/1951). On Thought Connection. In: D. Rapaport (ed.), *Organization and Pathology of Thought,* pp. 81–92. New York: Columbia University Press.

Bühler, K. (1934). *Sprachtheorie. Die Darstellungsfunktion der Sprache.* Stuttgart/New York: Gustav Fischer.

Cameron, D., McAlinden, F., and O'Leary, K. (1988). Lakoff in Context: The Social and Linguistic Functions of Tag Questions. In: J. Coates and D. Cameron (eds.), *Women in Their Speech Communities,* pp. 74–93. London: Longman.

Chesire, J. (2009). Syntactic Variation and Beyond. In: N. Coupland and A. Jaworski (eds.), *The New Sociolinguistics Reader,* pp. 119–135. Basingstoke: Palgrave Macmillan.

Chomsky, N. (1957). *Syntactic Structures.* The Hague: Mouton.

Chomsky, N. (1966). *Cartesian Linguistics: A Chapter in the History of Rationalist Thought.* New York: Harper & Row.

Clopper, C. G. and Pisoni, D. (2004). Some Acoustic Cues for the Perceptual Categorization of American English Regional Dialects. *Journal of Phonetics* 32: 111–140.

Coates, J. (1986). *Men, Women, and Language: A Sociolinguistic Account of Gender Differences in Language.* London: Longman.

Crawford, M. (1995). *Talking Difference: On Gender and Language.* Thousand Oaks, CA: Sage.

Crystal, D. (2006). *Language and the Internet,* 2nd ed. Cambridge: Cambridge University Press.

Crystal, D. (2008). *Txtng: The gr8 db8*. Oxford: Oxford University Press.

Danesi, M. (2013). *La comunicazione verbale al tempo di Internet*. Bari: Progedit.

Danesi, M. (2017). The Bidirectionality of Metaphor. *Poetics Today* 38: 15–33.

Dawkins, R. (1976). *The Selfish Gene*. Oxford: Oxford University Press.

Deacon, T. W. (2004). Memes as Signs in the Dynamic Logic of Semiosis: Beyond Molecular Science and Computation Theory. In: *International Conference on Conceptual Structures*, pp. 17–30. Berlin: Springer.

Deuze, M. (2010). *Media Life*. Cambridge: Polity Press.

Duranti, A. and Goodwin, C. (eds.) (1992). *Rethinking Context: Language as an Interactive Phenomenon*. Cambridge: Cambridge University Press.

Dyen, I. (1975). *Linguistic Subgrouping and Lexicostatistics*. The Hague: Mouton.

Eckert, P. and McConnell-Ginet, S. (2003). *Language and Gender*. Cambridge: Cambridge University Press.

Ekka, F. (1972). Men's and Women's Speech in Kurux. *Linguistics* 81: 25–31.

Emantian, M. (1995). Metaphor and the Expression of Emotion: The Value of Cross-Cultural Perspectives. *Metaphor and Symbolic Activity* 10: 163–182.

Frye, N. (1981). *The Great Code: The Bible and Literature*. Toronto: Academic Press.

Goddard, I. (2001).The Algonquian Languages of the Plains. In: *The Handbook of North American Indians*. Washington, DC: Smithsonian Institution.

Goffman, E. (1959). *The Presentation of Self in Everyday Life*. New York: Anchor.

Gray, R. D. and Atkinson, Q. D. (2003). Language–Tree Divergence Times Support the Anatolian Theory of Indo–European Origin. *Nature* 425: 435–439.

Gumperz, J. (1971). Dialect Differences and Social Stratification in a North Indian Village. *American Anthropologist* 60: 668–681.

Haas, M. (1944). Men's and Women's Speech in Koasati. *Language* 20: 142–149.

Hall, K. and Bucholtz, M. (1996). *Gender Articulated: Language and the Socially Constructed Self*. London: Routledge.

Holmes, J. (1984). Hedging Your Bets on Sitting on the Fence: Some Evidence for Hedges as Support Structures. *Te Reo* 27: 47–62.

Honeck, R. P. and Hoffman, R. R. (eds.) (1980). *Cognition and Figurative Language*. Hillsdale, NJ: Lawrence Erlbaum Associates.

Huls, E. (1989). Directness, Explicitness and Orientation in Turkish Family Interaction. In: K. Deprez (ed.), *Language and Intergroup Relations in Flanders and in the Netherlands*, pp. 145–164. Dordrecht: Foris.

Humboldt, W. V. (1836 [1988]). *On Language: The Diversity of Human Language-Structure and Its Influence on the Mental Development of Mankind*. Trans. P. Heath. Cambridge: Cambridge University Press.

Johnson, M. (1987). *The Body in the Mind: The Bodily Basis of Meaning, Imagination and Reason*. Chicago: University of Chicago Press.

Johnson, M. (2007). *The Meaning of the Body: Aesthetics of Human Understanding*. Chicago: University of Chicago Press.

Kay, P. (1975). Synchronic Variability and Diachronic Change in Basic Color Terms. *Language in Society* 4: 257–270.

Kay, P. (1997). *Words and the Grammar of Context*. Cambridge: Cambridge University Press.

Kramer, C. (1974). Folk Linguistics: Wishy-Washy Mommy Talk. *Psychology Today* 8: 82–85.

Labov, W. (1963). The Social Motivation of a Sound Change. *Word* 19: 273–309.

Labov, W. (1973). The Boundaries of Words and Their Meanings. In: C. Bailey and R. Shuy (eds.), *New Ways of Analyzing Variation in English*, pp. 340–373. Washington, DC: Georgetown University Press.

Lakoff, G. (1979). The Contemporary Theory of Metaphor. In: A. Ortony (ed.), *Metaphor and Thought*, pp. 203–251. Cambridge: Cambridge University Press.

Lakoff, G. (1987). *Women, Fire, and Dangerous Things: What Categories Reveal About the Mind*. Chicago: University of Chicago Press.

Lakoff, G. and Johnson, M. (1980). *Metaphors We Live By*. Chicago: University of Chicago Press.

Lakoff, G. and Johnson, M. (1999). *Philosophy in the Flesh: The Embodied Mind and Its Challenge to Western Thought*. New York: Basic Books.

Lakoff, R. (1975). *Language and Woman's Place*. New York: Harper & Row.

Langer, S. (1948). *Philosophy in a New Key*. New York: Mentor Books

Lees, R. (1953). The Basis of Glottochronology. *Language* 29: 113–127.

Lestari, W. (2019). Irony Analysis of Memes on Instagram Social Media. *PIONEER: Journal of Language and Literature* 10(2): 114–123.

Levine, L. and Crockett, H. (1967). Speech Variation in a Piedmont Community: Postvocalic R. In: S. Lieberson (ed.), *Explorations in Sociolinguistics*, pp. 76–98. Bloomington, IN: Indiana University Press.

Lewis, C. and Fabos, B. (2005). Instant Messaging, Literacies, and Social Identities. *Reading Research Quarterly* 40: 470–501.

Lindenfeld, J. (1969). The Social Conditioning of Syntactic Variation in French. *American Anthropologist* 71: 890–898.

Lunde, P. (2004). *Organized Crime: An Inside Guide to the World's Most Successful Industry*. London: Dorling Kindersley.

Macaulay, R. (2009). *Quantitative Methods in Sociolinguistics*. New York: Palgrave Macmillan.

Malinowski, B. (1923). The Problem of Meaning in Primitive Languages. In: C. K. Ogden and I. A. Richards (eds.), *The Meaning of Meaning*, pp. 296–336. New York: Harcourt, Brace & World.

Morris, C. W. (1938). *Foundations of the Theory of Signs*. Chicago: University of Chicago Press.

Nazir, B. (2012). Gender Patterns on Facebook: A Sociolinguistic Perspective. *International Journal of Linguistics* 4: 252–265.

Nicaso, A. and Danesi, M. (2013). *Made Men: Mafia Culture and the Power of Symbols, Rituals, and Myth*. Lanham: Rowman & Littlefield.

Norris, S. (2004). *Analyzing Multimodal Interaction: A Methodological Framework*. London: Routledge.

Ortony, A. (ed.) (1979). *Metaphor and Thought*. Cambridge, MA: Cambridge University Press.

Peirce, C. S. (1931–1958). *Collected Papers*. Cambridge, MA: Harvard University Press.

Pollio, H., Barlow, J., Fine, H., and Pollio, M. (1977). *The Poetics of Growth: Figurative Language in Psychology, Psychotherapy, and Education*. Hillsdale, NJ: Lawrence Erlbaum Associates.

Rahn, J. (2002). *Painting Without Permission*. South Hadley, MA: Bergin and Garvey.

Reeves, M. (2008). *Somebody Scream: Rap Music's Rise to Prominence in the Aftershock of Black Power*. London: Faber & Faber.

Richards, I. A. (1936). *The Philosophy of Rhetoric*. Oxford: Oxford University Press.

Sapir, E. (1921). *Language*. New York: Harcourt, Brace, & World.

Schwartz, H. A., Eichstaedt, J. C., Kern, M. L., Dziurzynski, L., Ramones, S. M., Agrawal, M., et al. (2013). Personality, Gender, and Age in the Language of Social Media: The Open-Vocabulary Approach. *PLOS ONE* 8: 1–15.

Smitherman, G. (2000). *Black Talk: Words and Phrases from the Hood to the Amen Corner*. Boston, MA: Houghton-Mifflin.

Swadesh, M. (1951). Diffusional Cumulation and Archaic Residue as Historical Explanations. *Southwestern Journal of Anthropology* 7: 1–21.

Swadesh, M. (1959). Linguistics as an Instrument of Prehistory. *Southwestern Journal of Anthropology* 15: 20–35.

Swadesh, M. (1971). *The Origins and Diversification of Language*. Chicago: Aldine-Atherton.

Thomas, E. R. (2007). Phonological and Phonetic Characteristics of African American Vernacular English. *Language and Linguistics Compass* 1: 450–475.

Tilley, C. (1999). *Metaphor and Material Culture*. Oxford: Wiley-Blackwell.

Trudgill, P. (1974). *The Social Differentiation of English in Norwich*. Cambridge: Cambridge University Press.

Van den Broek, J. (1977). Class Differences in Syntactic Complexity in the Flemish Town of Maaseik. *Language and Society* 6: 149–181.

Vandergriff, I. (2013). Emotive Communication Online: A Contextual Analysis of Computer-Mediated Communication (CMC) Cues. *Journal of Pragmatics* 51: 1–12.

Weaver, W. (1955). Translation. In: W. N. Locke and A. D. Booth (eds.), *Machine Translation of Languages*, pp. 15–23. New York: John Wiley.

Werner, A. (1919). *Introductory Sketch of the Bantu Languages*. New York: Dutton.

Wescott, R. (1980). *Sound and Sense*. Lake Bluff, IL: Jupiter Press.

Winner, E. (1988). *The Point of Words: Children's Understanding of Metaphor and Irony*. Cambridge, MA: Harvard University Press.

Wolfram, W. (1969). *A Sociolinguistic Description of Detroit Negro Speech*. Washington, DC: Center for Applied Linguistics.

Wundt, W. (1901). *Sprachgeschichte und Sprachpsychologie*. Leipzig: Eugelmann.

Yang, Y. (2019). A Review of Multimodality Research: Origins and Development. *Language and Semiotic Studies* 5: 119–141.

Young, R. (2000). *The Navajo Verb System: An Overview*. Albuquerque: University of New Mexico Press.

Zappavigna, M. (2012). *Discourse of Twitter and Social Media*. London: Bloomsbury.

Zappavigna, M. (2018). *Searchable Talk*. London: Bloomsbury.

3   Variation in Geographical Space

A primary objective of sociolinguistics is to study language variation in all kinds of spaces, physical and social—geographical, social, cultural, pragmatic, and mediated (online versus offline). Traditionally, the investigation of geographical variation has come under two branches: (1) *dialectology*, the scientific study of dialects, and (2) *contact linguistics*, the investigation of languages in contact, such as Spanish in contact with English in the US, producing what is colloquially called "Spanglish," a mixture of Spanish and English.

A *dialect* is a variant of a language that is recognizable in terms of specific differential features (phonological, grammatical, lexical, semantic, pragmatic) that evolve according to where it is spoken and who speaks it. But the line between a "dialect" and a "language" is rarely clear-cut. The term "English" is now interpreted as referring to a "language," rather than a "dialect." But there are many versions of "English" according to the areas in which the language is spoken (British English, American English, Canadian English, Australian English, and so on). However, these are hardly considered dialects of one another any longer, even though historically speaking they are. In other words, the language spoken in territories that achieved nationhood at some point after British colonization is no longer perceived as a dialect of British English (the source language) for sociopolitical reasons. Only the variants within each English-speaking nation are now considered to be regional dialects (Cajun American, Newfoundland Canadian, Cockney, and so on).

This chapter looks at the sociolinguistic study of geographically based linguistic variation. This includes not only the investigation of regional dialects per se, which falls more specifically under the rubric of dialectology, as mentioned, but also phenomena such as language admixture within the speech of certain communities, bilingualism, the assignment of prestige to specific dialects, known as diglossia, and the relation of dialect speech to social perceptions generally.

3.1 Dialects and Other Regional Variants

The term *dialect* comes from the Greek word *dialektos*, meaning "speech." It referred in antiquity to the actual ways in which people spoke in conversations. It is often the case that what we call a "national," or "standard language" is historically a dialectal variant that became the standard or norm at some point in time because of social, literary, or political reasons. For example, in France the language spoken in Paris, known as Parisian French, is today considered to be the standard language. Speech communities that do not use it routinely, having historically lived away from Paris, are said to speak a regional variant or dialect of this standard. But Parisian French was, once, just one among many dialects. The reasons why it became the official (national) standard are connected to the social, political, and economic prestige of the city of Paris. Initially, there was no perception of the Parisian variant as being prestigious with respect to other variants of French. But the instant that it became so, the other variants took on dialect status.

This historical pattern applies to the linguistic histories of most nations. The emergence of Florentine Tuscan as the basis for the standard language of Italy, for instance, had nothing to do with the quality of its pronunciation or grammar, but rather, with the fact that three famous and influential medieval writers (Dante, Petrarch, and Boccaccio) used it to promote an incipient literary style written in a vernacular tongue, rather than Latin, that people from all over Italy admired and wanted to emulate. Also, Florence had become a major political and economic center within Italy and, thus, speaking the vernacular of the Florentines was perceived as politically and socially beneficial; this reality led, over time, to making the Florentine vernacular a "standard" one for all Italians.

3.1.1 Mutual Intelligibility

As discussed in the opening chapter, determining whether two variants are dialects or distinct languages is guided by the notion of mutual intelligibility (Gooskens 2017). This means essentially that if speakers understand one another, then they likely speak dialects of the same language; if they do not, then they are probably speaking different languages. As Chambers and Trudgill (1998: 3) state, this view "has the benefit of characterizing dialects as subparts of a language and of providing a criterion for distinguishing between one language and another." There are, however, problems with this notion, as mentioned, because many levels of mutual intelligibility exist (even among unrelated languages), making it sometimes difficult to decide whether certain speech varieties should be considered dialects or distinct languages. In practice, however, it has proved to be a useful notion for the simple reason that most people can tell whether variants are related or not. As a trivial example, Americans recognize the speech variants that are characteristic of southern states, such as Alabama and Mississippi, as versions of Standard American English (SAE), because they can understand them, more or less, no matter what part of the US they live in. The differences (lexical, phonological, etc.) are thus perceived as peculiar to a specific group of speakers, not as reflective of a different language.

Dialect features allow us to pinpoint the region where a variant is spoken. For example, the variant of English spoken in various parts of New York and New England is typically characterized by the dropping of the /-r/ phoneme at the end of words (*car* pronounced /kah/), and the use of a short close /o/ instead of an open /ɔ/ (*fog* = /fog/). Some southern American dialects are distinguished by a broad /a/ (*time* = /ta^{h}m/), and a short /i/ in place of /e/ before a nasal sound (*pen* = /pi^{h}n/) (see Appendix D for a summary of the phonetic classification of English vowels.). These dialects are also marked by use of a plural form of the pronoun *you*—namely, *y'all*. Documenting differences in pronunciation, grammar, and vocabulary is a basic task of dialectology proper. The goal of sociolinguistics is more properly to examine the social perceptions that these differences entail.

The notion of *asymmetric intelligibility* is sometimes employed in place of mutual intelligibility. This refers to the fact that one group of speakers of mutually comprehensible dialects (or languages) experience more difficulty understanding the other code than the other way around. Speakers of Scottish English have greater facility in understanding speakers of American English; the reverse, however, is not necessarily so. Indeed, speakers of American English typically have to listen very carefully to a speaker of Scottish English in order to grasp the contents of an utterance. The likely reason for this is that Scottish English speakers are exposed daily to TV programs and movies based on American English, and thus become relatively more familiar with its features. The reverse is not normally the case.

The concept of *dialect continuum* is also employed by dialectologists to explain why some dialects are mutually intelligible and others perceived to be separate languages. The term refers to an interconnected group of geographically adjacent or historically related variants, some of which are mutually intelligible to different speakers, whereas others, over time, have become less comprehensible as distance between the speakers increased through migration or social events (such as intermarriages). For example, the Romance languages—Portuguese, Spanish, Catalan, Provençal, French, Romanian, Italian, and a few others—originally formed a dialect continuum with a relatively high degree of mutual intelligibility. Gradually these became national languages, leading to increasing incomprehensibility. Although there still are varying levels of mutual intelligibility between speakers of, say, Italian and Spanish today, distance and historical events have made it increasingly more tenuous.

Isolation, geographical or social, from the speakers of the standard language also fosters higher levels of incomprehensibility, as regional communities tend to adopt and preserve the linguistic features of their group rather than absorb those of the standard language for their daily affairs. The standard language for many regional communities is a code learned at school and used for official purposes; the dialect is the one used for daily communication among members of the group, constituting a code of identity.

3.1.2 *Dialect Atlases*

To study dialects, a number of research tools and methods have been developed by linguists. One of these is the *dialect atlas*. This is, as its name implies, a collection of maps of specific regions recording their actual speech features. The first to construct a dialect map was, as already discussed (Chapter 1), the German linguist Georg Wenker in 1876. He sent out questionnaires asking people to indicate how they would pronounce specific German words. He then recorded the various pronunciations on different maps, compiling them into an atlas. The atlas allowed him to subdivide Germany into distinct dialect areas according to their phonological characteristics.

In the last decade of the nineteenth century, the Swiss linguist Jules Gilliéron devised a similar questionnaire for eliciting 1,500 core vocabulary items. He chose a fieldworker, named Edmond Edmont, to compile the relevant data from the designated regions of France. From 1896 to 1900, Edmont conducted 700 interviews at 639 sites. Known as the *Atlas linguistique de la France*, publication of the atlas got under way in 1902 and was completed in 1910. It became a model for subsequent atlases. The map in Figure 3.1 is taken from this atlas. It shows how the lexeme for "Wednesday" varies according to region.

The map provides a snapshot of how a linguistic item is distributed according to dialect region. If one were to hear *mècres* spoken in a conversation, then it is highly probable that the speaker comes from a central region of France; if a speaker uses *dimècres* instead then we can assume that the interlocutor is speaking a southern version of the language; and so on. In addition to containing such information related to the speaker's regional background, the differential forms can also be examined as markers of social identity. If a southern speaker were to be conversing with a northern one and desire to reveal regional identity, consciously or unconsciously, the use of *dimècres* would do the trick rather well.

There has been some criticism of traditional dialect interview methods. First, it is pointed out that the collection of data was guided by the belief that the "real speakers" of a dialect lived in rural areas, untainted by influences from urban life. A second presupposition was that older male speakers were the authentic bearers of the dialect, whereas the speech of younger and female speakers might deviate from it. This male-centered view of the "ideal speakers" may have reflected the social biases of the era. Needless to say, the situation has changed today, as dialectologists sample balanced populations of speakers, males and females, young and old, rural and urban, alike.

Dialect maps provide a relatively precise empirical tool for describing variation along the dialect continuum. Today, data collection is carried out more and more via phone surveys, rather than physically on site. For example, Labov, Ash, and Boberg in 2005 used a telephone survey of 762 local speakers to compile their authoritative *Atlas of North American English: Phonetics, Phonology and Sound Change*, which has recast the distribution of regional

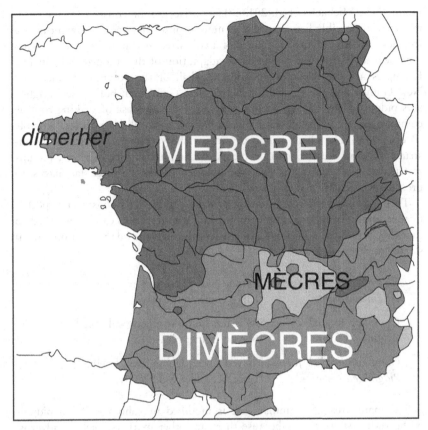

Figure 3.1 Geographical Distribution of French Lexemes for "Wednesday"
Source: *L'Atlas Linguistique del la France,* 1902–1910

dialects on the basis of phonological changes that were taking place in the 1990s. Dialectologists also have at their disposal a wide array of new and powerful research methods, including computer software, that allow them to analyze large amounts of data quickly and to produce linguistic maps with a greater degree of accuracy (Kretschmar 2017; Rabanus 2017; Upton, Widdowson, and Stewert 2017). They can also use social media to glean from the conversations on, say, Facebook or Twitter, features that relate to dialect usage and its social implications (Eisenstein 2017).

3.1.3 Pidgins and Creoles

Not all geographical variants are dialects, in the traditional sense of the word. The *pidgin* and *Creole* tongues spoken in various parts of the world are examples of nondialectal region-based variants of a language (Hall 1966;

Holm 1989; Michaelis et al. 2013). They arise spontaneously to make communication possible between two or more groups that speak different native tongues. Usually, it is the language of a colonizer that an indigenous denizen must learn, creating the pidgin as an adaptation of the colonizer's language. Examples are the Melanesian Pidgin English of the Solomon Islands and New Guinea and the English of Papua New Guinea. In both cases, English was pidginized by the indigenous people for the purpose of making routine communication with officials and monolingual English speakers possible (Bruce 1984). The phenomenon of pidgins shows that people respond constructively and creatively to problems of communication. In effect, pidgins restructure the grammars and vocabularies of their source languages to produce new creative versions of them.

To grasp what the pidginization process entails, let's construct hypothetical examples of how certain complex English utterances can be modified so that they retain their meaning nonetheless through the adaptive grammatical strategies:

> *Complete English form:* I would like to come tomorrow.
> *Pidginized form:*   *I like come tomorrow.

> *Complete English form:* She is not home so please call her later.
> *Pidginized form:*   *She no home; please call later.

> *Complete English form:* I haven't been feeling well lately.
> *Pidginized form:*   *I not been feel well, lately.

The main area of grammar that is modified morphologically in pidgins is the verb system; this is because there are other markers, such as adverbs, that can be used to indicate tense relations. Other common mechanisms in pidginization include: an SVO word order (subject-verb-predicate), preverbal negation ("I not been feel well"); and copula verb deletion: "I well" rather than "I am well."

There are three main outcomes for a pidgin. It may eventually disappear, if it loses its original social-communicative functions, which is what happened to Hawaiian pidgin, now almost entirely replaced by standard English in Hawaii. It can remain in use for generations, or even centuries, as has happened with some West African pidgins, but then it gradually drops out of use. A third possibility is when people in a pidgin-using community continue to use the pidgin routinely, passing it on to their own children, who become its first native speakers. The pidgin in such cases is called a *Creole* (McWhorter 2018). The word likely comes from the Spanish word *criollo*, meaning "native to the place," or Portuguese *crioulo* ("Brazilian speaker of Portuguese"). Creole speakers develop their own cultures and narrative traditions, some of which can become renowned beyond the Creole-speaking territory. The Creole music of Louisiana, for example, is now an important artistic musical form, as is its cuisine.

In theory, the descendants of any language family can be classified as pidgins themselves that developed into Creoles after the speech community gained autonomous nationhood. The colonization of many parts of the Mediterranean and adjacent territories by the Romans involved getting the local residents to speak Latin as best they could. Their attempts produced "Latin pidgins," even though they are not called in this way. These became "Creoles" when the Roman Empire collapsed, eventually becoming official languages (Spanish, French, Italian, and so on). This is why in early Romance texts, there is a lot of variation and uncertainty with respect to lexical and grammatical forms. Over time, these were standardized by various political, social, and literacy movements. All this reveals, perhaps, is that pidginization is an unconscious force in all language change.

3.1.4 Lingua Francas

Dialect variation implies the existence of a norm, which is essentially a code against which the dialects can be defined. Nations develop and use standard languages for their official purposes. Now, the question becomes: Which language is used for cross-national or international communications? On the Internet, the tendency is to use English as a common code among speakers of different languages. In such usage, English is technically what linguists call a *lingua franca*, a language conventionally, rather than casually, used to make communication possible among people not sharing the same native language (Ostler 2010).

Lingua francas have arisen throughout human history, often for commercial, scientific, or other cross-national official reasons. Thus, the question of what kind of characteristics English is developing as a lingua franca and the social roles that it plays in people's lives across the globe is becoming ever more important as an area of sociolinguistic research. Susan Cook (2004) has argued that the impact of global English on the non-English-speaking world is, however, hardly a hegemonic one, because it actually reproduces the social, political, and economic relations that exist in the real world. She also points out that there is growing evidence that the new electronic landscape, unlike the real landscape, is not playing by the expected sociolinguistic rules. So, non-native speakers shape English according to the semantic and grammatical mechanisms of their native tongues.

In this global environment, native speakers of English might incorrectly assume that if someone speaks their language they will instinctively understand the cultural presuppositions inherent in it. This can have negative effects on interpersonal communications between speakers who come from different cultural backgrounds. This situation is, however, not unique to the Internet age. From the writings of the ancient Romans, it is obvious that they believed that those who spoke Latin after conquest would understand the world as they themselves did. But they did not at first, a fact that led to various political and military conflicts. Over time, however, the imposition of Latin and its evolution into the Romance languages installed many of the values and beliefs of the Romans throughout the empire. The mutual intelligibility in this case is at the level of cultural meaning.

3.2 Diglossia, Bilingualism, and Multilingualism

In some countries, some dialects are considered to be more prestigious than others. The term *diglossia* is used to refer to such differential social perceptions (Ferguson 1959). Diglossia may also characterize the perception of the two codes that are associated with situations of social bilingualism and multilingualism. For reasons such as these, the notion of diglossia has received considerable attention from sociolinguists (Fishman, Cooper, and Ma 1971; Haugen 1972; Hudson and Fishman 2002). Significantly, the term comes from Greek *diglōssos* meaning "bilingual."

As discussed, the rise of a regional variant to national language status is due to nonlinguistic factors, which assign prestige to that variant. For example, the current Italian dialects are all equal descendants of the same mother tongue, Latin. During the Middle Ages, they prospered in their own territories as so-called *volgari*, meaning the tongues of common folk *(il volgo)*. But this situation changed with the rise of Tuscany as a political and cultural power broker in that era. By the late medieval period, the Florentine Tuscan *volgare* became, by force of circumstances, a *volgare illustre* (an illustrious tongue) and thus a prestigious code throughout the Italian peninsula, becoming the basis for the standard language. The other *volgari* became localized codes for use in region-based communication and interaction. To this day, there is an emotional attachment on the part of many Italians to their local dialectal speech. Even the inevitable push for assimilation into the linguistic mainstream, which gained unswerving momentum in the middle part of the twentieth century, has not completely severed the crucial emotional links that many Italians maintain to their dialectal past. There continues to be a profound sense of pride in people from across the peninsula in their dialect speech and culture.

3.2.1 Diglossia

Charles Ferguson (1959) was the one who initially put forth the notion of diglossia after researching speech communities in which dialectal variants were historically assigned levels of prestige according to their specific social functions. This is now called *classic diglossia*. Ferguson noted that one of the variants was the code for everyday, informal conversations; and the other for formal ones and literacy practices. He designated the former low (L) and the latter high (H). Two widely known examples of classical diglossia are found in Greek and German (see Table 3.1).

In speech communities where diglossia exists, the distinction between H and L forms is never straightforward. It all depends on the historical functions of each code and how the mainstream society evolved linguistically. Recall that

Table 3.1 Two Examples of Diglossia

	High	*Low*
Greek	Katharévousa	Dimotiki (Demotic)
German	Hochdeutsch (High German)	Schweizerdeutsch (Swiss German)

the Florentine Tuscan dialect became the standard language in Italy over time, because it boasted an emerging literary tradition starting in the medieval era. It was, in other words, a high dialect, emulated by many throughout the peninsula, even though there were, and still are, many dialects with their own literary traditions. In fact, a measure of diglossia is the ability of a dialect such as Florentine to migrate beyond its speech community and become used in other areas (Clivio, Danesi, and Maida-Nicol 2011). Wherever diglossia exists, H forms are used typically for formal purposes (education, official communications, etc.); L forms are employed instead for everyday talk and informal discourse (humor, folk stories, and the like) (Trudgill 1983). In Greek, for example, *demotiki* refers to the code that evolved naturally from Ancient Greek, whereas *katharévousa* was a code that was artificially raised to the official standard until 1976, at which time *demotiki* became the official standard language of Greece, leading to a breakdown in the classical diglossic situation in that country. Table 3.2 summarizes the foregoing discussion.

Diglossia implies that the perception dialect speech is hardly arbitrary; it is interpreted socially (Sayahi 2014). It is thus an important sociolinguistic notion. Today, the notion of *critical diglossia* has become a target of sociolinguistic research (Saxena 2014). In contrast to classical diglossia, which involves a historical assessment of dialect prestige, critical diglossia maintains that the assignment of prestige is an ideologically-based process that creates tensions among speakers. It thus studies the reasons why asymmetrical social relationships emerge between speakers of language variants. It also looks at

Table 3.2 Classical Diglossia

Low dialect	*High dialect*
low prestige	high prestige
intimate communication	formal communication
group solidarity	social authority and power
mainly spoken	part of literacy traditions
informal	formal
usually a native code	usually a learned code
passed on in community	passed on through schooling

lifestyle factors that influence the language choices made by individuals. This approach to diglossia can be traced to the American sociolinguist Joshua Fishman (1972, 1987), who pointed out that differences in language structures invariably evoke different perceptions where diglossia exists and this may lead to social imbalances; so, the objective of the sociolinguist in this area is to document them, relating them to the broader social system in which the variants exist.

3.2.2 *Bilingualism and Multilingualism*

Bilingualism refers to the ability of an individual, or a society, to speak two languages to varying degrees. When more than two are involved the ability is called multilingualism. In regions where two languages (or dialects) are in contact (for example, French and dialectal German in Alsace, German and Italian in the Dolomite valleys), bilingualism becomes the norm, rather than the exception. Bilingualism emerges typically in immigrant communities, where the native (or ancestral) language is spoken in the home and the language of the host society outside of the home.

The main forms of bilingualism are summarized below:

1   *Individual and social.* Individual bilingualism is used in reference to children who are reared in bilingual environments, acquiring two languages in tandem. It is also called *early bilingualism.* Social bilingualism refers to a society that is officially bilingual, even though speakers within it may not necessarily be reared as bilinguals. An example is Canada, where English and French are official languages, but citizens of the country may not necessarily be raised as French-English bilinguals.
2   *Productive and receptive.* Productive bilingualism is employed to describe an individual who can speak two languages fluently and receptive bilingualism, to someone who does so only partially, being fluent primarily in one of the two codes. Second or third immigrant children are typically receptive bilinguals, understanding (to varying degrees) the language of ancestry because of exposure in their immigrant communities, but generally unable to speak it fluently.
3   *Primary and secondary.* Primary bilingualism refers to a child who is exposed to two languages in a rearing context and who uses them both for daily communicative reasons and secondary bilingualism to anyone who acquires a second language later in life—also called *late bilingualism.*
4   *Additive and subtractive.* Additive bilingualism refers to a situation where bilingual children are allowed to use both languages at school; subtractive bilingualism refers instead to a situation that does not allow (and may even discourage) the use of both languages at school.

The broader sociolinguistic study of bilingualism and multilingualism covers several areas, including how bilingual communities form their own social networks within the mainstream society and what this implies for cultural assimilation processes. It also involves examining the role of colonization in the production of bilingualism. In the United States, English became the mainstream language from coast to coast, largely replacing colonial French and Spanish as well as the languages of Native Americans; but these continue to be spoken by various citizens of the country along with English.

As discussed previously, Basil Bernstein (1971) distinguished between elaborated and restricted codes in reference to the ways in which speech varieties reflect different social classes. Extending Bernstein's terminology, it can be said that in immigrant situations, the restricted code is typically the native tongue, which might present problems for the immigrant children if they enter monolingual schools. However, research has shown that by allowing the native language to become a basis upon which to develop the elaborated code at school, many of the problems faced by immigrant children seem to dissipate on their own. This is the goal of bilingual education systems (see, for example, Cummins and Danesi 1990; Tuan 1991; Vertovec 2007).

The sociolinguistic study of bilingualism and multilingualism has gained a new impetus in cyberspace. Cunliffe, Morris, and Prys (2013) found that young bilinguals (Welsh-English) on Facebook used code switching (see the next section in this chapter) strategically to garner mutual empathy for their particular ethnic identity, which goes back considerably in time in that region. In other words, bilingual speech manifestations online are strategies to convey pride in one's past (Danet and Herring 2007). So it would seem that online speech reveals the same kinds of social relations that are implied in offline speech. Paolillo (2011) examined the use of English, Hindi, and Punjabi in four Internet communication contexts. He found that the same pattern of mixing of English and Hindi or English and Punjabi that occurred in ethnically homogenous conversational F2F contexts also occurred online. Paolillo suggested that social communication in any medium or space (real or virtual) retains its historically based distinctions and social meanings.

3.2.3 Code Switching

Bilinguals often display a peculiar conversational habit—switching between their two codes as they communicate. This is called, logically, *code switching*. It occurs more typically during oral conversations than in writing, but it is found in all media and modes of communication, including in digital media (Zentella 1997; Gardner-Chloros 2009).

Code switching is often a strategy for signaling allegiance to the speaker's ethnic background. Gumperz and Cook-Gumperz (1982) found, for example, that in a small bilingual Puerto Rican community (Spanish-English) in New Jersey, the members would code switch in casual and formal gatherings to convey an unconscious allegiance to their Hispanic identity, often using an admixture of English and Spanish, called colloquially "Spanglish." The main finding of the project was that the use of Spanglish between parents and children was a strategy of endearment and an unconscious expression of pride in their Hispanic heritage (see also Guzzardo et al. 2016).

Box 3.1 Examples of Code Switching in Spanglish

(From Stavans 2004)

> "What is *esa cosa* (this thing) in Spanish?"
> "Hey, *chica* (girl), you have a bad *mancha* (spot) on your *camiseta* (blouse)."
> "My *padrito* (dad) likes to watch *el beisból* (baseball)."
> "Hey, *amigo* (friend, dude) *dónde* (where) are you going?"
> "He is really *loco* (crazy)."

Code switching is also a way to signal social distinctiveness. Research has found that young and socially mobile African Americans, who switch to AAVE (African American Vernacular English) during peer conversations conducted primarily in SAE (Standard American English) are using an unconscious strategy of identity bonding. Reverse switching, from AAVE to SAE, frequently has a different objective; it implies that speakers aim to project themselves advantageously into the mainstream via SAE; this happens especially during such official events as employment interviews (Hopper and Williams 1973; Akkinaso and Ajiritutu 1982), in educational settings (Smitherman 2003), and in legal situations (Ray 2009).

There are two main types of code switching: *intersentential* and *intrasentential*. The first refers to switching codes between separate sentences and the second within sentences. An example of an intersentential code switch by a speaker of Spanglish might be: "How are you? *Estás bien* ("Are you well")?" An intrasentential switch might be: "I want to go out *solo contigo* ("only with you")." Intersentential code switching requires a high level of competence in both languages, since it implies the ability to avoid violating the grammatical rules of either language that would make utterances difficult to interpret. Intrasentential code switching occurs typically when a bilingual starts a message in one language (say English) and ends it in the other (Spanish); or else when the speaker inserts words within the message from Spanish (Romaine and Kachru 1992). The distinction between the two is, however, a blurred one. And indeed some sociolinguists prefer to use the term *code switching* broadly to indicate any form of switching from one code to the other.

Overall, code switching has been found to serve four main cognitive or social functions (Goldstein and Kohnert 2005; Brice and Brice 2009):

1   It allows bilinguals to fill in conceptual gaps in one language from the other one. Bilinguals have access to two language systems and so when a conceptual-referential gap occurs in one, as they speak, they can easily fill it with an item from their other (if it exists). For example, an Italian-English bilingual might use the word *simpatico* in a sentence such as "I think he is *molto simpatico*," because the Italian term covers a broader range of meanings than do English equivalents such as "nice," "charming," and "sweet."

2   It allows the speaker to show allegiance to a group, as, for example, when a Hispanic speaker switches to, or mixes in, Spanglish when speaking to other Hispanics in English or even to monolingual English speakers: "I love being a *mexicano* (Mexican)."

3   It implies that certain topics are felt to be more appropriately expressed in one or the other code. For example, Hispanics discussing matters related to the family tend to use Spanish switches more than they do for other, more abstract topics.

4   It allows bilingual peers to share a common ground of unconscious understanding and worldview.

Code switching also manifests itself among dialect speakers, who may switch back and forth between the dialect and standard language for the same reasons as those listed above. Code switchers choose, in effect, the language that marks their feelings, beliefs, and obligations best during conversations (Myers-Scotton 1993; Sebba and Wooton 1998; Wei 1998; Cromdal 2001). Peter Auer (1984) has even suggested that code switching does not simply mirror social relations in conversational settings, but rather that it creates them. So, when the code switcher chooses one or the other language for a conversational turn, it influences the subsequent choices of all interlocutors, like a chain reaction. Rather than the social values inherent in the code chosen, the speaker concentrates on the meaning that the act of code switching itself creates, and this sets off the domino effect.

Code switching is now used in a broader sense in different media contexts. For instance, National Public Radio (NPR) in the United States established a blog called Code Switch to examine the "frontiers of race, culture and ethnicity." The site allows people to confront the challenges of the world they live in (racism, culture wars, and so on) through code switching between points of view. In this case, code switching occurs not between languages but between ideologies, views, and even media.

3.3 Languages in Contact

In immigrant bilingual communities the two languages of the members—the ancestral and the host one—are said to be in *contact* (Weinreich 1953, 1954). The branch of linguistics that studies languages in contact is called, logically, *contact linguistics*; its aim is to document the influences that languages in contact have on each other and, consequently, on their speakers. The kind of "mixed" language that crystallizes when languages are in contact, such as Spanglish, is of particular relevance to the study of how immigrant communities cope with linguistic diversity. Contact linguistics can also be used to examine how basic units and structures of a language affect the overall construction of meaning in language, including figurative meaning (Zenner, Backus, and Winter-Froemel 2019).

A term often used for describing a mixed language such as Spanglish is *koiné*. This was used in Ancient Greece to describe the speech based on the Attic language that became the common vernacular of the Hellenistic world, and from which later stages of Greek are descended. A case-in-point of a koiné is Spanglish, which is characterized not only by switches to Spanish, but also by American English words that have been "Hispanized," that is, adapted in pronunciation and word structure to resemble native Spanish words. This process is called technically *nativization*, as will be discussed in section 3.3.2.

3.3.1 Borrowing

The term *borrowing* refers to the taking-in and incorporation of the lexemes of another language into one's own native lexicon. It occurs typically when languages are in physical proximity (Spanish and English in the United States), when they are in intellectual contact historically (such as Latin and English), and when immigrant languages are in contact with the language(s) of the host country.

Borrowing in the last situation is particularly interesting to sociolinguistics. First-generation immigrants tend to borrow extensively from the host language, because the relevant lexemes allow them to carry out the tasks of naming the things and events of everyday life in the new society in a more direct and meaningful way (Betz 1949; Haugen 1950; Weinreich 1953, 1954; Scotton, Myers, and Okeju 1973; Poplack, Sankoff, and Miller 1988). Borrowing in this case is a strategy for either filling-in lexical gaps present in the native ancestral language or else for using the lexical items of the host language to better describe the new reality. The words that are borrowed are called *loanwords*. But borrowing is not just characteristic of immigrant speech. In English, words such as *naïve* (borrowed from French) and *memorandum* (borrowed from Latin) entered the language ostensibly because no English word existed at the time (and still does not) for expressing the concepts that such foreign words encode. Borrowing is thus a practical conceptual gap-filling strategy. When speakers of a language do not have a word for something that they wish to identify, they can either create one for it or else borrow the word from a language that does. The latter happens more frequently than one might think.

If gap filling is the reason behind a loanword, then it is called a *necessary loan*; if the reason is not to fill in a gap, but for some socially advantageous reason, such as a sign of erudition, then the loanword is called a *luxury loan*. Necessary loans allow immigrants to refer to the objects and ideas in their new physical and social environments with facility and concreteness. Not knowing the native word for *mortgage*, immigrants who came the US from Italy after World War II, adopted the English word and made it their own linguistically. The result was *morgheggio*. Of course, some speakers might have known the Italian equivalent—but it was not the same conceptually. The loanword *morgheggio* not only refers to a specific referent, but also bears a whole set of connotations that are specific to the borrower (Danesi 1985). The word alludes unconsciously to a world to which the immigrants relate emotionally. In *Italese* (the Italian spoken in immigrant communities in English-speaking host societies and similar to *Spanglish*), *morgheggio* refers not only to a "mortgage," but also to what it entailed socially. It meant "something to be paid off at any cost" which, in turn, implied the need "to work overtime or at several jobs" which, in its turn, implied "to save, save, save, so as to ensure the future well-being of one's offspring." In effect, *morgheggio* for the immigrants was a codeword for describing a reality that Standard Italian counterparts, *mutuo* or *ipoteca*, did not imply.

In addition to loanwords, a phenomenon that characterizes languages in contact is called *calquing*. Calques are phrases that have been translated literally from the source language—hence they are also called *loan translations*. Table 3.3 contains some examples of calques in North American Italese (Danesi 1985).

As can be seen, each calque reflects the structure and meanings of the English expression. So, "down" = *bassa* and "town" = *città* in *bassa città*. Calques exist in all languages. A classic example of a calque in English is the translated title by which the Russian novel written by Fyodor Dostoyevsky *The Brothers Karamazov* (1880) is known. We no longer realize that this is a calque of the Russian title, in which the adjectival name (*Karamazov*) follows the noun (*Brothers*). In proper English it should be *The Karamazov Brothers*, a word order that is reflected commonly in such parallel phrases as the *Smith Brothers*, the *Carpenter Brothers*, and so on.

3.3.2 Nativization

English has an extensive loanword component in its lexicon, which is no longer recognized as such because of nativization—the unconscious process of shaping the foreign lexeme to sound like a native one. In fact, on almost every

Table 3.3 Calques in Italese

English source	Calque	Standard Italian form
it looks good	*guarda bene*	*gli/le sta bene*
downtown	*bassa città*	*centro*
to make a call	*fare il telefono*	*telefonare*

page of a dictionary of the language one can find evidence of nativization. If one were to remove from the dictionary just the words borrowed from Latin and its descendants (Italian, French, Spanish, and so on), everyday speech would become rather impoverished from a lexical perspective. One cannot handle an object or talk about some abstract concept without recourse to some nativized loanword. For example, all nouns ending in -*tion* (*attention, education, nation*) have their roots in the Latin lexicon, as do most of the nouns ending in -*ty* (*morality, sobriety, triviality*). Why did this happen?

About 1,500 years ago three closely related tribes (the Angles, the Saxons, and the Jutes) lived alongside one another on the north shore of what is now northern Germany and southern Denmark. They spoke a language that was similar to the current West German dialects. Known as Old English, it allowed the tribes to establish social autonomy from their Germanic ancestry. Old English had grammatical cases that resemble those of modern German, and it formed the new words it needed largely by rearranging and recombining those present in its lexical stock. It borrowed infrequently from other languages.

However, the situation changed after the invasion and conquest of England by the Normans from northwestern France in 1066. Although they were originally of Viking extraction, by the middle of the eleventh century, the Normans had adopted French as their language. They imposed their French-speaking ways on the Anglo-Saxons. As a consequence, the English spoken by the latter became saturated with French-based words, which have survived in common speech to this day. Their French (and thus Latin) origin is no longer consciously recognized because of the fact that they have become completely nativized in pronunciation and word structure.

English came subsequently to adopt Latin-based synonyms for many of its native words. There are several reasons for this, but perhaps the most important was the fact that Latin was a prestige language (and, *ipso facto*, a lingua franca) in the medieval world. To borrow its words was perceived as a means of enriching the speech level of any emerging vernacular. This is, in fact, one of the reasons for the coexistence of such synonymous pairs in English as *clap* and *applaud, fair* and *candid, wedding* and *matrimony*, of which the second item in each pair is of Latin descent.

As the foregoing discussion implies, when a loanword is adopted by a language, gaining communicative currency, it is restructured to be in conformity with native words. Thus, for example, in Italese, borrowed nouns that become common in the speech community of the immigrants are assigned a grammatical gender through the addition of final vowels: "garbage" → *garbiccio*, "mortgage" → *morgheggio*, "switch" → *suiccia*, "fence" → *fenza*; borrowed verbs are assigned to the first conjugation, the most regular of the three conjugations of Italian: "push" → *pusciare*, "squeeze" → *squizare*, "smash" → *smesciare*. And each word is pronounced according to Italian phonology (in any of its variants). Once a loanword has been nativized, it enters the speakers' lexicon where it is no longer perceived as a foreign word, but rather as an item like any other native lexeme.

Box 3.2 Examples of Nativized Loanwords in Spanglish

parquear = to park (Standard Spanish: *aparcar*)
troca = truck (Standard Spanish: *camion*)
caro = car (Standard Spanish: *coche*)
sinco = sink (Standard Spanish: *lavabo*)
flora = floor (Standard Spanish: *piso*)

If the social prestige of an immigrant koiné increases, so too does its range of communicative functions. Spanglish, for example, is particularly attractive to young people who might use it in everyday interactions for reasons of self-identification with their Hispanic peers. This is particularly noticeable on social networking sites such as Facebook among speakers of Spanglish, where it seems to imply allegiance to ethnic identity.

3.4 Language Loyalty, Language Planning, and Literacy

Recall that, in Italy, the Florentine vernacular became the basis for the standard language because of the literary prestige of medieval writers in Florence, the central position of the city within Italy, and its expanding commercial power. The first official grammars and dictionaries of Italian were thus based on the Florentine vernacular. The *Accademia della Crusca* founded in 1583 in Florence, the first language academy, was established to promote the new standard to the rest of Italy. Modern-day Standard Italian is based on its Florentine predecessor, but it has also undergone modifications to reflect a broader use of the language throughout Italy.

When a linguistic variant on a dialect continuum becomes the standard language of a society, various sociolinguistic mechanisms are activated in tandem. One of these is the continued usage of the local dialect for reasons of cultural solidarity—a mechanism called *language loyalty*. Another is the set of official reactions that language variation or diversity within a society tends to evoke and the actions undertaken accordingly. This falls under the rubric of *language planning*. A third one is the notion of *literacy*, which is a derivative of the latter, implying that the standard language is to be imparted through education and various institutions as the official one.

3.4.1 Language Loyalty

The term *language loyalty* refers to the proclivity of groups and communities to remain loyal to their native language, dialect, or group-based code in the face of social, cultural, and linguistic change (Fishman 1972; Stoessel 2002). For instance, first-generation immigrants who live in ethnic communities tend to be very loyal to their native (ancestral) languages for the simple reason that they live in a linguistically unfamiliar society and such loyalty allows them to feel emotionally stable. This type of loyalty tends to be especially strong among refugees who may have left their countries of origin for political reasons or because of persecution. When the children of first-generation immigrants start going to school and developing acquaintances outside the home and ethnic community, they start assimilating the dominant host language and its culture. But feelings of language loyalty persist even in subsequent generations. This is colloquially called "returning to the roots," whereby the subsequent generations of immigrant communities feel a desire to recover their ethnic identities through a recovery of the ancestral language. Many seek instruction in that language in school settings, in order to satisfy this desire.

Language loyalty implies affiliation with a speech community. This now extends to online communities. As Wilson and Peterson (2002) have observed, the Internet has brought together dispersed groups of people with shared interests, even if they have different linguistic and social backgrounds. These communities might be mobilized to further particular political agendas, to bring together members of familial or ethnic groups, or they might be organized around specific interests. In traditional sociolinguistics, a speech community is a circumscribed entity in geographical space which is complete and self-contained. But this situation does not hold up in the online world, where physical space boundaries do not exist. The Internet seems to have developed its own types of language loyalty. A more fluid concept of speech community is thus emerging. Those belonging to a specific Twitter community, for instance, will adopt the language code of that community and use it for communications within it. This means that interlocutors can insert themselves into a virtual community, without any of the traditional expectations of group identity of real speech communities.

The term "tribal communities" is often applied to these online sociolinguistic formations. The tribe in this case is not based on historical cultural affiliations, but on political interests, work, and hobbies (Bryden, Funk, and Vincent, 2013). This is researched via algorithms that collect the Twitter feeds of all the users from the tribes, analyzing word usage in the tweets and then assigning them to corresponding lifestyles, ideologies, and the like.

3.4.2 Language Planning

The term *language planning* refers to the kinds of measures taken by official (usually governmental) agencies to preserve the standard language for formal communications. Sociolinguist Joshua Fishman (1987: 49) defines language planning as "the authoritative allocation of resources to the attainment of language status and corpus goals, whether in connection with new functions that are aspired to, or in connection with old functions that need to be discharged more adequately." There are four main varieties:

1   *Status planning*, whereby the government takes measures (such as legislation) to guarantee that the status of a standard language remains stable.
2   *Corpus planning*, whereby official institutions (such as academies and official dictionary makers) assign social prestige to the standard language.
3   *Language-in-education planning*, which is designed to privilege the standard language through education.
4   *Prestige planning*, which involves getting the different speech communities to accept the standard language as the prestige code through literacy practices and media promulgation.
5   *Revitalization and maintenance*, which occurs in countries that were previously colonized; such nations must decide what indigenous language(s) to designate as the standard language for one and all.

A common strategy in multilingual regions is for the power brokers to simply declare one of the languages as the official one. But this often leads to internal conflicts and social strife, as is witnessed in certain areas such as in Catalonia, an autonomous region in northeastern Spain, whose capital is Barcelona. The region has a longstanding separatist tradition, and has fought for use of its native language of Catalan, not only for everyday purposes, but also for official ones.

There are four general ideologies that motivate language planning (Nahir 2003). One is *linguistic assimilation*, which is the belief that every member of a society should learn to use the standard language and shed their linguistic heritage. In the United States, this is known as the "English-only" movement, which espouses the belief that only English reflects the mainstream social ethos of the country, ignoring the indigenous languages, as well as Spanish and French, in the history of the nation. In contrast, the ideology called *linguistic pluralism* espouses the use of multiple languages within a society. Examples include the coexistence of German, French, Italian, and Romansh in Switzerland, and English, Tamil, Malay, and Chinese in Singapore. In such areas, however, one of the languages is still perceived to be the primary one for official social purposes. A third ideology, called *vernacularization*, supports the restoration or development of an indigenous language along with its institutionalization as the standard code. Examples include Quechua in Peru and Hebrew in Israel. A fourth ideology, known as *internationalization*, is the adoption of a nonindigenous language as the official one in order to connect a country to the global village. Examples are the use of English in areas such as India, Singapore, the Philippines, and Papua New Guinea.

3.4.3 Literacy

At a basic level, literacy is simply the ability to read and write a language. This is called *pure literacy*. At another level, it is the ability to use a language for knowledge-based and various intellectual purposes. This is called *functional literacy*.

The social role of literacy, pure and functional, cannot be overstated. Before the fifteenth century and the advent of cheap print technology, most people in Europe were illiterate, never having had the opportunity to learn to read and write. There were few schools, perhaps because literacy was not required to work in farming villages and in many of the trades of the medieval towns. Most literate people belonged to the nobility, the upper classes, or the clergy. But the printing press changed this. The late Marshall McLuhan (1962, 1964) characterized the new world order brought about by the advent of the printing press in the fifteenth century as the "Gutenberg Galaxy," after its European inventor, the German printer Johannes Gutenberg (1400–1468). Through cheaply available books, the printed word became the chief means for the propagation and recording of knowledge and ideas. And because books could cross national boundaries, they set in motion the globalization of knowledge and the internationalization of commerce, thus encouraging literacy across the globe and paving the way for such events and movements as the European Renaissance, the Protestant Reformation, and the Enlightenment. With the spread of literacy and with industry becoming a dominant part of economic life during the eighteenth and nineteenth centuries, great numbers of people started migrating to cities. In order to find employment they had to learn how to read instructions and perform other tasks that required pure literacy. Governments began to value education for everyone more, and systems of public schooling cropped up everywhere. By the late 1800s, formal elementary education had become obligatory in many countries.

Today, new forms of literacy are cropping up because of the Internet (Ivkovic and Lotherington 2009; Varnhagen, Mcfall, and Pugh 2010). As Benson Mandwire (2018: 38) aptly observes, today the term *literacy* encompasses a broad range of meanings, including "conventional or basic literacy, functional literacy, digital literacy, media literacy, legal literacy, computer literacy, medical literacy and information literacy." In a relevant study, Greenhow and Gleason (2012) explored tweeting as a literacy practice, finding that it amalgamated traditional and new modes of writing (netlingo). They found that it is now impacting both informal and formal registers. Alongside so-called *twitteracy*, different literacies are evolving in different social media or online venues (Verheijen 2013). Black (2008) had called this "global literacy" a few years back, because it cuts across national borders, with its incorporation of common cultural artifacts, as well as multimodal pastiches of text, image, and sound. Davies (2012) found that self-presentation and friendship management were the primary concerns of social media users. Using tags, hashtags, emoji, and other digital communication strategies is having an impact on how we view literacy outside of the most formal of channels, such as in academic and scientific writing (Alvermann 2008).

Twitter is of particular relevance to the theme of global literacy. Tweets are conversational in style and function—exchanges between friends, associates, colleagues, and acquaintances. Some have designated Twitter as a venue for "social grooming," that is, for presenting oneself in a favorable way to others in order to gain attention and to gather followers. It is also used to promote one's personal agenda and political views. Institutions of various kinds, from NASA to universities, now use Twitter as a source of contact with clients and colleagues. The limited length of each tweet and the constant flow of tweets are all part of twitteracy (Gee 1999; Kress 2003; Hull and Nelson 2005; Lankshear and Knobel 2006; Perkel 2008; Coiro et al. 2008; Livingstone, Van Couvering, and Thumim 2008). Bryden, Funk, and Jansen (2013) found that tweeting constitutes not only a new form of literacy, but also a discourse strategy, involving how to self-present to the Twitter community, participate in it (*mentions*), distribute information (*retweets*), and organize conversations (*hashtags*). Haas and Takayoshi (2011) have introduced a useful distinction between "standard literacies," which are characteristic of formal offline contexts, and online "everyday literacies," which entail knowledge of text messaging and tweeting style. The two are dynamically intertwined, leading to a new form of diglossia. They may also complement one another in covert ways. Barden (2012) noticed an increase in standard literacy competence in dyslexic middle school subjects, after they had engaged with multimodal digital text structures. This led the subjects to a better understanding of sequence and relation in linear texts. In other words, their everyday literacy was enhanced via engagement with online literacy. A speech community, as discussed, traditionally implies a geographical locus defined by a language or a dialect. Twitter has enabled people to become part of a speech community without such a locus. This means that "connections on Twitter depend less on in-person contact, as many users have more followers than they know" (Gruzd, Wellman, and Takhteyev 2011: 1294). In terms of theories of conversation (to be discussed in Chapter 6), tweeting has significant implications, especially in how speech communities and tribal communities are meshing together more and more.

References and Further Reading

Akkinaso, F. N. and Ajiritutu, C. S. (1982). Performance and Ethnic Styles in Job Interviews. In: J. J. Gumperz (ed.), *Language and Social Identity*. Cambridge: Cambridge University Press.

Alvermann, D. E. (2008). Why Bother Theorizing Adolescents' Online Literacies for Classroom Practice and Research? *Journal of Adolescent and Adult Literacy* 52(1): 8–19.

Auer, P. (1984). *Bilingual Conversation*. Amsterdam: John Benjamins.

Barden, O. (2012). If We Were Cavemen We'd Be Fine. Facebook as a Catalyst for Critical Literacy Learning by Dyslexic Sixth-Form Students. *Literacy* 46: 123–132.

Benson Mandwire, S. (2018). Literacy versus Language: Exploring their Similarities and Differences. *Journal of Lexicography and Terminology* 2: 37–55.

Bernstein, B. (1971). *Class, Codes and Control: Theoretical Studies Towards a Sociology of Language*. London: Routledge.

Betz, W. (1949). *Deutsch und Lateinisch: Die Lehnbildungen der althochdeutschen Benediktinerregel*. Bonn: Bouvier.

Black, R. W. (2008). Just Don't Call Them Cartoons: The New Literacy Spaces of Anime, Manga and Fanfiction. In: J. Coiro, M. Knobel, C. Lankshear, and D. Leu (eds.), *Handbook of Research on New Literacies*, pp. 538–610. New York: Lawrence Erlbaum Associates.

Brice, A. and Brice, R. (eds.) (2009). *Language Development: Monolingual and Bilingual Acquisition*. Old Tappan, NJ: Prentice Hall.

Bruce, L. (1984). *The Alamblak Language of Papua New Guinea (East Sepik)*. Canberra: Australian National University.

Bryden, J., Funk, S., and Jansen, V. (2013). Word Usage Mirrors Community Structure in the Online Social Network Twitter. *EPJ Data Science* 2: 3. www.epjdatascience.com/content/2/1/3.

Chambers, J. K. and Trudgill, P. (1998). *Dialectology*, 2nd ed. Cambridge: Cambridge University Press.

Clivio, G. P., Danesi, M., and Maida-Nicol, S. (2011). *Introduction to Italian Dialectology*. Munich: Lincom Europa.

Coiro, J., Knobel, M., Lankshear, C., and Leu, D. (2008). Central Issues in New Literacies and New Literacies Research. In: J. Coiro, M. Knobel, C. Lankshear, and D. Leu (eds.), *Handbook of Research on New Literacies*, pp. 1–21. New York: Lawrence Erlbaum Associates.

Cook, S. E. (2004). New Technologies and Language Change: Toward an Anthropology of Linguistic Frontiers. *Annual Review of Anthropology* 33: 103–115.

Cromdal, J. (2001). Overlap in Bilingual Play: Some Implications of Code-Switching for Overlap Resolution. *Research on Language and Social Interaction* 34(4): 421–451.

Cummins, J. and Danesi, M. (1990). *Heritage Languages: The Development and Denial of Canada's Linguistic Resources*. Toronto: Garamond Press.

Cunliffe, D., Morris, D., and Prys, C. (2013). Young Bilinguals' Language Behaviour in Social Networking Sites: The Use of Welsh on Facebook. *Journal of Computer-Mediated Communication* 18(3): 339–361.

Danesi, M. (1985). *Loanwords and Phonological Methodology*. Montreal: Didier.

Danet, B. and Herring, S. C. (eds.) (2007). *The Multilingual Internet: Language, Culture, and Communication Online*. Oxford: Oxford University Press.

Davies, J. (2012). Facework on Facebook as a New Literacy Practice. *Computers & Education* 59: 19–29.

Eisenstein, J. (2017). Identifying Regional Dialects in On-Line Social Media. In: C. Boberg, J. Nerbonne, and D. Watt (eds.), *Handbook of Dialectology*, pp. 368–383. New York: Routledge.

Ferguson, C. (1959). Diglossia. *Word* 15: 325–340.

Fishman, J. (1972). *The Sociology of Language: An Interdisciplinary Social Science Approach to Language in Society*. Rowley, MA: Newbury House.

Fishman, J. (1987). *Ideology, Society and Language: The Odyssey of Nathan Birnbaum*. Ann Arbor, MI: Karoma.

Fishman, J. A., Cooper, R. L., and Ma, R. (1971). *Bilingualism in the Barrio*. Bloomington, IN: Indiana University Press.

Gardner-Chloros, P. (2009). *Code-Switching*. Cambridge: Cambridge University Press.

Gee, J. (1999). *An Introduction to Discourse Analysis: Theory and Method*. London: Routledge.

Goldstein, B. and Kohnert, K. (2005). Speech, Language and Hearing in Developing Bilingual Children: Current Findings and Future Directions. *Language, Speech and Hearing Services in Schools* 36(3): 264–267.

Gooskens, C. (2017). Dialect Intelligibility. In: C. Boberg, J. Nerbonne, and D. Watt (eds.), *Handbook of Dialectology*, pp. 204–218. New York: Routledge.

Greenhow, C. and Gleason, B. (2012). Twitteracy: Tweeting as a New Literary Practice. *The Educational Forum* 76: 464–478.

Gruzd, A., Wellman, B., and Takhteyev, Y. (2011). Imagining Twitter as an Imagined Community. *American Behavioral Scientist* 55(10): 1294–1318.

Gumperz, J. J. and Cook-Gumperz, J. (1982). Language and the Communication of Social Identity. In: J. J. Gumperz (ed.), *Language and Social Identity*. Cambridge: Cambridge University Press.

Guzzardo, R. E., Tamargo, C. M., Mazak, M. and Couto, C. F. (2016). *Spanish-English Code-Switching in the Caribbean and the US*. Amsterdam: John Benjamins.

Haas, C. and Takayoshi, P. (2011). Young People's Everyday Literacies: The Language Features of Instant Messaging. *Research in the Teaching of English* 45(4): 378–404.

Hall, R. A., (1966). *Pidgins and Creoles*. Ithaca, NY: Cornell University Press.

Haugen, E. (1950). The Analysis of Linguistic Borrowing. *Language* 26: 210–231.

Haugen, E. (1972). The Stigmata of Bilingualism. In: S. A. Dil (ed.), *The Ecology of Language: Essays by Einar Haugen*, pp. 307–324. Stanford, CT: Stanford University Press.

Holm, J. A. (1989). *Pidgins and Creoles*. Cambridge: Cambridge University Press.

Hopper, R. and Williams, F. (1973). Speech Characteristics and Employability. *Speech Monographs* 40: 296–302.

Hudson, A. (2002). Outline of a Theory of Diglossia. *International Journal of the Sociology of Language* 157: 1–48.

Hudson, A. and Fishman, J. (2002). Focus on Diglossia. *International Journal of the Sociology of Language* 157: entireissue.

Hull, G. and Nelson, M. E. (2005). Locating the Semiotic Power of Multimodality. *Written Communication* 22(2): 224–262.

Ivkovic, D. and Lotherington, H. (2009). Multilingualism in Cyberspace: Conceptualising the Virtual Linguistic Landscape. *International Journal of Multilingualism* 6: 17–30.

Kress, G. (2003). *Literacy in the New Media Age*. New York: Routledge.

Kretschmar, Jr., W. (2017). Linguistic Atlases. In: C. Boberg, J. Nerbonne, and D. Watt (eds.), *Handbook of Dialectology*, pp. 57–72. New York: Routledge.

Labov, W., Ash, S., and Boberg, C. (2005). *The Atlas of North American English: Phonetics, Phonology and Sound Change*. Berlin: Mouton de Gruyter.

Lankshear, C. and Knobel, M. (2006). *New Literacies: Everyday Practices and Classroom Learning*, 2nd ed. New York: Open University Press.

Livingstone, S., van Couvering, E., and Thumim, N. (2008). Converging Traditions of Research on Media and Information Literacies: Disciplinary, Critical, and Methodological Issues. In: J. Coiro, M. Knobel, C. Lankshear, and D. Leu (eds.), *Handbook of Research on New Literacies*, pp. 103–132. New York: Lawrence Erlbaum Associates.

McArthur, T. (2005). *Concise Oxford Companion to the English Language*. Oxford: Oxford University Press.

McLuhan, M. (1962). *The Gutenberg Galaxy: The Making of Typographic Man*. Toronto: University of Toronto Press.

McLuhan, M. (1964). *Understanding Media: The Extensions of Man*. London: Routledge.

McWhorter, J. (2018). *The Creole Debate*. Cambridge: Cambridge University Press.

Michaelis, S., Maurer, P., Haspelmath, M., and Huber M. (2013). *The Survey of Pidgin and Creole Languages*. Oxford: Oxford University Press.

Myers-Scotton, C. (1993). *Social Motivations for Codeswitching: Evidence from Africa*. Oxford: Clarendon.

Nahir, M. (2003). Language Planning Goals: A Classification. In. C. Paulston, C. Bratt, and R. Tucker (eds.), *Sociolinguistics: The Essential Readings*. Oxford: Wiley-Blackwell.

Ostler, N. (2010). *The Last Lingua Franca: English until the Return of Babel*. New York: Walker and Company.

Paolillo, J. C. (2011). Conversational Codeswitching on Usenet and Internet Relay Chat. *Language@Internet* 8, article3.

Perkel, D. (2008). Copy and Paste Literacy? Literacy Practices in the Production of a MySpace Profile. In: K. Drotner, H. S. Jensen, and K. C. Schroeder (eds.), *Informal Learning and Digital Media: Constructions, Contexts, and Consequences*, pp. 203–224. Newcastle: Cambridge Scholars Publishing.

Poplack, S., Sankoff, D., and Miller, C. (1988). The Social Correlates and Linguistic Processes of Lexical Borrowing and Assimilation. *Linguistics* 26: 47–104.

Rabanus, S. (2017). Dialect Maps. In: C. Boberg, J. Nerbonne, and D. Watt (eds.), *Handbook of Dialectology*, pp. 348–367. New York: Routledge.

Ray, G. B. (2009). *Language and Interracial Communication in the United States: Speaking in Black and White*. New York: Peter Lang.

Romaine, S. and Kachru, B. (1992). Code-Mixing and Code-Switching. In: T. McArthur (ed.), *The Oxford Companion to the English Language*, pp. 228–229. Oxford: Oxford University Press.

Saxena, M. (2014). Critical Diglossia and Lifestyle Diglossia: Development and the Interaction between Multilingualism, Cultural Diversity and English. *International Journal of the Sociology of Language* 225: 91–112.

Sayahi, L. (2014). *Diglossia and Language Contact: Language Variation and Change in North Africa*. Cambridge: Cambridge University Press.

Scotton, C., Myers, M., and Okeju, J. (1973). Neighbors and Lexical Borrowing. *Language* 49: 871–889.

Sebba, M. (1997). *Contact Languages: Pidgins and Creoles*. New York: Palgrave Macmillan.

Sebba, M. and Wooton, T. (1998). We, They and Identity: Sequential Versus Identity-Related Explanation in Code Switching. In: P. Auer (ed.), *Code-Switching in Conversation: Language, Interaction, and Identity*, pp. 263–286. London: Routledge.

Smitherman, G. (2003). *Talkin That Talk: Language, Culture, and Education in African America*. London: Taylor & Francis.

Stavans, I. (2004). *Spanglish: The Making of a New American Language*. New York: HarperCollins.

Stoessel, S. (2002). Investigating the Role of Social Networks in Language Maintenance and Shift. *International Journal of the Sociology of Language* 153: 93–131.

Trudgill, P. (1983). *Sociolinguistics*. Harmondsworth: Penguin.

Tuan, Y. F. (1991). Language and the Making of Place: A Narrative-Descriptive Approach. *Annals of the Association of American Geographers* 81: 684–696.

Upton, C., Widdowson, J., and Stewert, S. (2017). *Word Maps: A Dialect Atlas of English*. New York: Routledge.

Varnhagen, C., Mcfall, P., and Pugh, N. (2010). Lol: New Language and Spelling in Instant Messaging. *Reading and Writing* 23(6): 719–733.

Verheijen, L. (2013). The Effects of Text Messaging and Instant Messaging on Literacy. *English Studies* 94(5): 582–602.

Vertovec, S. (2007). Super-Diversity and Its Implications. *Ethnic and Racial Studies* 30: 1024–1054.

Wei, L. (1998). The "Why" and "How" Questions in the Analysis of Conversational Codeswitching. In: P. Auer (ed.), *Code-Switching in Conversation: Language, Interaction, and Identity*, pp. 156–176. London: Routledge.

Weinreich, U. (1953). *Languages in Contact*. New York: Linguistic Circle of New York.

Weinreich, U. (1954). Is a Structural Dialectology Possible? *Word* 10: 388–400.

Wenker, G. (1881). *Sprachatlas des Deutschen Reichs*. MS folio: Marburg University.

Wilson, S. M. and Peterson, L. C. (2002). The Anthropology of Online Communities. *Annual Reviews in Anthropology* 31: 449–467.

Zenner, E., Backus, A., and Winter-Froemel, E. (eds.) (2019). *Cognitive Contact Linguistics*. Berlin: Moutone de Gruyter.

Zentella, A. C. (1997). *Growing Up Bilingual*. Malden, MA: Wiley-Blackwell.

4 Variation in Social Space

The previous chapter dealt primarily with geographical or regional dialect variation. Starting with the empirical studies of Labov and Fischer (mentioned in Chapter 1), another primary target of sociolinguistic research is the kind of variation that emerges in social spaces. The variants in these are called *social dialects* or *sociolects*. The latter term is the one that will be used throughout this chapter.

This chapter looks at sociolectal variation, including such phenomena as slang, jargon, registers, styles, and speech codes. The relation between geographical and social dialects is an intrinsic one. Variation occurs simultaneously along the two axes—the geographical and the social—as does the social perception of the variants. Those who have a high level of competence in the standard variety of a language, or the sociolectal norm, generally have subtle or implicit social advantages over those who speak regional variants or dialects, indicating that the type of language used is crucial in social interactions (Carlson and McHenry 2006):

- Dialect speakers, or speakers of nonstandard variants, are perceived as more likely to be less educated (whether true or not).
- Dialect speakers are also more likely to be underrepresented in official social institutions and in politics.
- Speakers of the standard variety, by way of contrast, are perceived as more educated (again, whether true or not).
- They are also more likely to be represented positively in official social institutions and in politics.

As in other domains of sociolinguistics, the world of social media is now affecting how we perceive and use sociolectal variants, from slang and jargon to styles of delivery. These will be discussed at the end of this chapter. Particularly worrisome is the emergence of hate speech in the social media universe (Ferrini and Paris 2019). Internet platforms allow anyone to use harmful language and fear-inducing rhetoric, which seems to correlate with a rise in mass violence outbreaks across the globe—the dehumanization of people makes violence against them all too common (Mathew et al. 2019). It is little wonder that hate speech has become an important concern of sociolinguistic research. In this case the tools of conversation analysis will be of primary importance (see Chapter 6).

4.1 Slang

Ferdinand de Saussure (1916) was the first to use the term *speech community* to indicate a group of people sharing a common language (Chapter 1). As discussed in the previous chapter, traditionally this term designates a geographically and culturally circumscribed group of speakers. Today, it has been extended to include speakers connected to each other in a socially specific way, which may or may not have a geographical basis. This is known more specifically as a *speech network*. A network could be a group of lawyers, a group of sports fans, and the like. To be a member of a speech network an individual needs to use the appropriate linguistic *code* of the network in an appropriate way; that is, the individual must become familiar with the type of vocabulary, specific form of literacy, etc. that characterizes verbal interaction in the network. The code allows individuals to convey a connection to the network, from professional organizations, who speak a *jargon*, to groups such as cliques and gangs, who speak a *slang*. Using the dichotomy of high (H) and low (L) that applies to geographical dialects (Chapter 3), it can be said that slangs are L sociolects and professional jargons H sociolects. Although this is a highly reductive assessment, it can be used in a generic way to make practical comparisons among sociolects.

The slang code used in speech networks is not random, but rather part of linguistic behavior that connects speakers to their networks emotionally and socially. *Code* is an important concept within sociolinguistics. It was introduced initially by Saussure (1916: 31), implying the type of speech used in specific situations that allows speakers to align themselves with each other in some way. In theory, all speech variants are codes; in practice, however, the term is used to refer to a set of marked speech features that characterize communication within a particular social group.

4.1.1 Slang Codes

The topic of *slang* is a major one in sociolinguistics. Defining it, however, has always constituted a problem and, to this day, there is no clear definition for this form of speech (Dumas and Lighter 1978). Michael Adams (2009) questions the typical standard-versus-nonstandard and formal-versus-informal dichotomies made by linguists to define slang, arguing that it really is a matter of what a particular society perceives as slang or non-slang. Indeed, an item that may have emerged in the domain of slang can evolve over time into an item accepted as part of standard speech. An example is the word *jazz* (Danesi 1994). The term surfaces as a slang item around 1915 in reference to sexual activities, gradually referring to an exciting new musical style. When we use it today, however, it is unlikely that the original meaning comes to mind.

Rather, we tend to think of jazz as a refined genre of music that has a high cultural value. Its origin in the realm of slang is now largely a lost memory.

There are two main slang codes—*generic* and *group based*. An example of the former is the kind of vocabulary that comes out of popular culture or (today) the social media world, where it is perceived as part of shared cultural knowledge. Words such as *selfie* belong to this category of slang. Group-based slang, by the same token, refers to the type of coded speech used by cliques, gangs, and other social enclaves. Generic slang bespeaks of friendliness and commonality. When slang expressions gain broad currency, they are called *colloquialisms*, that is, expressions used in everyday informal conversations that are no longer perceived as slang. Group-based slang bespeaks instead of insider savvy. It arises within cliques and special groups for reasons of solidarity and ingroup communication.

We are hardly aware that many words in the standard lexicon originate as slang, as just mentioned. For example, the word *scuffle* used as a noun designating a fight comes from Shakespeare's play *Antony and Cleopatra* (Act I, Scene 1). It was, at the time, a slang word presumably used by Shakespeare to recreate street talk on the stage, enhancing his script in a realistic way. The term spread more broadly, no doubt because of the prestige and value of Shakespearean theater and, thus, of its linguistic content. So, a particular word (*scuffle*) started out as slang, but given the influence of Shakespeare on the development of English, it gained currency, becoming over time a colloquialism, a part of ordinary or familiar vocabulary.

Group-based slang codes arise, instead, within specific groups, such as teen cliques, but some expressions may migrate beyond the group to become part of generic slang. Words such as *jock, cool, chick, dude, sloshed, chill out*, among many others, started out this way, having subsequently become colloquialisms and part of common lexical knowledge. For example, the word *jock*, referring to a "strong athletic male," goes back to the 1950s and the teen slang of that era; and *cool*, meaning "relaxed" or "attractive," goes back to the 1940s' slang used by young jazz musicians. The fact that these words have remained as colloquialisms bespeaks of the influence of the mass media and popular culture in spreading and reinforcing everyday speech habits.

4.1.2 Emotives

The defining features of slang are not restricted to the domain of vocabulary. Slang involves the deployment of other systems, from phonology to pragmatics, in specific ways. An example of how these might coalesce is in teen slang, an area that has received much attention from sociolinguists (Davie 2019). One feature of teen slang, at least in the past, is its basis in communicative *emotivity* (Jakobson 1960; Reddy 1997). An *emotive* is defined as an expression or verbal mannerism that overtly reveals the feelings or attitudes that a speaker possesses (consciously or unconsciously) with regard to an event, another person, a situation, etc. Emotives are communicative devices that involve the direct expression of emotional states and feelings. If these become part of regular communicative behavior within groups, such as teen communities, then they come to characterize the slang used by the group.

The main emotives are *tags, hedges, fillers, commentators,* and *quotatives.* Tag expressions—"Right?," "You follow?," "Got it?"—show a need to secure consensus or reassurance (Danesi 1994). Fillers and hedges—"uhmmm," "like," etc.—allow the speaker to keep speaking without interruption. As a hedge, *like* became part of generic slang in the 1980s: "I, like, wanna come but, like, I'm a little busy now." Some emotives have a commentary function, usually of a satirical nature. These can be called *commentators.* For example, *duh* allows speakers to undercut mindless talk or insulting repetition. With its perfectly paired linguistic partner, *yeah right,* it constitutes a means for conveying savvy and sarcasm.

Box 4.1 Tags, Hedges, Fillers, Commentators, Quotatives

Tag question

A sentence that ends with a "tagged on" phrase that is designed to seek approval, agreement, or consent:

"You agree with me, don't you?"
"This is the truth, isn't it?"
"This is how to do it, right?"

Hedge

A word or phrase that makes utterances less forceful.
"It's kinda good to say this."
"She sort of said that."

Filler

A word or phrase that indicates to interlocutors that the speaker has not finished speaking, but has simply paused to gather further thoughts. Common fillers are:

"like"
"you know"
"well"
"so"

Commentator

A word or phrase that makes a comment on a situation (usually satirical):

"duh"
"no way"
"no kidding"

> **Quotative**
>
> A word or expression that introduces a quotation:
>
> "He's like: I didn't say that"
> "And she's like: Oh yes, you did."

Interestingly, *like* has several communicative functions. It is often used as a *quotative*, an expression replacing such phrases as "she said" or "he repeated" followed by a quotation (Romaine and Lange 1991; Blyth, Recktenwald, and Wang 2000). A slang (or colloquial) version of "Mike said: 'What are you doing?'" would be "Mike was like: 'What are you doing?'" Another function of *like* that has spread broadly to all levels of speech is that of a *quantifier*, replacing such expressions as "nearly," "approximately," and "very:" "The ticket's, like, 20 dollars, "It's, like, late, ya know," and so on. Another function is as an *exemplifier* word: "They're, like, OK!" (Siegel 2002). Some of these predate contemporary slang, surfacing in the 1950s, as evidenced by the title of a 1954 *Time* magazine article: "You Wanna Hear Some Jazz, Like?"

Needless to say, emotives characterize informal non-slang language as well; but they seem to be particularly prevalent in slang-using situations as strategic communicative devices. So, emotivity in speech networks is a matter of degree rather than of substance.

Slang is often symbolic of specific social trends, peculiar or otherwise, and thus is open to a critique of those trends. The use of *like* as an emotive construction was satirized in 1982 by the late rock musician Frank Zappa with his song *Valley Girl*, using it to satirize the slang that was in vogue at the time. It was also used as a hedge in the *Scooby-Doo* comics and cartoons of the late 1960s, functioning as an indirect comedic comment on human foibles. The story of *like* is a case-in-point of how slang terms spread to the mainstream via the media. Laroche (2007: 48) provides the following relevant commentary:

> The media not only help spread new language from all quarters, they also produce it when they coin terms to describe themselves and their activities. Media-related words are especially interesting because they often have social resonance. They're not just appropriate or imaginative describers of a certain medium, but also say something important about our larger world. The hybrid "infotainment," for example, merges information and entertainment, just as some media increasingly do. The hybrid word not only reflects the fact, but it also tells us something about our society and our society's values, pressures, trends.

As Laroche's last sentence indicates, slang is often a gauge of social trends or perceptions. Consider the word *dude*, which started out as a slang item referring to a generic male person with no distinctive qualities, and having emotive commentator function. It is now used in greetings ("What's up, dude?"), in exclamations ("Whoa, dude!"), as a means to convey commiseration ("Dude, I'm so sorry"), and to one-up someone ("That's so lame, dude"). In the late 1800s, a *dude* was a dandy, meticulously dressed man, in contrast to a virile man. The current meaning of *dude* began with the 1982 movie *Fast Times at Ridgemont High*, and then reinforced by the movie, *The Big Lebowski* (1998). The same kind of sociolinguistic story can be drafted for many other slang terms. The word *cool* (meaning "nice, attractive, stylish, fashionable") was used in the fifteenth century as a term of approval, suggesting calm and refrain. But its modern meaning comes from jazz musician Charlie Parker's 1947 *Cool Blues*, referring to a lifestyle and attitude that was associated with jazz culture, and which has since spread to mainstream culture.

4.1.3 Vocabulary

Slang emerges most prominently at the level of vocabulary. Below is an etymological (historical) sketch of some terms that were born as slang forms, but have become colloquialisms over time (Morrish 1999):

- *Geek:* designating a gamer or a computer aficionado, referred initially to a young male individual with an odd personality. In Victorian times, it meant a fool or dupe. Shakespeare used it in *Twelfth Night* and *Cymbeline* with this sense. Today, geek can refer to a male or female ("Hey, Jeannie is a real geek; she loves computer games").
- *Gross:* meaning disgusting, came into prominence in the Valley Girl talk of the 1980s, although it was already around in early 1970s' adolescent slang to express a dislike of something ("Eww, how gross"). It derives originally from Latin *grossus*, "big." In the fifteenth century, it was used to refer to people who stand out because of their body proportions and were thus perceived to be unattractive. It was used in this way by Shakespeare.
- *Icon:* meaning celebrity ("Marilyn Monroe is a true icon"), is of religious origin and used for the first time in celebrity culture to describe the American pop singer Madonna. The first users were aware of the irony behind this use of the term, given that the name Madonna refers to the Virgin Mary in Christian tradition. But it caught on broadly right after, and is now used in reference to any widely known celebrity, male or female.
- *Nerd:* started out as an insult used by teens in the 1980s against a socially awkward male peer ("He's unpopular because he's a nerd"). It may come from a Dr. Seuss rhyme of 1950: "And then I'll show them, I'll sail to Ka-Troo,/And bring back an It-Kutch, a Preep and a Proo,/A Nerkle, a Nerd, and a Seersucker, too!"

Slang terms may document socially or historically relevant events or perceptions. A word such as *hip* is actually a time capsule of socially-significant meaning. John Leland (2004) has dated the origin of the word to 1619 when the first African Americans arrived off the coast of Virginia as slaves. Without them, Leland maintains, there would be no "hip culture" in America, including jazz music, the blues, rock-and-roll, and rap. Hip is all about a nonchalant but subtly transgressive attitude. It is something that one feels, rather than understands, and that is why it has always been associated with musical styles. In a 1973 tune, the funk group Tower of Power defined *hip* as follows: "Hipness is—What it is! And sometimes hipness is, what it ain't." Hip is about a flight from mainstream conformity, a way to stand out, to look and be different. It is also a way to give a voice to underprivileged people. As Rapper Chuck D stated in a 1992 interview with *XXL* (a rap magazine): "This is our voice, this is the voice of our lifestyle, this is the voice of our people. We're not going to take the cookie cutter they give us let them mold us."

Hip is a metaphor that resonates with unconscious nuances of lifestyle meaning. Many slang terms are metaphors. Words like *hottie, babe, player,* for instance, are figurative sketches that depict specific individuals; other words are comedic or ironic portraits—for example, *crib* (home, emphasizing the childish treatment young people tend to receive at home) and *issues* (personal problems). Slang can thus function as part of social protest or transgression.

4.1.4 Cryptolects

Criminal organizations use group-based slang as an insider code. This type of slang is known more specifically as a *cryptolect* (literally, a secretive sociolect), arising in a criminal group as a means to keep outsiders out of the communicative and social loop of the group. The most common cryptolects are called *argots* and *cants*, as already discussed. Argots are used by street criminals on a temporary basis, so they come and go quickly; cants, in contrast, are codes that emerge in durative criminal gangs, such as the Sicilian Mafia, and thus have continuity across generations of gang members. Starting in the late 1800s, Mafia gangs began using a lexicon based on older dialectal forms (Sicilian or Calabrian) which virtually no one other than the criminals themselves knew (Nicaso and Danesi 2013). This allowed the gangs to declare themselves as connected to the original traditional languages of the region, thus legitimizing themselves culturally.

So-called "thieves' cants" were widespread in sixteenth-century England, attesting to the rise in street crime and alluding, in turn, to the abject quality of life for many poor people. The cants thus bore social and political connotations. For this reason, the leading Elizabethan playwrights and pamphleteers of the day, such as Thomas Harman, Thomas Dekker, and Christopher Marlowe, invented a literary genre known as the "literature of roguery," depicting the dismal conditions of the underworld, incorporating cant in plays and other publications (Chandler 1907). Thomas Harman, who included samples of cant in his *Caveat for Common Cursitors* (1566), claimed that he collected his information from the "vagabonds" (as he called them) whom he had interrogated at his home in Essex. His book might be the first record of a criminal cant in history. In 1591, Robert Greene produced five pamphlets on various aspects of the criminal underworld, followed by similar pamphlets by Thomas Middleton (*The Black Book*, 1604) and Thomas Dekker (The *Bellman of London*, 1608; *Lantern and Candlelight*, 1608). The cant of the thieves was included in these works together with (alleged) descriptions of the social lives of beggars, the robbery techniques of the thieves, and descriptions of the underworld, making them quite popular. Shakespeare also used thieves' cant in his *As You Like It* (1623) and *The Winter's Tale* (1623), thus bringing social realism into his plays through the appropriate street language he crafted for his villainous characters.

Box 4.2   Thieves' Cant

Examples of the cant used by pickpockets in England are as follows (from Lunde 2012: 129):

bung	the targeted purse
cuttle	the knife used to cut the purse
drawing	taking the purse
figging	pickpocketing
foin	a pickpocket
nip	someone who cuts the strings of the victim's purse
shells	the money in the purse
smoking	spying on the victim
snap	a pickpocket's accomplice
stale	an accomplice who distracts the victim
striking	the act of pickpocketing

In excluding outsiders, cant creates a sense of unity among its speakers. To become a "made man" in the Mafia an individual has to undergo an identity transformation; this includes "talking the talk," among other symbolic behaviors. One cannot be a mafioso without speaking like one. As far as can be told, most criminal cants are marked for gender; they aim to emphasize the gender of the members—that is, male gangs use codes where the masculine gender is the default one in the lexicon, and female gangs use a code with the reverse markedness. In the Mafia, originally a woman was called *panza lenta* ("loose guts") because she was seen as being too talkative and gossipy and thus "spilling her guts out." Men, however, were called *uomini di panza* ("men of the gut") because they could be trusted not to talk and spill their guts out. Ironically, it has always been the men who, as *pentiti* ("repentant ones"), have talked willingly to the authorities. By and large, women are perceived to be supplementary role players by the Mafia.

Michael Halliday (1976) refers to cryptolects as "anti-languages," because they are designed to pit speakers against the social mainstream. He identifies several criteria that a code must meet to be considered an anti-language. These are worth paraphrasing here.

- The simplest form taken by an anti-language is to assign new meanings to existing words—a process called *relexicalization.*
- Effective communication depends on ensuring that the code is inaccessible to the outsider.
- The anti-language is not just an option, it is central to the existence of the group.
- It is a vehicle for the resocialization of members.
- There must be continuity, grammatical and lexical, between the anti-language and the mainstream language, otherwise understanding would be blocked.

4.2 Register

The use and significance of specific linguistic forms (lexical, grammatical, phonological, semantic, pragmatic) according to social context is studied under the rubric of *register,* discussed briefly in the opening chapter. A register is defined as a level of speech that is guided by codes of formality, by communicative purpose, or by the social status of the users. A trivial, yet insightful, example is the register that academics and scientists use, when speaking formally, which has more technical words in it, more passive than active sentences, and so on. This type of register imparts a sense of formality and objectivity to the speech act. To say "Yesterday, I conducted an experiment that didn't work out" implies a lower register and, thus, perceived to be less objective than "The experiment conducted yesterday did not produce the anticipated results."

Registers are synchronized to speech situations. Take, for example, saying goodbye to another person in English. This might vary somewhat as follows:

Highly formal	Goodbye!
	Have a nice day!
	I'm looking forward to our next encounter!
Mid-formal	Bye!
	See you later!
	I must be going!
	Take care!
Informal	See ya'!
	Take it easy!
	I'm off!

I'm outta here!

I gotta split!

The choice of one expression or the other is not random or optional. The highly formal register is perceived to display politeness and is used with strangers and superiors. The mid-formal one is used with those whom we see frequently and with whom we have developed a degree of familiarity (coworkers, peers, and so on). The informal register is used with those with whom we are on the friendliest of terms. The misuse of one register or the other is felt to be a breach of social etiquette or as anomalous communication. It would be considered rude to address a superior at work with an informal mode of speech (unless the superior permits it); and it would be considered to be aberrant or strange to address a close friend with a highly formal register.

Incidentally, the term *register* was first used with this technical sense in 1956 by Thomas Bertram Reid in order to distinguish sociolectal variants determined by variables such as age, gender, class, and geography. Halliday and Hasan (1976) subsequently defined it as the set of linguistic features that encode social variables, guiding relations and behaviors among interlocutors during verbal interactions in a specific context.

4.2.1 Levels of Formality

Native speakers of a language recognize some usage as formal or informal through the specific linguistic forms. Consider the following list of expressions that are synonymous:

Formal	Informal
abode	house, place
alcoholic beverage	drink, booze
offspring	children, kids
currency	bucks

The formal lexemes typify such speech acts and written texts as government forms, academic lectures, communications with people in high authority, and so on. The informal items instead typify common everyday speech among friends, family members, colleagues, and acquaintances. In formal speech, clipped or abbreviated words tend to be avoided:

Formal	Informal
goodbye	bye
hello	hi
yes	ya'
thank you	thanks

It is the context that determines the degree of formality that is appropriate. In formal conversations, aspects of informal speech may be incorporated for various reasons, such as establishing a friendly tone or suggesting a shift to an informal register. Moreover, as the linguist Martin Joos argued in his classic 1967 book titled *The Five Clocks: A Linguistic Excursion Into the Five Styles of English Usage*, we all move unconsciously up and down the register scale in regular daily conversations. Consider the different kinds of speech used by average individuals who work in, say, an office environment. How would they speak in the morning when they get up with family members? How would they speak at a place of work with coworkers? How would they speak at a place of work with superiors? How would they converse with friends at a pub after hours? How would they communicate late at night with a romantic partner? Answers to these questions would show how speech registers are synchronized with daily life routines and interpersonal interactions. Although there is much leeway in the grammatical, lexical, and pragmatic choices that can be made to carry out conversations successfully, these are nonetheless constrained by factors such as situation and social relationship. For example, the utterances below convey anger, but in different ways:

1   Don't say that, idiot!
2   It is best that you not say that!

The first one might be uttered by someone who is on close or intimate terms with an interlocutor; the second one by someone who is instead on formal terms. The latter could also be intended as ironic with someone with whom we are familiar. The choices are constrained by situation and social relationship. Rather than *register*, the term *diatype* is sometimes used to describe the situation when the speaker intentionally changes the register for some effect, such as irony (Gregory 1967).

Joos described five main types of register styles:

1   *Frozen* or *static*. This is characterized by formulaic speech including archaisms, aphorisms, Biblical quotations, and so on. Examples are the oath taken in a courtroom, the Pledge of Allegiance ("I solemnly swear to tell the truth, …"), and the expressions used for official purposes in public spaces: "Everyone must latch their seatbelts for takeoff," "You are requested to turn off your cellphones during the movie." The wording is similar every time and the speech act does not require a response.

2   *Formal*. This register is marked by conventional speech strategies that are designed to convey politeness, objectivity, respect, etc. It is used at business meetings, classroom settings, courtrooms, and the like: "I would like to call this meeting to a close," "Would everyone please come at the established time?" It is also indicative of formal relationships: "Hello. My name is Mark Smith. Glad to make your acquaintance."

3   *Consultative.* This register is largely informal and characterizes situations where advice, help, or assistance might be needed. It also typifies interactions between a superior and a subordinate, between an expert and apprentice, a teacher and student, a lawyer and client, and so on: "Please, listen very carefully," "Let's not make any assumptions."

4   *Casual or informal.* This register is the one used mainly between friends and peers; it is usually replete with slang items, incomplete sentences, and colloquialisms: "I'm off!" "Get your act together!"

5   *Intimate.* This register is used among individuals who have a close relationship, including family members, close friends, and romantic partners. It has a relaxed and friendly style, even in situations where conflict is implied: "Are you upset at me?" "Come off it!"

Register styles both reflect and guide speech acts according to situation, time of day, and relationships among interlocutors. Joos' book was truly significant for the era in which it appeared, dovetailing with the research of other linguists in the mid- to late 1960s that eventually led to the establishment of sociolinguistics as an autonomous branch of linguistic science. It showed that *parole* lends itself to systematic analysis as much as does *langue* and, more importantly, that there is a dynamic interrelationship between the two.

4.2.2 Politeness

The ways for saying "goodbye" mentioned above involve the conveyance of levels of *politeness*. The choice of one or the other phrase is determined by an overarching sociolinguistic pattern: the highly formal register is used with social superiors or strangers; the mid-formal one with colleagues, instructors, professionals such as doctors; and the informal register with close friends and intimates. As mentioned, there is flexibility between the registers in modern-day social interactions. But in traditional societies, such as in Java (as already discussed in Chapter 1), politeness registers are tied much more strictly to a hierarchy of social distinctions: the aristocrats (at the top); the townsfolk (in the middle); and the peasants (at the bottom). Politeness forms are obligatory when an individual at a lower class level addresses someone at higher levels.

We all use politeness protocols unconsciously. They indicate the type of relation we have with an interlocutor. The violation of these protocols might lead to misinterpretation and even conflict, especially in situations of intercultural communication. If speaker A (a non-native speaker of English) were to use a register that is highly formal with a friend, B (a native speaker), then A might be misconstrued by B as attempting to be ironic or emotionally distant. By the same token, if A uses informal speech with a superior, also a native speaker, miscommunication would likely result, because the language does not match the expected register. Using the *tu* (familiar) forms of address to a stranger in Italy, rather than the *Lei* (polite) forms, would be perceived as an act of impoliteness or rudeness, unless the speaker reveals that they are a foreigner either directly or indirectly. Saying *ciao* ("hi"), rather than *scusi* ("excuse me") to, say, police officers in order to get their attention will tend, initially at least, to prompt a negative response (or no response at all). Breaking a rule of politeness speech protocols is perceived as breaking social manners, not a lack of linguistic knowledge.

Politeness will be taken up in more depth in Chapter 6. Suffice it to say here that there are various registers that are deployed to convey politeness. For example, to express uncertainty and ambiguity in a polite way, several strategies are available to native speakers, including the use of hedges ("I think that, maybe, this can be interpreted, hmm, in a different way"), euphemisms ("She has passed on"), and tags ("This is what you mean, isn't it?"). Studies have shown that politeness speech is marked not only for class, but also for age and gender (Holmes 1995).

4.2.3 Honorifics

Politeness also involves a correct use of titles and other terms of respect, known as *honorifics* (*Mr., Ms., Sir, Madam, Professor, Doctor, Reverend*). In some languages there exist complex honorific systems, which are sensitive to class, gender, and even age. Korean politeness protocols, for example, are sensitive to age differences among the speakers, even very young ones. It is not surprising, therefore, that Korean speakers will try to learn the age of a new acquaintance as soon as possible or at least to estimate it as accurately as possible: this is necessary in order to be able to choose the proper honorifics to address the interlocutor.

There are three main types of honorifics. One is the *addressee honorific* which is designed to allude to the social status of the person addressed. In Javanese, there are three different words for "house," to be used in accordance with the social level of the addressee. If the person has social superiority then the word for "house" will reflect this—it is analogous to using the word *domicile* rather than *house* in English. If the addressee has lower social status, then the speaker would use a different form analogous, more or less, to English *hut*. A second type of honorific is called *referent* because it designates the level of formality expected to be used among speakers. In French, this can be seen in the use of the *tu* versus *vous* forms of address (both meaning "you"). The former references a speaker with whom an interlocutor is on informal terms: *Qu'est-ce que tu veux* ("What do you want")? The latter references instead a speaker with whom an interlocutor is on formal terms: *Qu'est-ce que vous voulez?* A third type is called *bystander* because the protocol is designed to allude to the status of a bystander, not a participant, in the conversation. This involves typically an avoidance strategy, whereby a speaker switches to a different register in the presence of, say, a relative.

4.3 Style and Genre

Style is a distinctive form of speech that corresponds to specific situations. In many instances, it is governed by the context or by the degree of formality that is called for. An example is the difference between active and passive sentences. They are not alternatives; they are reflective of different styles that may be required in certain contexts. Consider the sentences below:

1   The apple was eaten by Rebecca. It was not eaten by me, neither was it my intention to do so. The eating action was accomplished quickly. The apple was devoured by her.
2   I put sodium together with chlorine. I knew I was going to get a reaction. I thought I would get salt. But it didn't work out for some reason.

If told that (1) was written by one friend to another and (2) by a scientist in a professional journal, we would immediately think that something is amiss in either one. The reason is that stylistic practices dictate that (1) should be phrased mainly in active sentences and (2) in passive ones, along with other syntactic and lexical adjustments. Active sentences are used to emphasize the speaker as the actor in a direct relation with the goal (the person spoken to or the object involved), whereas passive ones are used to de-emphasize the speaker as actor and highlight the goal as the object of interest. This style is typical of scientific and other types of formal speech, where the "goal–object" is highlighted over the "subject–actor" relationship. Reformulating both sentences by reversing their voice (active-to-passive and vice versa, as the case may be) rectifies the stylistic anomalies:

1   Rebecca ate the apple. I didn't eat it, neither did I intend to do so. She ate it quickly. She devoured it.
2   Sodium and chlorine were mixed, in order to attain the expected reaction. The anticipated outcome was salt. However, this outcome was not achieved for some reason.

4.3.1 Style

When we receive a card (by mail or electronically) sent to us by a friend, rather than by, say, a dentist, we can easily formulate specific hypotheses as to the nature of the card's content and style even before reading it. The friend might have sent it to wish us a happy birthday, to congratulate us for having achieved something, and so on. A card from a dentist would hardly have a similar type of content, unless the dentist is a friend or family member. Its purpose is, usually, to remind us about an appointment or to request payment for some service. In the former case, the style used will be casual or intimate ("Congrats on getting your degree"); in the latter, it will be formal or formulaic ("You are reminded that payment for services rendered is overdue").

Style correlates with social and political functions. In communist Poland, for example, the *podanie* style of Polish flourished for a specific reason—it allowed common people to write their requests to the authorities in a strategic fashion (Wierzbicka 1991). Petitioners were expected to ask the authorities for favors and to portray themselves as highly dependent on their good will. *Podanie* style would be unusual in English-speaking societies, because the practice of asking favors from authorities does not have the same significance that it had in communist Poland, where people's lives "were dominated, to a considerable degree, by their dependence on the arbitrary decisions of bureaucratic despots" (Wierzbicka 1991: 193). As Wierzbicka (1991: 195) puts it: "a person who is writing an *application* is *applying*, not *asking for* or *requesting*." In an English-speaking society an application can be unsuccessful, but not refused or rejected, as with *podanie*.

Style is also symbolic of specific communities or social networks. For example, there are urban styles versus rural styles of speaking English. This is mirrored in the speech of several humorous Looney Tunes characters. Bugs Bunny, for example, used an ironically tinged urban hip style; his catchphrases ("What's up, doc?") and tics ("What's cooking?") came from the hip slang of the 1940s. It showed great savvy. His nemesis, Elmer Fudd, spoke with an unclassy, unhip style ("Be vewy vewy quiet, I'm hunting wabbits"). Today, Bugs Bunny would be called a "badass" and Elmer Fudd a "loser." In effect, comedians, announcers, writers, lecturers, motivational speakers, and so on adopt a certain style that makes them recognizable and identifiable.

4.3.2 Genre

A speech *genre* is a mode of speaking or writing that people recognize as distinctive—letters, lectures, job interviews, medical consultations, comedy routines, and so on (Bakhtin 1981; Fairclough 2003). As Charaudeau, Maingueneau, and Adam (2002: 278–280) have observed, an utterance's genre can be identified by the particular phrasal style and choice of vocabulary. Lack of the ability to distinguish among genres is a major cause of interactional breakdowns. As Russian literary critic Mikhail Bakhtin (1981: 80) observed: "Many people who have an excellent command of a language often feel quite helpless in certain spheres of communication because they do not have a practical command of the generic forms used in the given spheres." A native speaker of English, who is perfectly fluent in the language, might still not be able to write an academic paper according to the proper conventions of that genre. Conversely, someone may well be able to write such a paper, but be strikingly awkward when it comes to telling jokes.

Speech genres serve many social functions, including ritualistic ones. The purpose of language in rituals is not to create new meanings, but to assert communal sense making and to ensure cultural cohesion. People typically love to hear the same speeches, songs, and stories at specific times during the year (at Christmas, at Passover, and so on) in order to feel united with the other members of the community. Genre-based communication tends to be predictable and rely on widely known and accepted conventions and linguistic constructions. These help people understand what is relevant in a ritual, because they can rely upon the style and content to satisfy their expectations.

Genres are formulaic or quasi-formulaic in their forms and functions. One can recognize something as a joke in English culture according to the following traits and cues (Sacks 1974; Raskin 1985).

1   It narrates a situation that is typical, but it violates expectations at the end of the narration (called a "punch line"); without knowing this, the joke will not succeed.
2   A joke tells of events and people that are familiar to listeners, caricaturizing them in a specific way. This means that there is a mutual understanding between the joke teller and the listener that the narration is a joke. This is reinforced by the sequential structure of the joke: the framing—the telling—the punch line. Framing often involves a formulaic expression ("Have you heard the one about ...")? "Reminds me of a joke I once heard ...").
3   The context is crucial in allowing people to identify a narration as a joke, rather than something else. This includes who is telling the joke and to whom. Some are identified as specialized joke tellers (comedians and comics); others are assumed to make a joke at some point, such as motivational speakers or politicians. This is known as a "performance frame." Both the performer and audience understand that the joke sets the story apart from the real world. So, when someone says "A hippo walks into a bar ..." both performer and audience recognize this as the start of a joke.
4   The telling of the joke is succinct; the longer the telling, the less likely the joke will produce laughter.

The foregoing discussion aimed to illustrate that we unconsciously possess knowledge of what a speech genre is. When we read a thriller novel, we anticipate what is involved, from its framing and telling to its denouement. So, the treatment of, say, murder in the novel will be different than how it will be treated scientifically or philosophically, as in criminological treatises. The two approaches reflect different genres, treating the same subject matter in differential ways (Arntfield and Danesi 2017).

4.3.3 Jargon

Jargon refers to the type of speech genre distinguished by the terms used by specialized groups or by anyone for specialized reasons. Jargon allows its speakers to communicate with each other effectively and unambiguously. As a case-in-point, consider medical jargon, as we can see in Table 4.1.

Table 4.1 Medical Terms

Medical term	Common term
hematoma	blood clot
coronary thrombosis	heart attack
pruritis	itchiness
verruca	wart
furuncle	boil, pimple
rectum	bum
pustule	pus
varicella	chickenpox
posology	dosage
hemeralopia	impaired vision
strabismus	squinting
contusion	bruise

Although the medical terms can always be converted to more common descriptive ones, the latter do not have the specialized function of the former. Recall from Chapter 2 that denotation is the primary (literal) meaning of a lexeme, whereas connotations are the meanings that the lexeme accrues from its uses in social contexts. Denotative meaning does not generally vary, connotative meaning does. Jargon is largely denotative, when used among the members of the specialized group—that is, it is typically precise and invariable as to what it designates. This is critical among professionals and scientists, where ambiguity in meaning can lead to disastrous results. When doctors use the term *verruca*, they are referring to something physiological; it does not bear any social connotations per se. The descriptive equivalent *wart* does, as it can evoke negative social perceptions. Similarly, a *coronary thrombosis* indicates a medical condition resulting from a blockage of a coronary artery by a blood clot, which, in turn, obstructs the blood supply to the heart muscle, resulting in death of the muscle. This is called a *heart attack* in everyday speech, that is, an "attack on the heart." The medical term for this is *infarction*, which literally denotes the effects of a coronary thrombosis, with no social connotations. The common term, *heart attack,* on the other hand, often implies connotations connected with lifestyle or diet.

Box 4.3 Denotation Versus Connotation

Denotation

This is the referential (literal) meaning of a word. The word *cat* when used denotatively refers to a "mammal with four legs, long tail, whiskers, and retractile claws."

Connotation

This is the variable meanings that a word takes on in social context. The connotative meanings of *cat* can be seen in expressions such as "He's a cool cat" (an attractive person); "You let the cat out of the bag" (secret); and so on.

In her significant book *Illness As Metaphor* (1978), the late American writer Susan Sontag cogently argued that socially embedded connotations in medical terms might even predispose people to interpret specific illnesses in self-destructive ways. Sontag argued that the word *cancer* has historically been perceived as more than just a dangerous physical disease (Sontag 1978: 7): "As long as a particular disease is treated as an evil, invincible predator, not just a disease, most people with cancer will indeed be demoralized by learning what disease they have." Common examples of how we refer to cancer to this day bring out the validity of Sontag's main argument:

1   Cancer is a *killer*.
2   Cancer is a *predator*.
3   It's an uphill *battle* to beat cancer.
4   Cancer is a *scourge*.

These metaphors instill the unconscious perception that cancer is an "enemy" that must be defeated, rather than a clinical condition per se. There are, actually, many metaphorical expressions that connect cancer to fate, lifestyle, and other culturally-based perceptions ("He didn't deserve it;" "Smoking habits and cancer are connected;" etc.). Sontag's point that people suffer as much from the judgments about their disease in cultural terms than from the disease itself is, indeed, a well-taken and instructive one.

Jacalyn Duffin (2005) has also argued that throughout history illness is often what we define it to be. She points out that "lovesickness" was once considered to be a true disease, even though it originated in the poetry of antiquity and reinforced in the poetry of the medieval period. Its elimination as a disease from medical practice is due to twentieth-century skepticism and scientific research, which finally exposed it as a cultural myth. She also pointed out that hepatitis C—a major cause of cirrhosis that might result from contaminated needles for injecting drugs, tattooing, or body piercing—has also been enmeshed in mythic-metaphorical connotations. It was finally defined as a disease by discoveries in virology and by tragedies in transfusion medicine. The same kind of story can be told with regard to diseases such as AIDS and various STDs (sexually transmitted diseases), which (also in the past) carried moral stigmas. The point is that, at any given point in time, concepts of disease are shaped by social, linguistic, and cultural connotations.

Jargons serve important functions. For example musical jargon, which comes largely from the Italian language (see Table 4.2) must be learned by anyone desiring to study music professionally.

It is relevant to note that some jargons migrate to common discourse. Because everybody studies mathematics starting in elementary school, a basic mathematical jargon is widely used in common speech. Terms such as *equation, coordinate, factoring*, and *prime number* are part of jargon, but also part of common vocabulary. Only terms with a more specialized usage are perceived to be restricted to mathematical jargon: *matrix, fractal, parameter, imaginary number*. The line between jargon and common vocabulary is obviously a thin one, given the fact that people have had some degree of formal education.

4.4 Speech Codes

The department store study by Labov, mentioned in the opening chapter, is an example of how a specific linguistic feature—the pronunciation of final /-r/—is perceived by people to correlate with social class and social mobility. In effect, it showed how perceptions of class are encoded in a particular phonemic cue.

The term *community of practice*, rather than *speech community*, is sometimes used in order to put the focus on everyday language practices that relate to the use of speech codes that reflect social variables. Relevant to sociolinguistic analysis in this domain of inquiry is the concept of *prestige*, already discussed in the previous chapter with respect to diglossia. Certain

Table 4.2 Musical Jargon

Musical term	*Meaning*
a piacere	freely
a tempo	with the original tempo
adagio	slowly
allegro	quickly, brightly
andante	slowly, but not too slowly
cadenza	a virtuosic solo passage
coda	tail end of a part or piece
da capo	from the beginning
forte	loud
largo	very slow, deliberate
moderato	at a moderate pace
presto	fast
vivace	vivacious, lively
cantabile	in a singing manner

sociolects are seen as having a positive or negative prestige. In the case of /-r/ the positive value assigned to its pronunciation meant working at a more prestigious store. The study of speech codes is another important area of sociolinguistic research.

4.4.1 Class

A classic study on the relation between social class and language is the one by Basil Bernstein (1971), discussed in the first chapter, in which he elaborated the theory of elaborated and restricted speech codes. The meaning of code in this theoretical framework is a "set of organizing principles behind the language employed by members of a social group" (Littlejohn 2002: 278). Bernstein used this notion to show how the language people use in everyday life both reflects and influences the their expectations and social assumptions. Bernstein found that the reason for the relatively poor performance of working-class students in language-based subjects, at the same time that they scored as high as their middle-class counterparts in mathematics, was that fact that the restricted code excluded them from the learning process. It was only when they gradually controlled the elaborated code did they improve their grades in these subjects. As Bernstein (1971: 76) puts it: "Forms of spoken language in the process of their learning initiate, generalize and reinforce special types of relationship with the environment and thus create for the individual particular forms of significance." The forms of a specific speech code and how they are used within a speech community affect the way people assign meaning to the things about which they are speaking. In a phrase, the code that individuals use symbolizes and enacts their social identities and influences their worldviews.

The restricted code is for ingroup interaction, and thus involves a great deal of shared and embedded group-based knowledge and beliefs. It is economical and to the point, conveying a vast amount of information and meaning with minimal linguistic resources. It functions like an index finger, pointing implicitly to a whole set of social nuances, background knowledge, and shared beliefs to which the group members have direct and constant access. This is why it is often called *indexical*. Conversely, the elaborated code uses a more complicated lexicon and grammar that allow interlocutors to indicate their intentions and opinions explicitly, not assume them. It also works better in situations where there is no prior or shared knowledge system. As Bernstein (1971: 135) puts it: "Clearly one code is not better than another; each possesses its own aesthetic, its own possibilities. Society, however, may place different values on the orders of experience elicited, maintained and progressively strengthened through the different coding systems."

In small speech communities, a restricted code tends to emerge as the primary form of communication. It is generally within the broader community of practice that an elaborated code arises. In a society that values individuality, elaborated codes tend to be used for advancement, whereas in a community that values conformity, restricted codes are the rule. Restricted codes are characterized by abbreviated syntax and an abundant use of tag questions and hedges: "you know," "you know what I mean," "right?" and "don't you think?" Elaborated codes have a longer, more complicated sentence structure that incorporates uncommon vocabulary and turns of phrase. Phonological differences also keep the codes distinct. For instance, Dubois and Horvath (1998) found that speakers of English in one Cajun Louisiana community were more likely to pronounce English "*th*" /θ/ as /t/ (*thing* as *ting*), or /ð/ as /d/ (*that* as *dat*) if they participated in what they called "a relatively dense social network" (that is, a speech community that demonstrated strong local ties among the members), and less likely if the networks were looser (that is, had fewer local ties). This is because not only class, but also class aspirations, are important. (See Appendix A for phonetic symbols.)

4.4.2 Race and Ethnicity

The terms *race* and *ethnicity* come up frequently in sociolinguistics. Human beings the world over typically think of themselves as members of *races* or *ethnic* groups, that is, as belonging to groups of people that have a common genetic-evolutionary origin. But racial or ethnic classifications are often misleading. No two human beings, not even twins, are identical genetically. Geneticists have yet to turn up a single group of people who can be distinguished from others strictly by their chromosomes. Moreover, because of interbreeding, DNA sequences are common to all humans (Sagan and Druyan 1992: 415). Nevertheless, from ancient times people have, for some reason or other, always felt it necessary to classify themselves in terms of racial or ethnic categories.

The systematic study and classification of races and ethnic groups was a consequence of the worldwide explorations of the sixteenth and seventeenth centuries. The Swedish botanist Carolus Linnaeus (1707–1778) was among the first to classify humans as primates, alongside apes and simians. The German scholar Johann Friedrich Blumenbach (1752–1840) then gave the world its first racial taxonomy. After examining the skulls and comparing the physical characteristics of different peoples, Blumenbach concluded that there were five races: Caucasians (West Asians, north Africans, and Europeans except the Finns and the Saami), Mongolians (other Asian peoples, the Finns and the Saami, and the Inuit of America), Ethiopians (the people of Africa except those of the north), Americans (all aboriginal New World peoples except the Inuit), and Malayans (peoples of the Pacific islands). These divisions remained the basis of most racial classifications well into the modern era. But population scientists now recognize the indefiniteness and arbitrariness of these demarcations. Indeed, many individuals can be classified into more than one of Blumenbach's racial categories or, indeed, into none. All that can be said is that the concept of race makes sense, if at all, only in terms of lineage: that is, people can be said to belong to the same race or ethnicity if they share the same pool of ancestors. But, as it turns out, even this seemingly simple criterion is insufficient for rationalizing the classification of humans into discrete racial or ethnic groups because, except for brothers and sisters, no individuals have precisely the same array of ancestors. This is why, rather than using genetic, anatomical, or physiological traits to study human variability, anthropologists today prefer to study them in terms of social criteria and cultural aspects, not biological ones.

Language plays a fundamental role in perceptions of race and ethnicity. Consider a hypothetical example. The author of this book is of Italian origin, born of parents who lived and spoke Italian even after immigrating to Canada after World War II. As such, their only child (myself) spoke Italian first and would be easily classified by people even today as an "Italian," given that he speaks Italian fluently. Now, if the same person (the author) were born of the same parents in France, but abandoned post partum and raised in France, speaking French as his native language, how would he then be perceived? He would be identified as French, not Italian. The gist of this hypothetical story is that language and culture are more important in determining people's identity than are abstract racial or ethnic categories.

Sociolinguistic research has shown, in fact, that we tend to ascribe race or ethnicity according to the speech used by individuals. Some studies have demonstrated that participants exposed to voice recordings will tend to pigeonhole certain vocal features as indicative of a specific ethnicity or race. But this could be misleading as well. In one such experiment (Purnell, Idsardi, and Baugh 1999), subjects were exposed to hidden speakers articulating only the word *hello* and on that basis to identify the speaker's race. The hidden speakers were Chicanos, African Americans, and White Americans. The subjects were surprisingly accurate at identifying the race of the speaker as Chicano or White, but a sizable portion was not able to classify the African American English (AAE) speaker correctly. In a subsequent study, the researchers had 50 African American men and 50 white men record a single vowel. Subjects then heard the vowel pronounced by each. They were told ahead of time that one was articulated by a white man and the other by an African American man and that they had to decide which was which. On average, they successfully identified the speaker barely about 60 percent of the time. So, when looked at together, these studies suggest that people are not really that good at detecting speech patterns as racially coded.

The problem with associating language and race is that it often results in a covert form of racial profiling, called *linguistic profiling*. The notion was first developed by John Baugh (2003) to describe discriminatory practices in the housing market influenced by the type of language spoken by clients.

4.4.3 *Online Sociolects*

Twitter communities, as discussed previously, tend to emerge on the basis of a common interest among members, rather than in terms of the traditional geographically based communities. As a result, social media networks have developed their own distinctive sociolectal codes.

Participants in F2F conversations tend to converge to one another's communicative behavior, by synchronizing the style (choice of words, syntax, utterance length, pitch, and gestures) and register of communication—known as *accommodation*. The question of how accommodation applies to sociolectal speech in social media networks is becoming increasingly important, because the virtual social network involved is unlike any other in which accommodation has been observed. Do Twitter users adapt to the style and register of their community? The answer appears to be yes and no. Danescu-Niculescu-Mizil, Gamon, and Dumais (2011) looked at style and register on Twitter. By comparing #followers, #followees, #posts, #days on Twitter, #posts per day, and ownership of a personal website, the researchers found that some stylistic features appear to be only weakly connected to the traditional social stratification of offline speech. Paolillo (2001) also documented weak ties between the two (online and offline speech) in chat relays, and Gilbert and Karahalios (2009) noted a poor correlation in Facebook sites. The reason would seem to be that unlike F2F, where physical contact is a factor in style adjustments, social media treat all users the same, whether they are trusted friends or total strangers, with little or nothing in between.

Ramage, Dumais, and Liebling (2010) looked at millions of Twitter posts, identifying four general registers, which they characterized as based on *substance, status, social,* and *style* variables: that is, on events, ideas, things, or people (substance), on some common goal (social), related to personal updates (status), or indicative of broader trends of language use (style). A primary factor in changing the sociolinguistic rules (or at least modifying them) is frequency of interaction. Twitter conversations are not time and situation dependent, unlike F2F ones, and thus conversations are more likely to be open,. This affects the nature of speech acts, making them more likely to be audience based rather dyadic (between two people). The gist is that register and style are adapting to new media and technologies.

In a comprehensive study of Twitter, Rao et al. (2010) looked at how social variables, such as gender, played out in Twitter conversations. They wanted to determine if it was possible to detect if a Twitter user was male or female simply by the linguistic cues in postings. Whereas many Twitter users use their real name, which can reveal their gender, many others choose nicknames that do not convey gender. So, the researchers concentrated on whether it was possible to infer gender exclusively from the content and style of the writing. But the results were ambiguous. A similar approach was used to identify age and regional origin variables. Age is also a difficult variable to detect in twitterlects. Not only does it change constantly, but also age-based communication behavior differs according to socioeconomic variables, and there is no known indicator for age on Twitter. The main finding of the project was that there are some commonalities between F2F sociolects and twitterlects, but also significant differences.

References and Further Reading

Adams, M. (2009). *Slang: The People's Poetry*. Oxford: Oxford University Press.

Arntfield, M. and Danesi, M. (2017). *Murder in Plain English*. New York: Prometheus.

Bakhtin, M. M. (1981). *The Dialogic Imagination*. Trans. C. Emerson and M. Holquist. Austin, TX: University of Texas Press.

Baugh, J. (2003). Linguistic Profiling. *Black Linguistics: Language, Society, and Politics in Africa and the Americas* 155: 155–163.

Bernstein, B. (1971). *Class, Codes and Control: Theoretical Studies Towards a Sociology of Language*. London: Routledge.

Blyth, C., Recktenwald, S., and Wang, J. (2000). I'm like, Say What? A New Quotative in American Oral Narrative. *Journal of American Speech* 65: 215–227.

Carlson, H. K. and McHenry, M. A. (2006). Effect of Accent and Dialect on Employability. *Journal of Employment Counseling* 43: 70–83.

Chandler, F. W. (1907). *The Literature of Roguery*. Boston, MA: Houghton-Mifflin.

Charaudeau, P., Maingueneau, D., and Adam, J. (2002). *Dictionnaire d'analyse du discours*. Paris: Seuil.

Clopper, C. G. and Pisoni, D. (2004). Some Acoustic Cues for the Perceptual Categorization of American English Regional Dialects. *Journal of Phonetics* 32: 111–140.

Danescu-Niculescu-Mizil, C., Gamon, M., and Dumais, S. (2011). Mark My Words! Linguistic Style Accommodation in Social Media. *International World Wide Web Conference Committee*, ACM 978-1-4503-0632-4/11/03.

Danesi, M. (1994). *Cool: The Signs and Meanings of Adolescence*. Toronto: University of Toronto Press.

Davie, J. (2019). *Slang across Societies*. London: Routledge.

Dubois, S. and Horvath, B. (1998). Let's Tink About Dat: Interdental Fricatives in Cajun English. *Language Variation and Change* 10(3): 245–261.

Duffin, J. (2005). *Disease Concepts in History*. Toronto: University of Toronto Press.

Dumas, B. and Lighter, J. (1978). Is Slang a Word for Linguists? *American Speech* 53(5): 14–15.

Fairclough, N. (2003). *Analysing Discourse: Textual Analysis for Social Research*. London: Routledge.

Ferrini, C. and Paris, O. (2019). *I discorsi dell'odio*. Roma: Carocci.

Gilbert, E. and Karahalios, K. (2009). Predicting Tie Strength with Social Media. In: *Proceedings of the SIGCHI Conference on Human Factors in Computing Systems*, pp. 211–220. New York: ACM.

Gillen, J. and Merchant, G. (2013). Contact Calls: Twitter as a Dialogic Social and Linguistic Practice. *Language Sciences* 35: 47–58.

Gregory, M. (1967). Aspects of Varieties Differentiation. *Journal of Linguistics* 3: 177–197.

Halliday, M. A. K. (1976). Anti-Languages. *American Anthropologist* 78: 570–584.

Halliday, M. A. K. and Hasan, R. (1976). *Cohesion in English*. London: Longman.

Holmes, J. (1995). *Women, Men and Language*. London: Longman.

Jakobson, R. (1960). Linguistics and Poetics. In: T. Sebeok (ed.), *Style and Language*. Cambridge, MA: MIT Press.

Joos, M. (1967). *The Five Clocks*. New York: Harcourt, Brace, & World.

Laroche, P. (2007). *On Words: Insight into How Our Words Work and Don't*. Oak Park, IL: Marion Street Press.

Leland, J. (2004). *Hip: The History*. New York: HarperCollins.

Littlejohn, S. (2002). *Theories of Human Communication*. Albuquerque, NM: Wadsworth.

Lunde, P. (2012). *The Secrets of Codes*. San Francisco: Weldonowen.

Mathew, B., Dutt, R., Goyal, P., Mukherjee, A. (2019). *Spread of Hate Speech in Online Social Media*. Boston: ACM WebSci.

Morrish, J. (1999). *Frantic Semantics: Snapshots of Our Changing Language*. London: Palgrave Macmillan.

Nicaso, A. and Danesi, M. (2013). *Made Men: Mafia Culture and the Power of Symbols, Rituals, and Myth*. Lanham: Rowman & Littlefield.

Paolillo, J. (2001). Language Variation on Internet Relay Chat: A Social Network Approach. *Journal of Sociolinguistics* 5: 180–213.

Purnell, T., Idsardi, W., and Baugh, J. (1999). Perceptual and Phonetic Experiments on American English Dialect Identification. *Journal of Social Psychology* 18: 10–30.

Ramage, D., Dumais, S., and Liebling, D. (2010). Characterizing Microblogs with Topic Models. *International AAAI Conference on Weblogs and Social Media*. Association for the Advancement of Artificial Intelligence, pp. 130–137.

Rao, D., Yarowsky, D., Shreevats, A., and Gupta, M. (2010). ACM 978-1-4503-0386-6/10/10.

Raskin, V. (1985). *Semantic Mechanisms of Humor*. Dordrecht: Reidel.

Reddy, W. M. (1997). Against Constructionism: The Historical Ethnography of Emotions. *Current Anthropology* 38: 327–351.

Reid, T. B. (1956). Linguistics, Structuralism, Philology. *Archivum Linguisticum* 8.

Romaine, S. and Lange, D. (1991). The Use of Like as a Marker of Reported Speech and Thought: A Case of Grammaticalization in Process. *American Speech* 66: 227–279.

Sacks, H. (1974). An Analysis of the Course of a Joke's Telling in Conversation. In: R. Bauman and J. Sherzer (eds.), *Explorations in the Ethnography of Speaking*, pp. 337–353. Cambridge: Cambridge University Press.

Sagan, C. and Druyan, A. (1992). *Shadows of Forgotten Ancestors: A Search for Who We Are*. New York: Random House.

Saussure, F. de. (1916). *Cours de linguistique générale*. Paris: Payot.

Siegel, M.E.A. (2002). Like: The Discourse Particle and Semantics. *Journal of Semantics* 19: 35–71.

Sontag, S. (1978). *Illness as Metaphor*. New York: Farrar, Straus & Giroux.

Wierzbicka, A. (1991). *Cross-Cultural Pragmatics: The Semantics of Human Interaction*. Berlin: Mouton de Gruyter.

5   Language, Personality, and Identity

Language varies not only along geographical and social axes, but also according to individual speaker characteristics. The particular type of style that individuals use (and which identifies them) is called an *idiolect*, defined as a form of *parole* shaped by the categories of the specific language used, the personality of the speaker, and the sense of identity that the speaker brings to a verbal interaction. The study of idiolectal speech constitutes a broad area of sociolinguistic research today, especially since identity construction in social media venues offers significant insights into the traditional relations among personality, identity, and language.

Identity is the awareness of one's distinctiveness, psychologically and socially. Some psychologists see the sense of identity as a psycho-biological endowment, a fixed quality of Selfhood and character that is nevertheless susceptible to adaptation according to situation. Others argue that it is largely constructed by individuals throughout life in response to the experiences they undergo. James Baldwin (1985: 23) encapsulates the latter perspective succinctly as follows: "An identity would seem to be arrived at by the way in which the person faces and uses his/her experience." The ongoing research in sociolinguistics suggests that the language one acquires in childhood is a major factor in shaping one's sense of identity, but that it changes throughout the stages of life, as mirrored in the style that characterizes an individual's speech during these stages. This chapter looks at this important area of sociolinguistic research.

Needless to say, there is more to personality and identity than the specific grammatical and lexical categories of the language acquired in a rearing context. These are shaped as well by cultural, religious, and other influences on a person's life. For this reason, the term *linguistic identity* is used here when alluding specifically to the impact of language on one's sense of identity. This is defined as the sense of Self that is embedded in patterns of linguistic behavior that are felt as meaningful to individuals (Bucholtz 1999; Bucholtz and Hall 2005). Linguistic identity is a kind of "Self-code" that varies according to context, stages of life, and the experiences individuals glean from using a language in interactional contexts.

5.1 Personality

The sociolinguistic study of the relation between a specific language and the development of personality in specific cultural contexts crosses disciplinary lines, involving psychology, anthropology, and other cognate disciplines. Research in linguistic anthropology in particular has emphasized that the two are intertwined in specific ways (as will be discussed further in Chapter 8). Our particular manner of speaking—our idiolect—certainly does not completely identify us. Moreover, correlating it with personality is always problematic, because people and circumstances of language use change constantly. An idiolect is as much a variable entity as are dialects and sociolects (Firth 1950). Nonetheless, it can be examined broadly in terms of the individual's speech style as it manifests itself in social contexts and at different stages of life.

It is relevant to note that the idea of an individualistic personality is a result of a paradigm shift that originated in the Renaissance. In medieval Europe the sense of Self was intertwined with the kinship network in which the child was reared and the adult person's role in either village life or life in the world of trades in the new cities. This changed, as Marshall McLuhan (1964) cogently argued, with the rise and spread of mechanical print technology in the mid-1400s, a period in which writing became an increasingly expanding mode for encoding and disseminating information and knowledge. This brought about what he called the "print age," an era of history shaped by the structure of the written word. People started to see themselves as separate from the orally based form of social life because of the simple fact that they read by themselves, forming opinions on their own without the guidance of some orator and without the pressures of groupthink. Over time, this encouraged individualism, abstract thinking, and the valorizing of literacy. As he so eloquently put it: "Literacy, the visual technology, dissolved the tribal magic by means of its stress on fragmentation and specialization and created the individual" (McLuhan and McLuhan 1998: 23).

5.1.1 Age Factors

Idiolectal patterns are connected, first and foremost, to stage of life. This means that we speak differently at different stages. Some speech patterns are based in brain development, but others are social in origin. Language acquisition in infancy bears this out (see, for example, Clark 1993; Saxton 2017). At first, infants emit cooing sounds. Around 20 weeks of age, they start producing phonetically suggestive sounds. When they reach six months, they start to emit monosyllabic utterances (*mu, ma, da, di,* etc.), called *holophrastic* (one-word) phrases. These have been shown to serve three psycho-social functions: (1) naming an object; (2) expressing an action or a desire for some action; and (3) conveying emotional states. Holophrases are typically imitations of adult words—*da* for *dog, ca* for *cat,* etc. During the second year children typically double their holophrases—*wowo*, "water," *bubu*, "bottle," *mama*, "mother," etc. They also start to use language more and more during play to accompany their movements, to simulate the sounds they hear in their environment, and to refer to what they are doing.

Around the age of 2 or 3, children have acquired the ability to use language for social reasons and to display a personal style that differentiates them from other children. As Russian psychologist Lev Vygotsky (1961) showed in his pioneering research, children become aware of the social power of language the instant they realize that using it allows them to accomplish various things—for example, the instant they discover that the word *no* allows them to express displeasure and to achieve a relevant reaction from interlocutors, they start using it repetitively.

When children reach puberty, they become increasingly aware of the power of language to regulate and influence social interactions, as well as a means to construct their own sense of self. Adolescent speech concretely reveals how this manifests itself at puberty (Gusdorf 1965; Labov 1972; Eble 1989, 1996; Rampton 1995). At this stage of life slang in particular is a means of asserting or constructing a linguistic identity differentially from the one developed in childhood that is sensitive to new social conditions.

Young people in western societies have typically resorted to slang words since the medieval Ages in order to strengthen group identity and to set themselves apart from adults. Medieval university students, for instance, used the word *lupi*, "wolves," to refer to spies who reported other students for using the vernacular instead of Latin to their professors (Eble 1989). In effect, adolescent slang has psychological and social functions—it can hardly be considered a form of aberrant communicative behavior. It is an age-based sociolect that is highly variable according to individual and situation. As Hudson (1984: 46) aptly observes, this type of sociolect is "used by teenagers to signal the important difference they see between themselves and older people" (Hudson 1984: 46). Adults frequently resort to slang for the various reasons discussed in the previous chapter. But for adolescents slang typically becomes a strategic form of speech that allows them to gain access to meaningful social interaction with peers. So, whereas generic slang is a speech option available to the population at large, adolescent slang is a sociolect that is specific to the teenage group.

The whole gamut of emotional responses that teenagers have to their social environments, as well as the linguistic strategies they employ to handle specific social situations, are reflected in the ways in which they program their discourse, in the kinds of words they coin, and generally in the highly emotive style of delivery they use, as discussed (Chapter 4). Emotivity often verges on irony, allowing teens to interpret the world in wry and satirical ways. Words such as *vomatose* (a combination of *vomit* + *comatose*), *thicko* (slow-brained), *burger-brain* (version of *thicko*), *knob* (hard-headed) of a few years ago are cases-in-point. They are ironic comments of others and specific social situations.

Box 5.1 Examples of Teen Slang (circa 2019)

affluential   someone with money and power ("affluence" + "influence")
dope   cool, awesome
frenemy   duplicitous person ("friend" + "enemy")
Gucci   attractive, cool
lit   amazing
rides   sneakers, shoes
snatched   looks good
squad   group of friends
tope   very cool
YOLO   you only live once

As Cooper and Anderson-Inman (1988: 239) pointed out in a classic study, slang in adolescence is a control mechanism: "Gaining control over marked linguistic features shows a growing competence in the use of communicative strategies that both realize and regulate behavior and speech patterns appropriate to gender and peer group membership." Another classic study by Maltz and Borker (1982) connects slang to ingroup power dynamics. Teens with ineffectual verbal skills generally have to accept lower status within the clique hierarchy. Those with the greatest ability to "outtalk" the others are the ones who assert a leadership role within it. Eder (1990: 67) has labeled this *ritual conflict*:

> Ritual conflict typically involves the exchange of insults between two peers, often in the presence of other peers who serve as an audience. This activity is usually competitive in nature, in that each male tries to top the previous insult with one that is more clever, outrageous, or elaborate.

5.1.2 Frame Analysis

A research model that is useful in explaining and investigating the social role of language at specific stages of life is the one put forward by Erving Goffman (1974), which he called *frame analysis*. This is the technique of dividing human interaction into separate frames of behavior that can then be analyzed in terms of constituent units of Self-portrayal within them.

Taking his cue from Gregory Bateson (1936), Goffman called the sequence of actions that identify a person's Self-portrayal during speech a "strip" (in reference to the "comic strip" as a structured sequence of actions). Frame analysis consists in: (1) describing the strip (the actual behavioral scene), (2) reducing it to a basic typology (actions, language forms, and so on), and (3) interpreting the strategies deployed by the characters in the strip. With this technique, Goffman was able to draw attention to the fact that people seek to skillfully present themselves during speech as if they were delivering it on a stage. People see themselves as "character actors" in their own narratives, using language to impress or influence each other to obtain some goal. The Latin term for "cast of characters" is *dramatis personae*, literally, "the persons of the drama," a term revealing the theatrical origin of our concept of personhood. *Persona* was the "mask" in Greek theatre. We seem, in a phrase, to perceive life as a stage and our role in it as that of a "character." Goffman actually defined the frame space as if it were a real theater, with a front region in which the "actors" perform their scripts, and the background as constituting an audience situation. Frame analysis has been adopted and adapted by sociolinguists broadly to describe how communication unfolds in social situations.

This type of analysis can be used to understand, for example, how ideas are framed visually via social media channels such as Instagram, given that visual presentations on Instagram are laid out in a strip-like fashion. Using an implicit frame analytical approach, Hu, Manikonda, and Kambhampati (2014) surveyed and distinguished eight types of picture-framing sequences or clusters found on Instagram based on the following themes: friends, food, gadgets, captioned photos, pets, activities, selfies, and fashion. In all cases, the layout was a means to elicit a favorable impression or to obtain some goal. In another relevant study, Smith and Sanderson (2015) used Goffman's notion of Self-presentation to examine the Instagram feeds of 27 professional athletes. The researchers analyzed the framing of photographs, accompanying captions, and hashtags to establish what the objectives were and what meanings we can derive from them. The main finding was that, despite conventional belief that men are traditionally framed with closer power headshots and women from a distance, in their personal Instagram feeds, both male and female athletes posted photos that displayed their full bodies. What stands out to the present author is that the captions and hashtags revealed speech strategies based on figurative language analogies and cultural allusions. The study suggests overall that we can assess what social changes are occurring by examining how people present themselves via social media framing.

5.1.3 Bilingualism and Personality

As discussed in Chapter 3, bilingualism is an important area of research in sociolinguistics, extending to the investigation of the relationship between language and personality in bilingual speakers. Spanish-speaking communities in the US tend to develop a different sense of identity with respect to the broader English-speaking community by preserving their native linguistic heritage. Hispanics share many of the traditional values of English-speaking Americans, of course, but they are also typically proud of their own linguistic identities. Many feel that they should not lose contact with their cultures of origin or lose competence in Spanish. Bilinguals sometimes report "feeling" or "thinking" differently when they speak either one of their two languages. This raises a specific question: Do bilinguals unconsciously change their personality when they switch languages? It is known that people in general can switch between different ways of interpreting events and feelings—a phenomenon known as *frame shifting*. So, is bilingualism a form of frame shifting?

Bilingualism, as we have seen, is acquired in various ways according to context and thus implies different forms of code competence. Secondary bilinguals, for example, are those who have learned one language at home, and another later in life, usually at school. Their competence in one or the other language is variable. They rarely code switch, perhaps because they frame their conversations in one language or the other autonomously. But what about primary bilinguals, that is, speakers raised equally in two languages? Even if they do not usually have perfectly balanced bilingual competence, they still use both languages functionally, as is, for example, the case among Hispanic speakers in many parts of the US. Is there something about this form of bilingualism that shapes the individual's personality differentially from others? Do the vocabularies and grammars of the two languages guide the bilingual's thoughts and sense of Self along different cognitive and emotional paths? So far, there is no evidence that the perception of Self in bilinguals is different from that of monolingual speakers. It would be a striking finding indeed if such evidence were ever to emerge. However, in the case of languages in contact, whereby mixed languages or koines such as Spanglish emerge (Chapter 3), the question of the relation of language to identity is a legitimate one: Does Spanglish have an effect on Hispanics' sense of Self vis-à-vis other Spanish-speaking communities such as those in Spain? Rothman and Rell (2005) have argued that Spanglish involves an "emphasized" identity. In speaking Spanglish, individuals do not change their sense of Self as such; rather, they emphasize different aspects of their bilingual personality, according to context. For instance, those who identify themselves as Mexican among relatives might identify themselves as Americans at work or when away from the US. The question of language and identity in bilingualism is a complex one which has no easy answer, given the high variability of subjective experiences and ever-changing social perceptions about the role of specific languages in a society.

5.2 Identity

In an in-depth sociolinguistic study, John Edwards (2009) argued that the language we are born into and which we use habitually imparts to us an intuitive sense of who we are. Linguistic identity (LI) is thus a key factor in human psychological and social growth and development; it is forged both through upbringing and within a specific speech community, or communities (in the case of bilingualism). LI affects our sense of Self, because it allows us to build a model of ourselves through specific language structures and meanings, albeit a *distant* one, as Ochs (1993: 288) calls it, because it is not necessarily rendered obvious in the structures themselves:

Linguistic constructions at all levels of grammar and discourse are crucial indicators of social identity for members as they regularly interact with one another; complementarily, social identity is a crucial dimension of the social meaning of particular linguistic constructions. But no matter how crucial language is for understanding social identity and social identity for understanding the social meaning of language, social identity is rarely grammaticized or otherwise explicitly encoded across the world's languages. In other words, the relation between language and social identity is predominantly a sociolinguistically *distant* one.

Individuals who speak Italian as a native language tend to experience not only an emotional allegiance to Italian culture and society, but also to see themselves as different from others (whether or not this is sustainable). But LIs are highly variable. For one thing, LI is experienced differently in subsequent generations. Moreover, in cyberspace, the linguistic rules of identity formation have changed, as LIs are being constructed not only through the traditional "real" social structures of the world (including rearing and upbringing), but also through Self-construction strategies. A Facebook profile is a case-in-point, which includes not only basic background information about oneself (work, education, and so on), but also presentations of oneself (relationship status, significant life events, and so on). The way these are written and narrated allows users to recreate their offline identities in specific ways.

5.2.1 Theories

Sifting through the literature on identity in the social and cognitive sciences, one finding stands out: it evolves primarily during two periods in the life-cycle—in childhood and at adolescence. In the former, identity can be designated as an "indexical" system of Self-awareness, because it is imparted to children by and through the environment in which they are reared and, thus, in reference to it. The specific language and cultural codes (art, music, and so on) in the child's rearing environment constitute the indexical resources through which the child comes to develop an unconscious sense of Selfhood. The form of identity that emerges at puberty, in contrast, can be called "symbolic," because the adolescent interprets the world more consciously and adapts to it symbolically, that is, through symbolic resources such as slang and lifestyle. But in both stages—childhood and adolescence— it is through interaction with others from which one's sense of identity arises. It is largely unconscious in childhood, because it is imparted through situational factors (indexical); whereas it is conscious, or at least intentional, in the coming-of-age period (symbolic). The shifts in identity that come about subsequent to adolescence through job choices, education level, marriage, and other events need not concern us here.

The first attempt to understand how indexical identity evolves into a symbolic form through maturation is the one undertaken by Sigmund Freud

(1905, 1913, 1923). Although many now discard Freud's basic theory of development, it nevertheless continues to have many implications and applications, in spite of the relevant criticisms. Essentially, Freud saw the passage from childhood to adolescence as a period of difficult emotional adjustment because the passage may or may not be successful and, when it is not, it tends to lead to traumatic emotional results. At puberty, the maturing child must come to grips with sexual identity and body image at a symbolic level, given the hormonal and physical changes that take place during this critical developmental period. As a result, pubescent individuals may feel that they are inhabiting a strange new sexual body, which might make them feel awkward, anxious, guilty, or afraid of the desires and feelings that it generates. To cope with these, adolescents seek out peers and peer groups, which serve as sheltering social enclaves, into which adolescents can submerge themselves to gain emotional comfort and protection. It is within these enclaves that the adolescent seeks to forge a symbolic identity—an identity negotiated in large part through group membership. The manifestations of this "insider symbolic identity" can be seen in clothing preferences, hairstyle, various bodily decorations, and above all else in language. "Talking the talk" at this symbolic stage of development implies that the words are socially significant. Ironic uses of language emerge for this very reason, because irony is a linguistic defense mechanism, as discussed previously.

The psychologist who explored the emergence of symbolic identity as a crucial stage was the American Erik Erikson (1950, 1968). Although schooled in Freudian theory, Erikson proposed the non-Freudian concept of *identity construction*, which is now used broadly across the social and cognitive sciences. He defined it as the model of Self that adolescents construct in response to the strong need to belong to peer groups. Erikson stressed the continual development of human beings throughout the lifecycle. At adolescence, however, the individual experiences an "identity crisis" because of inner conflicts related to body image and social pressures, which eventually lead to a sense of Self-understanding or, as Erikson called it, "ego identity." The Russian psychologist Vygotsky (1961, 1978) similarly saw the advent of adolescence as a period of identity formation, with language playing a major role in the identity-making process.

In terms of Och's distance hypothesis, the social and the linguistic dimensions can be separated, of course, and kept distant if the case arose to necessitate this (such as in social upheavals), but by and large the distance between the two becomes minimal especially during adolescence. In the era of CMC, that distance seems to be decreasing even more, as contact through social media is bringing about a more proximate response to identity construction.

5.2.2 Linguistic Identity

Needless to say, the LI developed in childhood is critical in shaping the individual's perception of Self throughout life. For example, in Italy, most speakers have in the past acquired their LIs on the basis of dialects. The indexical identity was thus dialectally based; the symbolic one was developed in situations of contact (at school, in the broader society, and so on). The factors for facilitating the shift from indexical to symbolic identity included: (1) geographical isolation, (2) patterns of cultural independence, and (3) continuous contact with Standard Italian in various situations.

Don Kulick (1992) conducted ethnographic work in a village in Papua New Guinea called Gapun, in which they spoke Taiap, a language known only to the villagers. He was able to document how that language, although spoken solely by a small group of people, constituted a source of pride, constituting an index to identity by allowing the villagers to feel and claim autonomy from Tok Pisin speakers (the pidgin spoken by others). Taiap let the villagers express their shared values, especially during ritualistic situations that garnered a high level of emotional resonance.

Language is, as these example shows, a socializing agent, as the work of Elinor Ochs and Bambi Schieffelin has also brought out (Ochs and Schieffelin 1984; Ochs 1988; Schieffelin 1990, 1995, 2000, 2002; Ochs and Taylor 2001). The two researchers looked extensively at how children are socialized into belief systems and historical content through oral narratives. In one study, they found that the narratives told at dinner time in white middle-class households in southern California typically presented role structures, gender distinctions, and other socializing and enculturation themes to family members. These shaped the LI and worldview of the children. The interaction among LI, beliefs, and sense of Self is unmistakable, although it is difficult to make concrete correlations among them (Omoniyi and White 2006).

Sometimes worldviews can be changed by simply changing the meanings and use of a grammatical structure, such as pronouns, as already discussed. Using a gender-neutral pronoun—*they* rather than *he* or *she* in the singular as well as the plural—appears to boost positive feelings towards LGBTQ individuals. Margit Tavits and Efrén Pérez (2019) looked at the psycho-social impact of gender-neutral pronouns on the views of over 3,000 Swedes, given that the Swedish language has introduced the gender-neutral term *hen* alongside *hon* and *han*, corresponding to English *she* and *he*. Subjects were first shown the cartoon of an androgynous figure walking a dog. They were then split into three groups and asked to describe the picture. One group was told to use only neutral pronouns, another only female pronouns, and the third only male pronouns. Those who used gender-neutral pronouns for the task were more likely to use non-male names and in a follow-up questionnaire revealed improved positive feelings towards LGBTQ people.

As mentioned, In English, the word *they* is now similarly used as a gender-neutral pronoun, which according to the *Oxford English Dictionary* appears in singular form as far back as the fourteenth century in the medieval romance *William and the Werewolf*. There is now a growing awareness that non-binary gender identities are being reflected more and more in language and that language change can thus become a factor in the elimination of biases.

5.3 Names

A central aspect of indexical identity formation is name giving. Names transform human beings into legal persons. The study of names falls under the branch of linguistics called *onomastics* (from Greek *onoma*, "name"). Across cultures, neonates are not considered legal members of society until they are given a name. The act of naming a newborn infant is, in effect, a rite of passage. If a child is not given a name by the family, then society will step in to do so. A person taken into a family, by marriage, adoption, or for some other reason, is typically assigned a name by that family. The surname given to the child is part of establishing indexical identity and thus a trace to ethnic origins, whether or not this may be actually true. It is interesting to note that sometimes the surname may have been assigned to the family in reference to its ancestral origins. Some examples can be seen here.

Name	*Likely ancestral origin*
Johnny English	British
Mary Ireland	Irish
Marco Siciliano	Sicilian
Sally Israel	Israeli
Jack Berliner	Germanic
Jennifer Danish	Danish, Scandinavian

5.3.1 The Social Functions of Names

In traditional Inuit cultures, an individual is perceived to have a body, a soul, and a name; the individual is not seen as complete without all three. Across social and cultural spaces, people invest a lot of meaning in names. In western cultures, name giving is a largely unregulated process. But even so, it is shaped by several customs and trends, many of them implicit or unconscious. Common names assigned to neonates in European and Anglo-American societies come typically from Hebrew, Greek, Latin, or Teutonic languages, as can be seen below (and see Box 5.2).

Names	*Origin*
John	Hebrew
Mary	Hebrew
Alexander	Greek
Julius	Roman
Richard	Germanic, Teutonic
William	Germanic, Teutonic

Name giving is sometimes tied to the circumstances of birth, such as the time of birth, the birth order, or the parents' emotional reaction to the birth itself. In various native African languages, including the Kwa language of the Yoruba, an official language of Nigeria, names such as *Mwanajuma* (Friday), *Esi* (Sunday), *Khamisi* (Thursday), and *Wekesa* (harvest time) refer to the day on which the child was born. Names reflecting birth order include *Mosi* (first born), *Kunto* (third born), *Nsonowa* (seventh born), and *Wasswa* (first of twins). *Yejide* (image of the mother) and *Dada* (curly hair) are examples of names indicating reaction to the birth. Analogous naming practices exist in other societies. English names such as *June* (time of birth), *James the Second* (birth order), and *Felicity* (happy reaction) display an analogous naming pattern.

Box 5.2 English Names

Hebrew origin
  David ("beloved")
  Elizabeth ("oath of God")
  Hannah ("God has favored me")
  James ("may God protect")
  John ("gracious gift of God")
  Joseph ("the Lord shall add")
  Mary ("wished for")
  Michael ("who is like God")
  Samuel ("God has heard")

Greek and Latin origin
  Alexander ("helper of humanity")
  Barbara ("stranger")
  Clarence ("famous")
  Emily ("flattering")
  George ("farmer")
  Helen ("light")
  Margaret ("pearl")
  Patricia ("of noble birth")
  Philip ("lover of horses")
  Stephen ("crown or garland")
  Victor ("conqueror")
  Virginia ("maidenly")

Germanic, Teutonic origin
  Albert ("noble," "bright")
  Arnold ("eagle power")
  Edward ("rich guardian")
  Richard ("brave power")
  William ("will," "helmet")

Until the late Middle Ages, one personal name was generally sufficient as an identifier of people. Duplications, however, began to occur so often that additional identification became necessary. Hence, surnames were given to individuals (literally "names on top of a name"). These provided further indexical differentiation on the basis of such features as place (where the individual was from), parentage (to which family or kinship group the individual belonged), or occupation. For example, in England a person living near or at a place where apple trees grew might be called "John where-the-apples-grow," hence, *John Appleby*. Such names constitute a fairly large number of surnames in English—*Wood* or *Woods, Moore, Church, Hill*, etc. Descendant surnames, or names indicating parentage, were constructed typically with prefixes and suffixes—*McMichael* ("of Michael"), *Johnson* ("son of John"), *Maryson* ("son of Mary"). Surnames reflecting medieval life and occupations include *Smith, Farmer, Carpenter, Tailor*, and *Weaver*.

The Chinese were among the first to use more than one name indexically. The Emperor Fuxi is said to have decreed the use of family names about 2850 BCE. The Chinese customarily have three indexical names. The family name, placed first, comes from one of the words in the Chinese sacred poem *Baijia Xing*. It is followed by a generation name, taken from a poem adopted by each family, and a given name. The Romans had at first only one name, but later they also started using three names: (1) the *praenomen* stood first as the person's given name; (2) the *nomen*, which indicated the *gens*, or clan, to which the person belonged; (3) the *cognomen*, which designated the family. A citizen sometimes added a fourth name, the *agnomen*, to commemorate an illustrious action or remarkable event.

Family names (and surnames) gained currency in Europe in the latter half of the tenth century, becoming common by the thirteenth. Nobles at first adopted family names to set themselves apart from common people. They made these hereditary, passing them on to children. As a consequence, the use of a family name became the mark of a well-bred person. Throughout Europe, wealthy families adopted this naming practice. For example, the "son of Robert" might be known as *Henry Robertson*, or *Henry, son of Robert*. At times, someone might be given a descriptive nickname as their surname. Someone named *Robert* might be called *Robert, the small*, because of his height, abbreviated eventually to *Robert Small*. In such cases the nickname became the surname. Many surnames were formed in this way—*Reid, Reed*, and *Read*, for instance, are early spellings of *red*, referring to someone with red hair.

Names are perceived throughout the world to be much more than simple identifiers. They are laden with symbolic meanings. The ancient Egyptians believed that a name affected the bearer throughout life and even beyond. They also believed that if an individual's name was forgotten on earth, the deceased would have to undergo a second death. To avoid this danger, names were written many times on walls, tombs, and papyri. Political rulers would sometimes erase the names of previous monarchs as a means of rewriting history in their favor, because removal of a person's name meant the extinction of the person from memory. Numerologists in various parts of the ancient world believed that a person's name was an important clue to character. They changed letters in the name to numerals according to a code. The digits of the number were then added together to produce a "personality number" that was believed to describe the individual's personality and even destiny. The Romans thought names were prophetic—*nomen est omen*, a "name is an omen." Would the Roman view explain names such as Cecil Fielder who was a fielder in baseball, Rollie Fingers who was a pitcher, William Wordsworth a poet, Francine Prose a novelist, and Mickey Bass a musician? Perhaps such coincidences simply indicate that some people are inspired subliminally by their names to gravitate towards occupations suggested by them.

In a 2002 study, Pelham, Mirenberg, and Jones found that individuals were more likely to choose jobs, careers, and professions with names that were similar to their personal names. Similarly, in 2010, Abel and Kruger found that doctors and lawyers were more likely to have surnames that referred to their professions: people with the surname *Doctor* were more likely to be doctors than lawyers, whereas those with the surname *Lawyer* were more likely to be actual lawyers. And they found, remarkably, that the initial letters of their names were significantly related to a subspecialty: for instance, someone named *Raymond* was more likely to be a radiologist than a dermatologist. Frank Nuessel, a professor of linguistics at the University of Louisville, has coined the tongue-in-cheek term *aptonym* to refer to names that mirror the nameholder's profession, although he claims that aptonyms are more coincidental than psychologically motivated (Silverman and Light 2011). In fact, the claim that a name impacts on life decisions is an extraordinary one that will require exceptional evidence. Nevertheless, we seem to feel intuitively that there is a grain of truth in aptonyms.

Naming trends are remarkably stable in most societies. This is because, as mentioned, names link people to culture and tradition. According to the United States' Social Security Administration, one-fourth of the top 20 names given in 2004 in America were as traditional as those given way back in 1880. The top five names for girls and boys in the two eras, according to that governmental agency, are as shown in Table 5.1.

Little has changed since 2004 in this respect. Between 2010 and 2018, the most popular names given to children in America derived from the same historical sources mentioned above (see Table 5.2).

In some communities differential naming practices may be a declaration of autonomy from the mainstream and thus a system of individualistic identity formation. Prior to the middle part of the twentieth century, African Americans gave their children names that were consistent with those used in mainstream American culture. With the civil rights movement, this situation changed. Many continued to name their children in traditional ways, but others shifted to other strategies. Naming practices adopted by African American culture include the following:

Table 5.1 Naming Patterns in America, 1880–2004

Girls	
Mary	Emily
Anna	Abigail
Emma	Madison
Elizabeth	Olivia
Minnie	Hannah

Boys	
John	Jacob
William	Michael
James	Joshua
Charles	Matthew
George	Ethan

Table 5.2 Most Popular Names in America, 2010–2018

Girls	
Ava	Sophia
Grace	Emma
Victoria	Madison
Elizabeth	Olivia
Abigail	Charlotte

Boys	
Noah	Jacob
William	Michael
James	Liam
Daniel	Matthew
David	Benjamin

Source: Social Security Administration

1   Names such as *Chantal* and *Antoine* derive from French culture, which has been influential in areas such as Louisiana.
2   Names such as *Ashanti* and *Tanisha* have their origins in continental African culture.
3   Names such as *JaMarcus* and *LaKeisha* are new constructions; they show the blending of affixes with root names as well as creative spellings.

5.3.2 Nicknames

Nicknames are memorable and more likely to stand out than official indexical names. For organized criminals, they are part of how they define themselves, alluding to something in a gangster's character, appearance, or background that is thought to have significance. Mafioso Lucky Luciano, born Salvatore Lucania, was called *Lucky* because of the noticeable large scars around his neck that permanently recorded his fortuitous escape from death after being slashed and left dead by criminal rivals. The nickname of *Scarface* was given to American Mafioso Al Capone because he was involved in a fight that left him with three noticeable scars on his face. Such nicknames are personal brands, emphasizing toughness and fierceness. Frank Costello, known as the *Prime Minister* of Cosa Nostra in the 1930s and 1940s in the US, was quoted by *Time* magazine as stating this as follows (*Time*, November 28, 1949: 16):

> I'm like Coca-Cola. There are lots of drinks as good as Coca-Cola. Pepsi-Cola is a good drink. But Pepsi-Cola never got the advertising Coca-Cola got. I'm not Pepsi-Cola. I'm Coca-Cola because I got so much advertising.

Gangster Luciano Leggio's nickname of *La Primula Rossa* ("Scarlet Pimpernel") probably comes from the 1935 movie of that name, a remake of an early silent version, which revolves around an aristocratic hero during the French Revolution, called the Scarlet Pimpernel, who gallantly rescues aristocrats sentenced to death. Leggio was certainly gallant in appearance, but vicious in his life. Leggio was also nicknamed *The Professor* probably because of his inclinations to pontificate to other clan members. As Nicaso and Lamothe (2005: 41) aptly observe, all this shows that the nickname is part of the remaking of identity:

> Those who are brought into the formal underworld may have had nicknames in their former lives; however, when initiated they're given new names or allowed to choose one. Some names describe a physical characteristic—Vyacheslav Ivankov, for example, was called Yaponchik because of the Asiatic cast to his eyes. Others might be for a thief's attitude: Tank or Dashing. A home invader might be called Madhouse because of his single-minded wrecking of a victim's house.

Michele Greco, born in Palermo in 1924 into a family with strong Mafia ties, came to be known as *Il Papa* ("The Pope") because of the power he wielded as head of a prominent clan known appropriately with the religious epithet of *La Cupola* ("The Cupola"). His brother, Salvatore, was known as *Ciaschiteddu* ("Little Bird"), a Sicilian word, because he was raised on a citrus fruit grove where birds would flock. Mafioso Antonino Giuffrè got his nickname *Manuzza*

("Little Hand"), also Sicilian, because of his deformed right hand, mangled on account of a hunting accident. Gangster Totò Riina was nicknamed *U curtu* ("Shorty") in Sicilian for the self-explanatory reason that he was a short man. Pino Greco, a Mafioso hitman, was named *Scarpuzzedda* ("Little Shoe"), because he was the son of a Mafioso nicknamed *Scarpa* ("Shoe"). American racketeer Joseph Lanza was nicknamed *Socks* because of his tendency to settle disputes with his fists (as in *to sock someone*).

Nicknaming is not specific to Mafiosi, of course. It is found across social groups. The Vikings used nicknames to celebrate someone's achievements; Indonesians use nicknames as forms of politeness; in Indian society, people have at least one nickname as part of a system of affection (alluding to some interesting thing about the person). Among the motivating factors in nick-naming, the following can be highlighted:

- *Appearance:* As we saw, the nickname *Scarface* alluded to an aspect of Al Capone's appearance. Often, these have an ironic nuance, referring to weight (*Skinny*), height (*Shorty*), hair (*Blondie, Curly*), complexion (*Pinky*), etc.
- *Character and personality:* Some nicknames are descriptors of character or personality: *Chatterbox* (talkative person), *Sleepy* (tired person), *Brainiac* (smart person), *Sherlock* (logical thinking person), and so on.
- *Lifestyle:* Lifestyle is also a source of nicknaming practices: *Jock* (sports enthusiast), *Hottie* (attractive person), *Nerd* (odd lifestyle).
- *Emotive nuances:* Shortening a name can add emotive nuances to it: *Maggie* (friendliness), *Bobbie* (cuteness or shortness), *Ed* (familiarity).

5.4 Online Identities

The coinage of handles—the names that users create for themselves in order to enter and interact in various social media—and hashtags are cases-in-point of online nicknames. Whereas in the past nicknames were given to people by others, in cyberspace individuals rename themselves. Handles are personal brands that empower individuals to construct their LI on their own terms. In effect, the Internet is changing not only language itself in specific ways, but also assigning linguistic authority to people in new ways.

5.4.1 Identity Construction

A PBS documentary called *Growing Up Online* (January 22, 2008) brought out an important aspect of identity construction in online contexts. The filmmakers spoke to a number of teenagers about their online habits. One girl nicknamed *Autumn* was a 14-year-old who felt that she "never fit the mold" in her New Jersey town, and was horribly teased about it as a result. So, she reinvented herself online as *Autumn Edows*, a sexy model and creative artist. She took scantily clad photos of herself and posted them on her personal blog. She began to enjoy all the attention she was receiving, having attracted many new friends through her online persona, compiling numerous comments telling her she was beautiful, sexy, and artistic. She was constantly on her computer, and her parents had no knowledge of her online social life. She herself was somewhat unsure of her new identity, although she did feel empowerment: "I didn't feel like myself, but I liked that I didn't feel like myself." When the school principal found out, deeming her photographs inappropriate, her mother took action and forced her to delete every single file. The teen's popularity disappeared and she fell back into a depressive state. Autumn responded by saying that such intervention devastated her: "If you have something that is that meaningful to you, to have it taken away is like your worst nightmare."

The filmmakers also spoke to a group of teen girls who, in the fall of 2006, began trading insults on MySpace. They would post comments on their profiles, and argue for no reason other than to engage in a public conflict, paralleling the verbal dueling tactics previously mentioned. In reality, however, there was no real conflict, until a negative comment about one of the girls was left about her in a post. The girl then blurted out: "You can't say it to my face. I'm right here," which resulted in a brawl. The school principal later reported having seen students videotaping the fight, which was posted on YouTube. Afterward, both groups of girls reported feeling "famous." They were seemingly looking to get their "15 minutes of fame," as Andy Warhol famously put it.

Eckert and McConnell-Ginet (1999: 185) showed, at the threshold of Web 2.0 technologies, that online discourse is a powerful one in shaping relations. In relevant research (see Barton and Lee 2013) it has been found that online identity construction is fraught with emotional consequences, as the PBS documentary showed.

In a study of South Korean youth, Kyongwon Yoon (2003) discovered that there were three functions of identity construction in online venues. One was connecting primarily with those who were a part of their daily lives, for example, to keep in touch with school companions and friends in their immediate environments. A second was to maintain relationships with those who were a part of a broader social network, such as friends who attended other schools. The third was to develop and acquire new friendships and to strengthen initial F2F encounters (see also Wright 2017).

5.4.2 Twin Identity

The blending of online and offline LIs can be called a "twin identity" construction process (Rushkoff 1996; Tapscott 1998; Prensky 2001). As Gelder (2007: 143) has aptly put it, the Internet offers people "a realm where one's yearnings for community can at last find their realization." The identity construction process involves several main strategies:

1 *Impression management.* The refers to the use of the multimodal resources of the Internet and social media sites to ensure that the desired impression of oneself is communicated effectively.
2 *Friendship management.* This refers to the creation of profiles that will attract others in the social media world either to become a "friend" (Facebook) or a "follower" (Twitter).
3 *Network structure.* This determines what kind of personality-construction style is required to join a particular virtual community.
4 *Bridging.* This refers to the common requirement of bridging online and offline identities, much like what bilinguals are faced with (mentioned above).

Bazarova, Taft, and Choi (2013) examined online identity construction through an analysis of language styles on Facebook. They collected a corpus of status updates, wall posts, and private messages from 79 participants. The messages revealed that emotives correlated with Self-presentation concerns in status updates. They also found that specific emotive language cues served as markers to differentiate between more and less familiar partners in public wall posts. In other words, Self-presentation on Facebook (and likely other social media) involves a careful crafting of identity through emotivity.

Interestingly, Gruzd, Wellman, and Takhteyev (2011) discovered that online and offline Self-presentations and identity formations are not significantly different. Ross et al. (2009) used a five-factor model of personality to investigate identity construction on Facebook (see Box 5.3). They also found that it was not affected significantly by the online medium. Facebook actually allows individuals to reinforce and highlight aspects of the personality they have acquired in a real-world context.

Box 5.3 Five-Factor Model of Personality

A model of five personality types used commonly in psychology and sociolinguistics:

1. *Openness to experience.* Personality that displays a high degree of intellectual curiosity, creativity, and a preference for novelty and variety
2. *Conscientiousness.* Personality that displays a tendency to be organized, dependable and self-disciplined
3. *Extraversion.* Personality type that displays an outgoing, energetic, and positive approach to others, seeking their company regularly
4. *Agreeableness.* Personality type that displays friendliness, compassion, and cooperativeness
5. *Neuroticism.* Personality type that displays sensitivity and nervousness, with a tendency to experience unpleasant emotions easily

Individuals who were high on the trait of *extraversion* belonged to significantly more Facebook groups; but surprisingly levels of extraversion did not correlate with number of friends. This suggests that extraverts may use Facebook as a social tool, but not as an alternative to social activities offline. Overall, the researchers discovered that personality factors were not as crucial in Facebook contexts as many had previously thought, with users maintaining their profiles to match their offline personalities and identities.

Using the same five-factor model, Nakardni and Hofmann (2012) discovered, however, that those who are shy or have low self-esteem tend to be heavy Facebook users and reshape their identity through the site. In effect, they found that the same factors that influenced LI in real-world contexts played out in social media.

Page (2012) found that Twitter in particular is a "self-branding" marketplace. Analyzing approximately 92,000 tweets and comparing the discourse styles of the tweets of corporations, celebrity practitioners, and ordinary users, she discovered that self-branding practices correlate with social and economic hierarchies that exist in offline contexts. In other words, the offline world has simply migrated to the Twitterverse, with very few, if any, adjustments. The difference may be that cyberspace, as Walther (2012: 397) puts it, may neutralize prejudicial perceptions that occur in real space: "the expression of affect and immediacy online, the virtual presentation of self and gender, the management of online conversations, adaptation via visual grounding in electronic collaboration, and the employment of online interaction technology to reduce intergroup prejudice."

References and Further Reading

Abel, E. L. and Kruger, M. L. (2010). Athletes, Doctors, and Lawyers with First Names Beginning with "D" Die Sooner. *Death Studies* 34: 71–81.

Bakhtin, M. M. (1981). *The Dialogic Imagination*. Trans. C. Emerson and M. Holquist. Austin, TX: University of Texas Press.

Baldwin, J. (1985). *The Price of the Ticket*. New York: St. Martin's.

Barton, D. and Lee, C. (2013). *Language Online: Investigating Digital Texts and Practices*. London: Routledge.

Bateson, G. (1936). *Naven: A Survey of the Problems Suggested by a Composite Picture of the Culture of a New Guinea Tribe Drawn from Three Points of View*. Stanford, CA: Stanford University Press.

Bazarova, N., Taft, J., and Choi, Y. (2013). Managing Impressions and Relationships on Facebook: Self-Presentational and Relational Concerns Revealed Through the Analysis of Language Style. *Journal of Language and Social Psychology* 32: 121–141.

Bouissac, P. (ed.) (2019). *The Social Dynamics of Pronominal Systems*. Amsterdam: John Benjamins Publishing Company.

Bucholtz, M. (1999). Why Be Normal? Language and Identity Practices in a Community of Nerd Girls. *Language in Society* 28: 203–225.

Bucholtz, M. and Hall, K. (2005). Identity and Interaction: A Sociocultural Linguistic Approach. *Discourse Studies* 7: 585–614.

Clark, E. V. (1993). *The Lexicon in Acquisition*. Cambridge: Cambridge University Press.

Cooper, D. and Anderson-Inman, L. (1988). Language and Socialization. In: M. Nippold (ed.), *Later Language Development*, pp. 225–245. Boston: Little, Brown & Company.

Eble, C. (1989). *College Slang 101*. Georgetown, CO: Spectacle Lane Press.

Eble, C. (1996). *Slang and Sociability*. Chapel Hill, NC: University of North Carolina Press.

Eckert, P. and McConnell-Ginet, S. (1999). New Generalizations and Explanations in Language and Gender Research. *Language in Society* 28: 185–201.

Eder, D. (1990). Serious and Playful Disputes: Variation on Conflict Talk Among Female Adolescents. In: D. Grimshaw (ed.), *Conflict Talk*, pp. 67–84. Cambridge: Cambridge University Press.

Edwards, J. (2009). *Language and Identity*. Cambridge: Cambridge University Press.

Erikson, E. H. (1950). *Childhood and Society*. New York: Norton.

Erikson, E. H. (1968). *Identity: Youth and Crisis*. New York: Norton.

Firth, J. R. (1950). Personality and Language in Society. *The Sociological Review* 42: 37–52.

Freud, S. (1905). *Drei Abhandlungen zur Sexualtheorie*. Frankfurt am Main: Fischer.

Freud, S. (1913). *Totem and Taboo*. New York: Norton.

Freud, S. (1923). *The Ego and the Id*. New York: Norton.

Gelder, K. (2007). *Subcultures: Cultural Histories and Social Practice*. London: Routledge.

Goffman, E. (1974). *Frame Analysis*. New York: Harper and Row.

Gruzd, A., Wellman, B., and Takhteyev, Y. (2011). Imagining Twitter as an Imagined Community. *American Behavioral Scientist* 55(10): 1294–1318.

Gusdorf, G. (1965). *Speaking*. Evanston, IL: Northwestern University Press.

Hu, Y., Manikonda, L., and Kambhampati, S. (2014). What We Instagram: A first Analysis of Instagram Photo Content and User Types. In: *Eighth International AAAI Conference on Weblogs and Social Media*, pp. 595–598. AAAI Press.

Hudson, R. (1984). *Invitation to Linguistics*. Oxford: Robinson.

Kroskrity, P. V. (1998). Arizona Tewa Kiva Speech as a Manifestation of Linguistic Ideology. In: B. B. Schieffelin, K. A. Woolard, and P. Kroskrity (eds.), *Language Ideologies: Practice and Theory*, pp. 103–122. New York: Oxford University Press.

Kulick, D. (1992). *Language Shift and Cultural Reproduction: Socialization, Self and Syncretism in a Papua New Guinea Village*. Cambridge: Cambridge University Press.

Labov, W. (1972). *Language in the Inner City*. Philadelphia: University of Pennsylvania Press.

Maltz, D. and Borker, R. (1982). A Cultural Approach to Male-Female Communication. In: J. Gumperz (ed.), *Language and Social Identity*, pp. 196–216. Cambridge: Cambridge University Press.

McLuhan, M. (1964). *Understanding Media: The Extensions of Man*. London: Routledge.

McLuhan, M. and McLuhan, E. (1998). *Laws of Media: The New Science*. Toronto: University of Toronto Press.

Nakardni, A. and Hofmann, S. G. (2012). Why Do People Use Facebook? *Personality and Individual Differences* 52: 243–249.

Nicaso, A. and Lamothe, L. (2005). *Angels, Mobsters & NarcoTerrorists: The Rising Menace of Global Criminal Empires*. Toronto: John Wiley Canada.

Ochs, E. (1988). *Culture and Language Development: Language Acquisition and Language Socialization in a Samoan Village*. Cambridge: Cambridge University Press.

Ochs, E. (1993). Constructing a Social Identity: A Language Socialization Perspective. *Research on Language and Social Interaction* 26: 287–306.

Ochs, E. and Schieffelin, B. B. (1984). Language Acquisition and Socialization: Three Developmental Stories and Their Implications. In: R. Shweder and R. A. LeVine (eds.), *Culture Theory: Essays on Mind, Self, and Emotion*, pp. 276–320. New York: Cambridge University Press.

Ochs, E. and Taylor, C. (2001). The Father Knows Best Dynamic in Dinnertime Narratives. In: A. Duranti (ed.), *Linguistic Anthropology: A Reader*, pp. 431–449. Oxford: Wiley-Blackwell.

Omoniyi, T. and White, G. (eds.) (2006). *Sociolinguistics of Identity*. London: Bloomsbury.

Page, R. (2012). The Linguistics of Self-Branding and Micro-Celebrity in Twitter: The Role of Hashtags. *Discourse & Communication* 6: 181–201.

Pelham, B. W., Mirenberg, M. C., and Jones, J. T. (2002). Why Susie Sells Seashells by the Seashore: Implicit Egotism and Major Life Decisions. *Journal of Personality and Social Psychology* 82: 469–487.

Prensky, M. (2001). Digital Natives, Digital Immigrants. www.marcprensky.com/writing.

Rampton, B. (1995). *Crossing: Language and Ethnicity Among Adolescents*. London: Longman.

Ross, C., Orr, E. S., Sisic, M., Arsenault, J. M., Simmering, M., and Orr, R. (2009). Personality and Motivations Associated with Facebook Use. *Computers in Human Behavior* 25: 578–586.

Rothman, J. and Rell, A. B. (2005). A Linguistic Analysis of Spanglish: Relating Language to Identity. *Linguistics and the Human Sciences* 1: 513–536.

Rushkoff, D. (1996). *Playing the Future: How Kids' Culture Can Teach Us to Thrive in an Age of Chaos*. New York: HarperCollins.

Saxton, M. (2017). *Child Language: Acquisition and Development*. London: Sage.

Schieffelin, B. B. (1990). *The Give and Take of Everyday Life: Language Socialization of Kaluli Children*. Cambridge: Cambridge University Press.

Schieffelin, B. B. (1995). Creating Evidence: Making Sense of Written Words in Bosavi. *Pragmatics* 5(2): 225–244.

Schieffelin, B. B. (2000). Introducing Kaluli Literacy: A Chronology of Influences. In: P. Kroskrity (ed.), *Regimes of Language*, pp. 293–327. Santa Fe, NM: School of American Research Press.

Schieffelin, B. B. (2002). Marking Time: The Dichotomizing Discourse of Multiple Temporalities. *Current Anthropology* 43: 5–17.

Silverman, R. E. and Light, J. (2011). Dr. Chopp, Meet Congressman Weiner: What's in a Name? *The Wall Street Journal*. http://online.wsj.com/article.

Smith, L. R. and Sanderson, J. (2015). I'm Going to Instagram It! An Analysis of Athlete Self-Presentation on Instagram. *Journal of Broadcasting & Electronic Media* 59: 342–358.

Tapscott, D. (1998). *Growing Up Digital: The Rise of the Net Generation*. New York: McGraw-Hill.

Tavits, M. and Pérez, E. O. (2019). Gender-Neutral Pronouns and Gender Equality. *Proceedings of the National Academy of Sciences*. Article #19–8156

Vygotsky, L. S. (1961). *Thought and Language.* Cambridge, MA: MIT Press.

Vygotsky, L. S. (1978). *Mind in Society.* Cambridge, MA: Cambridge University Press.

Walther, J. B. (2012). Interaction Through Technological Lenses: Computer-Mediated Communication and Language. *Journal of Language and Social Psychology* 31: 397–414.

Wright, M. (2017). Online Identity Construction. In: *The International Encyclopedia of Media Effects.* Malden, MA: John Wiley.

Yoon, K. (2003). Retraditonalizing the Mobile: Young People's Sociality and Mobile Phone Use in Seoul, South Korea. *European Journal of Cultural Studies* 6: 328–343.

6   Conversation and Discourse

Consider the kinds of answers that might be given during routine conversations to questions such as the following:

Question: What does your sister love?
Answer: Hamburgers.
Question: Is it true that your sister loves hamburgers?
Answer: Yes, it is.
Question: Who loves hamburgers, you or your sister?
Answer: My sister.

The use of the single-word answer "Hamburgers" in the first Q&A sequence is sufficient to give the required information solicited by the questioner. Conversational style dictates that it is unnecessary to utter an entire sentence as the relevant response ("My sister loves hamburgers"). The answer in the second Q&A sequence is intended to confirm (or deny) what the questioner asks. And the answer in the third sequence identifies which of the two alternatives presented by the questioner is the appropriate one.

These responses are not random or disconnected; they are guided by what linguists call pragmatic rules of communication. The term *pragmatics*, as mentioned in Chapter 2, was coined by the American philosopher and semiotician Charles Peirce and applied to the study of communication by psychologist Charles Morris in the 1930s. It is now a branch of linguistics that deals with language as it is used in specific contexts, covering the study of such matters as how the answers above are connected logically and linguistically to questions, what social factors guide turn taking in conversations, what implications and presuppositions are at play in any conversational exchange—in a phrase, pragmatics studies the structure, functions, and maxims that characterize conversations. The term *maxims* was introduced by philosopher Paul Grice (1975), who claimed that without them conversations would make no sense. For example, there is an implicit maxim of *relevance* that guides conversations, by which interlocutors assume that anything spoken about is intended to be relevant (whether it is true or not). It is the expectation of relevance that is at play here. When we hear someone utter that they are not going to be doing the driving after a party because they intend to drink alcohol, we presume that the utterance is relevant to the immediate situation, which involves the dangers that drinking and driving pose.

The answers in the Q&A sequences above reveal knowledge of "how to answer," that is, knowledge of what selection of verbal forms applies in each instance. One of these is that complete sentences are not necessary in responding to questions of a certain type; it is sufficient to use a single lexeme that fits into the object slot of the complete sentence, because it is in this slot that the essential content of an answer lies. This kind of knowledge is called *communicative competence*. The study of this form of competence shows that language is an adaptive and context-sensitive instrument that is shaped by its uses in conversations and by the implicit rules of social interaction that these entail. The internal structures of language are pliable entities that are responsive to external social situations. The ways in which language is used in conversations constitute primary vehicles for establishing, maintaining, defining, and cueing social relations, roles, and agendas. This chapter will look at some of these ways.

6.1 Conversations

The responses above show that the choice of the linguistic structures that are utilized in conversations will vary, being governed by implicit pragmatic principles. This kind of practical knowledge is different from the knowledge of word formation or sentence structure in themselves (called, technically, *linguistic competence*). It constitutes communicative competence, a term coined by American linguist Dell Hymes (1971), as discussed in Chapter 1. A simple protocol such as making contact with someone requires a detailed knowledge of the appropriate speech forms and nonverbal cues that will enable a speaker to negotiate the interaction successfully. An infringement of any of the forms or cues might lead to a breakdown in a conversation, even if each word or phrase is formed perfectly at grammatical and lexical levels.

Starting in the 1980s and 1990s the scientific study of conversations, called *conversation analysis* (CA), has unraveled many aspects of the relation between linguistic and communicative competence—that is, between *langue* and *parole*. Research in CA has documented how people understand and respond to each another in conversations (Sidnell 2010; Sidnell and Stivers 2014; Clift 2016). The research in CA is consistent with the work on *speech acts*, which started in the early 1960s, after British philosopher John L. Austin (1961) suggested that speaking replaces physical actions or acts, so that the meaning of the speech event is to be found in what it actually brings about. If we tell someone to "Sit down" then we are anticipating that the physical act of sitting down will occur. Thus, the utterance is a substitute to physically getting someone to sit down. CA and speech act analysis share many theoretical and research objectives. A branch of linguistics, called *systemic linguistics*, developed in the 1970s and 1980s by Michael A. Halliday (1985), also shares many goals and research models with both. In all such approaches, the central premise is that the choices made during conversations, and their structure, are constrained by factors such as situation, social rules, style, and speaker intentions.

6.1.1 Conversational Devices

The overall aim of CA is to investigate the ways in which people talk in terms of a system of implicit social rules and patterns—a system that is both responsive to, and directive of, conversations. Hutchby and Wooffitt (1998: 14) define the goal of CA as follows:

> CA is the study of recorded, naturally occurring talk-in-interaction. Principally, it is to discover how participants understand and respond to one another in their turns at talk, with a central focus being on how sequences of interaction are generated. To put it another way, the objective of CA is to uncover the tacit reasoning procedures and sociolinguistic competencies underlying the production and interpretation of talk in organized sequences of interaction.

The tacit reasoning procedures to which Hutchby and Wooffitt refer are manifestations of communicative competence, suggesting that knowing how to use language during conversations is as systematic as knowing the grammar of the language being employed. The two are inextricably intertwined. In fact, in CA phonemes, lexemes, morphemes, and sentences are studied as units within conversational texts, not as separate abstract entities. Personal pronouns, for example, are viewed as trace devices, serving conversational rules, such as the desire to maintain the smooth flow of a conversation by connecting its parts in a streamlined fashion. Consider, for instance, the following two utterances, which tell the same story in different ways, both of which are well-formed linguistically, but only one of the two is appropriate communicatively:

1 Sophia went to the mall a few days ago. Sophia ran into an old friend at the mall. Sophia hadn't seen the friend in a while. Sophia and the friend were thrilled.
2 Sophia went to the mall a few days ago. *She* ran into an old friend *there*. Sophia hadn't seen *her* in a while. *They* were thrilled.

The first utterance is perceived as stilted and odd, even though each sentence in it is well-formed when considered in isolation. The second one reads more like ordinary conversation because in English, as in other languages, repetition is perceived as hampering the communicative flow. For this reason, several communicative devices are used that allow for the same information to be conveyed smoothly. Devices that refer back to some word or syntactic category are called *anaphoric*. In (2), *she* refers back to *Sophia*, *there* to *the mall, her* to *the friend,* and *they* to *Sophia and the friend*. Anaphora is a "repetition-eliminating" conversational strategy. The converse of anaphora is *cataphora*. This is a signal anticipating some word or syntactic category. For example, in the sentence "Even though she will deny it, I tell you that Mary did it," the pronoun *she* refers ahead to *Mary*. Pronouns, demonstratives, adverbs, locatives, and other kinds of morphemes and lexemes, are often used as anaphoric and cataphoric devices in conversations.

Box 6.1 Relevant Terms

Pronoun	any word that can replace a noun or noun phrase, such as *you, she, him, mine* ("*The students* love this course" → "*They* love this course")
Subject pronoun	a pronoun that functions as the subject of a sentence. Its form often indicates this function: *I, you, he, she, they* ("*I* love sitcoms; *you* also love them")
Object pronoun	a pronoun that functions as the object of a sentence. Its form often indicates this function: *me, him, her, them, it* ("The woman bought *that book* yesterday" → "The woman bought *it* yesterday")
Locative	any adverb that refers to place or location: *here, there, up, down* ("Hang that picture *here*")
Demonstrative	a word that specifies whether something or someone is relatively near or far: *this, that, these, those* ("I am going to buy *this* device, not *that* one over there")
Adverb	a word that indicates the manner, time, or location connected with some action: *often, slowly, clearly, there* ("My friends tend to walk *slowly*")

This type of analysis highlights the fact that the sentences in conversations have a different composition and function than if they were considered in isolation as part of *langue*. They are constructed in the service of communicative efficiency. The replacement process of the parts of speech in the two utterances above is called *deixis*. Consider the following stretch of conversation:

Speaker A: Jasmine is a lawyer.
Speaker B: Yes, Jasmine is a lawyer.
Speaker A: Jasmine always likes to talk about Jasmine.
Speaker B: Yes, Jasmine sure does like to talk about Jasmine.

Each sentence is well-formed grammatically, but the conversation as a whole is perceived as repetitious and thus as stilted. It does not lack grammatical structure; it lacks deictic structure. A communicatively appropriate version of the same conversation is one in which pronouns are used as deictic particles:

Speaker A: Jasmine is a lawyer.
Speaker B: Yes, *she* is.
Speaker A: *She* always likes to talk about *herself*.
Speaker B: Yes, *she* sure does like to talk about *herself*.

In general, the term *device* is used in reference to such conversational forms. Devices that convey intent, motive, aims, and other states indirectly are called *gambits*:

1 Uh huh ... yeah ... hmm ... aha ...
2 It's, like, she never meant it, you know, ...
3 You like this, don't you?
4 May I ask you something?
5 She arrived a few hours ago; sorry, I meant a few minutes ago.

The grunt-like expressions in (1) are hedges, as already discussed in Chapter 4; they are gambits that allow listeners to make it known to speakers that they are, in fact, listening, especially on the phone. The word *like* and the phrase *you know* in (2) are fillers (Chapter 4); they allow speakers to gather thoughts before proceeding to the next part of an utterance, thus maintaining the ground in a communicative situation, rather than conceding it to an interlocutor. Total silence is typically not a gambit in English, although it may be in other languages. The gambit in (3) is a tag question (Chapter 4); it is a strategy designed to seek approval, agreement, consent, not an answer as in the Q&A sequences at the start of this chapter. Utterance (4) is a gambit that allows an interlocutor to signal the start of a conversation, to take a turn within a conversation, or to enter into a conversation. In English, expressions such as "May I?," "Sorry, but could you tell me ...?," "Excuse me?" are all opening or interceding gambits. Utterance (5) is a repair gambit. When there is a minor breakdown in a conversation, or something is not explained properly, repairs allow a speaker to solve the problem. Expressions such as "sorry" and "I meant" are examples of repair gambits.

The classic work of Sacks, Jefferson, and Schegloff (1995) has revealed that gambits allow for a conversation to signal intents indirectly and are paired to other conversational devices in a cohesive way. Devices are thus said to form *adjacency pairs*—that is, connected by communicative intent and anticipated procedures. So when someone asks something, the interlocutor knows that an answer is the appropriate follow-up in the sequence. Not only that, but also, as we saw at the start of this chapter, the interlocutor knows how to articulate the answer appropriately. Q&A sequences are examples of adjacency pairs.

Another area of interest in CA concerns the social framing of speech acts. This means that conversations can be aggressive or subdued, competitive or cooperative, depending on situation. In the case of competitive speech, the devices used are typically intended to be adversarial, whereas in the case of cooperative speech, they indicate that the speakers are inclined to produce shared meanings. Cooperative speech is marked by features such as the following:

1   Speakers tend to build on one another's comments ("That's true," "I agree").
2   They tend to use well-placed hedges to indicate consent ("Uh-huh," "Yeah," "Sure," "Right").
3   Disagreement is rare, and when it surfaces, a difference of opinion is negotiated via hedges ("Yeah, but, maybe …").
4   Tag questions are used to ensure consent ("You agree, don't you?").

These devices impart a sense of togetherness. As Robin Lakoff (1975) has observed, speakers regularly refrain from saying what they mean in many situations in the service of the higher goal of cooperation in its broadest social sense, fulfilling the *phatic* function, to be discussed below (Watts 2003). Competitive or conflictual conversations are framed in markedly different ways:

1   Speakers tend to contradict one another's comments ("That's really not true," "I wouldn't say that").
2   They tend to use hedges to indicate dissent ("No, no," "No way," "Not true").
3   Difference of opinion is also indicated with various hedges ("Sure, but, maybe …").
4   Tag questions are used to challenge ("You really don't mean that, do you?").

6.1.2 Grice's Maxims

As stated briefly above, the notion of *maxims* is an important one in CA. It was first put forward by Herbert Paul Grice (1975, 1989), who came up with this idea after studying the intentions built into typical utterances. Essentially, Grice's claim is that people who enter into conversations assume the presence of shared maxims. Without these, we hardly would want to engage in them, although this happens occasionally, as in courtroom cross-examinations and in police interrogations, where people know from the outset that they may not apply or that they may apply differently. Grice's maxims can be paraphrased as follows:

1 *Maxim of quantity.* This asserts that interlocutors tend to make their message as informative as required, and not more so, for the purposes of efficiency of communicative flow.
2 *Maxim of quality.* This states that interlocutors expect the contents of an utterance to be true under normal circumstances. This is why when someone lies, it is assumed, initially, not to be a lie. Lying is something discovered, not assumed, in most situations.
3 *Maxim of relevance.* This claims that interlocutors enter into a conversation because they believe that it will be relevant.
4 *Maxim of manner.* This asserts that interlocutors will tend to be perspicuous by avoiding obscurity of expression, avoiding ambiguity, being brief, and being orderly.

These maxims remind us that we tend to perceive communication as part of ethical behavior. When a conversation turns out to violate the maxims, we react negatively to the speaker. In effect, conversations are fraught with danger when the maxims are violated. It is the expectation that is at play here, not necessarily the reality, because people break the maxims all the time for various reasons. Grice also pointed out that most of the meanings that are built into utterances are implicit, rather than explicit. He called the process *conversational implicature.* He illustrated it as follows (Grice 1989: 306):

Speaker A: How is John getting on at his new job at the bank?
Speaker B: Oh, quite well I think; he likes his colleagues, and he hasn't been in prison yet.

B's answer seems to contain an irrelevant remark about prison. A, however, likely infers that B was implying something more, such as, for instance, that John "is the sort of person likely to yield to the temptations provided by his occupation" and thus might easily end up in prison (Grice 1975: 306). How does A arrive at this conclusion? Grice proposed that it occurred through the assumption of a "common purpose, or set of purposes" upholding the reason behind the conversation. The interlocutors want to be cooperative, contributing meaningfully to the purpose of the exchange. So, A extracts from B's utterance that B wanted to communicate more than what he actually said. It is this pattern of inferential reasoning that characterizes utterance meaning and which, obviously, can be a source of misunderstanding in many conversations.

6.1.3 Speech Acts

The notion of *speech act* is a central one in pragmatics, because it provides a taxonomy for pigeonholing utterances in terms of their social functions. As mentioned, a speech act is an utterance that aims to bring about, modify, curtail, or inhibit some real action. The utterance "Be careful!", for instance, is intended to have the same effect as putting a hand in front of someone to block them from crossing the road carelessly. The statement "I sentence you to life imprisonment" uttered by a judge has the same effect as marching the accused directly to prison and locking him up.

There are three main types of speech acts:

1   *Locutionary*, a speech act aiming to convey information of some type ("The moon is a sphere"; "My name is Mark").
2   *Illocutionary*, a speech act indicating purpose or intent, such as asking and answering questions, conveying assurance, promising, ordering, and so on ("I'll do it, sooner or later"; "Come here!").
3   *Perlocutionary*, a speech act that aims to produce effects on the feelings, thoughts, or the actions of interlocutors ("I'm sorry"; "Don't worry").

Another commonly used typology of speech acts is the following one (Searle 1969; Nastri, Pena, and Hancock 2006):

1   *Representatives*. Utterances that stand for some action or some type of agency on the part of one or the other interlocutor ("I will do it for you"; "Let me try").
2   *Assertives*. Statements that assert facts and beliefs, often aiming to get an interlocutor to form or accept a belief ("What she said is a fact"; "That story is true").
3   *Effectives*. Statements designed to bring about change ("You're fired"; "They need to study more in order to succeed").
4   *Directives*. Utterances designed to get an interlocutor to do something ("Just do it"; "Be quiet").
5   *Commissives*. Statements committing the speaker to some future course of action ("Only a few days to go"; "I promise to help you out").
6   *Expressives*. Utterances revealing the psychological state of the speaker ("Your music is amazing"; "That movie sucks").
7   *Declarations*. Utterances connecting assumptions or beliefs to reality ("I am leaving this job because of what you said"; "She is doing this because of what she believes").
8   *Quotations*. Utterances reporting someone else's speech ("She said that she was coming too"; "I heard him say that they were moving").

Through such speech strategies, an individual not only "acts" within the world but also "interacts" with it. Speech act theory thus indirectly studies how the attitudes and actions of everyone involved in a situation can be influenced by specific types of utterances. Research suggests that the functions of speech as they are shown through these acts, manifest themselves already in childhood (Dore 1975). Among the functions that appear early on in childhood language, the following list stands out as being cross-cultural:

1 labeling
2 repeating
3 answering
4 requesting (action)
5 requesting (answer)
6 calling
7 greeting
8 protesting
9 practicing.

6.2 Communicative Competence

Speakers regularly refrain from saying what they mean in many situations in the service of the higher goal of politeness or cooperation in its broadest sense—that is, to fulfill one of the primary social functions of conversation, which has been called the *phatic* function (above). The following excerpt of conversation is typical of how we make contact using words and expressions phatically, rather than literally:

Speaker A: Hi, how's it going?
Speaker B: Great. And you? See ya' later.
Speaker A: OK!

A's question "How's it going?" is not intended to convey literal meaning. It is a polite form of contact, with a well-wishing subtext built into it. This fact is clearly understood by B, since his response ignores the literal meaning. Indeed, if B had said something different, such as "It is not going well," then the conversation would have taken a completely different turn. Clearly, knowing how to frame speech in specific conversations entails knowledge of how speech and situation intersect. The sequences that occur in conversations are thus strategies that "provide participants with resources for displaying evaluations of events and people in ways that are relevant to larger projects that they are engaged in" (Goodwin and Goodwin 1992: 181). As Goffman (1978: 814) perceptively remarked, our utterances often make "a claim of sorts on the attention of everyone in the social situation," and that each situation is grounded in cultural presuppositions that reveal themselves through the language used. In effect, most conversations are grounded in unstated cultural knowledge. This, as mentioned several times already, comes under the rubric of communicative competence.

Dell Hymes (1971) identified eight basic features that shape communicative competence. He cleverly named each one according to the initial letter in the word *speaking*:

S = *setting* and *scene*: the time, place, and psychological setting of a conversation

P = *participants*: the speaker, listener, or audience involved in a conversation

E = *ends*: the desired or expected outcomes of the conversation

A = *act sequence*: the sequence in which the parts of a conversation unfold

K = *key*: the mood or spirit (serious, ironic, jocular, etc.) of the speech act

I = *instrumentalities*: the linguistic variety used (dialectal, sociolectal)

N = *norms*: conventions or expectations about volume, tone, rate of delivery

G = *genres*: different types of speech (joke, lecture, sermon).

Hymes went on to claim that this type of competence develops in tandem with linguistic competence—that is, the child's development of grammar is tied to how language is used in context.

6.2.1 Modeling Communicative Competence

The Russian-born American linguist Roman Jakobson (1960) prefigured the current work on communicative competence, constructing a model of verbal communication that is still used to explain the way conversations unfold psychologically and socially. First, Jakobson claimed that there are six main constituents that make up any conversation or speech act:

1   the *addresser* is the one who initiates the conversation; the addresser can be an individual, an organization, or any entity capable of communicating something

2   the *message* is the information, commentary, annotation, etc. that the addresser constructs or formulates for some reason or in response to something

3   the *addressee* is the one to whom the message is addressed; the addressee can be an individual, an audience, or any other potential receiver of the message

4   the *context* is the situation and conditions in which the message is created and which makes it meaningful; for example, the utterance "Help me" would have a different meaning depending on whether it was spoken by someone lying motionless on the ground or by a student in a classroom working on a difficult math problem

5   the mode of *contact* is the means by which a message is delivered; this involves the physical, social, and psychological modalities that exist or are established between the addresser and addressee; it could be F2F, through an online social network, and so on; the mode can thus be

synchronous, occurring at the same time (as in oral conversation or through devices such as instant-messaging devices) or asynchronous, occurring in a delayed fashion (as in emails)

6 the *code* is the system(s) providing the expressive forms or resources (language, gesture, facial expressions, and so on) for constructing and deciphering messages meaningfully and efficiently.

Each of these constituents involves a different communicative function:

1 *emotive*, revealing the addresser's emotions, attitudes, social status, beliefs, or intents, which, no matter how literal or information-based the message might be, will invariably indicate the reason why the addresser entered into communication in the first place

2 *conative*, or the effect (physical, psychological, social) that the message has, or is expected to have, on the addressee

3 *referential*, is a message constructed to carry information unambiguously; it is also the term indicating that any message is perceived as referring to something other than itself

4 *poetic*, is a message constructed with poetic style, as can be seen in rhythmic or rhyming constructions such as "ping-pong," "Take a break"

5 *phatic*, is a message designed to establish, reaffirm, or routinely carry out continuous social contact ("Hi, how's it going?")

6 *metalingual*, is a message referring to the code being used ("The word I just used is a foreign word").

This model suggests that communicative competence involves unconscious knowledge of how the system of interrelated constituents and functions guide any speech act. Jakobson's notions of *phatic function* and *context* require further commentary. The former, as already discussed, is designed primarily to ensure fluid social contact and continuity. So, for example, when two office workers pass each other in the morning and say, "Hi, how's it going?" "Not bad, and you?" they are not literally inquiring about each other's health. The adjacency pairs in such instances are part of phatic speech and are intended for making contact and keeping the social relation going. All kinds of ritual and social practices are based on phatic communication, which is not intended to create new meanings but to reinforce existing ones. The term *context* in this model is not a synonym for setting. The context is the place (here, there), time (now, then), and specific indexical relation (this, that) that shapes a communication event. It guides what an utterance means in real terms. So, the expression "How are you?" will vary in meaning according to context. As discussed, if exchanged between coworkers habitually it is a phatic expression; if directed by a doctor to a patient during an examination, it has a different meaning, namely it asks about the patient's actual health.

6.2.2 Speech Functions

Already in the 1920s, anthropologist Bronislaw Malinowski (1922) saw verbal communication as fulfilling and serving specific social functions. He was the one who coined the term *phatic communion*, as the exchange of words and phrases that are important less for their dictionary meanings than for establishing social contact and enacting social rituals. From Malinowski's work came the notion of *speech function*, which was taken up by several linguists, including Benjamin Lee Whorf (1956) (see Chapter 8). Although it overlaps somewhat with the notion of speech act, the term speech function implies, more generally, that language permits the realization of social roles and psychological agendas.

Various typologies have been put forward as frameworks for studying speech functions. Some of these are as follows:

1   *instrumental*, the use of language to satisfy material needs: "May I have some water please? I'm thirsty"
2   *regulatory*, the utilization of language to control others or something: "Please shut the door"; How can I get this machine to work?"
3   *interactional*, speaking to maintain social ties and relations, filling in blanks in a conversation, making contact, and so on: "Hi, how's it going?"; also called *phatic* (as discussed)
4   *personal*, using language as a means to express oneself emotionally or intellectually: "Ouch!," "Hey, leave me alone!," "Let me tell you who I really am"
5   *heuristic*, employing language to gain information: "What's that?," "Can you explain the Pythagorean theorem to me?"
6   *imaginative*, the use of language to convey ideas creatively: "I wonder why time flies?"
7   *representational*, using language to represent things, that is, to classify the world in specific ways
8   *performative*, the use of language in rituals and performances (prayers, jokes, etc.)
9   *socialization*, utilizing language to indicate a connection to a society, community, or group.

6.2.3 Politeness: A Case-in-Point

Politeness is an important part of phatic communion—knowing how to be courteous, decorous, and respectful is critical knowledge in societies across the globe. Penelope Brown and Stephen Levinson (1987) have argued that politeness is not just part of communicative competence, but also part of Self-presentation, called generally "saving face" in reference to the work of Goffman (1955). So, the ways in which we express politeness is not only tied to social conventions, but also to personal agendas. In other words, it intersects between the emotive and phatic functions.

Generally, politeness speech is designed to show or convey deference in culture-specific ways, establishing or reinforcing a positive relationship among interlocutors. It is a form of cooperative speech. So, "Could you please pass the salt?" communicates respect in contrast to "Pass the salt"; similarly, "Excuse me, do you know where this building is?" is perceived as more courteous than "Tell me where the building is."

Box 6.2 Politeness Strategies

"If you don't mind ..."
"If it's no bother, ..."
"I hope this isn't too much trouble ..."
"Glad to make your acquaintance ..."
"Sir, you are right ..."
"Dr. Smith, my apologies ..."
"Please, can you help me out? ..."
"Excuse me, do you know where this street is? ..."

Research shows that politeness varies according to age, class, education, and gender variables (Leech 2014) and that the misuse of politeness protocols tends to produce negative or conflictual communication (Meyerhoff 2006). Brown and Levinson identified three variables that guide the choice of politeness protocols in specific situations: (1) the social distance of the interlocutors, (2) the relative power of one interlocutor over the other, and (3) the absolute ranking of impositions in the culture. The greater the social distance between the interlocutors, the more the use of polite speech is felt to be necessary in an interaction. Analogously, the greater the relative power of one interlocutor over another, the more it is expected that the lower ranking interlocutor use polite forms, even non-reciprocally. And the heavier the imposition made on interlocutors (the more time required, or the greater the favor asked), the more the politeness level of speech expected.

Brown and Levinson also identified two main kinds of politeness:

1 *Negative politeness*: This involves making a request less infringing with the use of negative devices: "If you don't mind..."; "If it isn't too much bother...". The intent is to show respect for someone's right to act freely.
2 *Positive politeness*: This seeks to establish a positive relationship among interlocutors. It is based on direct speech acts and Grice's maxims.

They also identified two subsidiary forms:

1   *Bald-on record*: This involves the use of abrupt or direct forms of speech, rather than a politeness strategy: "Yes, give it to me" rather than "Would you mind giving it to me?"
2   *Off-record*: This involves taking off the pressure on an interlocutor for doing, giving, or receiving something: "I tried to call you many times, but there was never any answer."

It has been found that some cultures prefer one or the other form of politeness—negative or positive; but these categories do not apply universally. In East Asian cultures, politeness is oriented towards acknowledging the positions or roles of all the participants as well as adherence to formality norms appropriate to the situation (Matsumoto 1988; Ide 1989). Japanese has two main politeness protocols: one for intimate acquaintances, such as family members and friends, and one for other people, each of which is marked by morphological subsystems—some verbs, nouns, and pronouns, for example, are used to reference the gender, age, rank, and degree of acquaintance of the interlocutors.

6.3 Discourse and Dialogue

Terms such as *conversation, dialogue*, and *discourse* are often used interchangeably. But there are sociolinguistically relevant differences. The main technical difference between *conversation* and *dialogue* is one of intentionality. Conversations are typically interactions, fulfilling the various functions discussed in the previous sections; they are unplanned and unscripted. The *dialogue*, by way of contrast, is a form of speech intended for achieving understanding, exploring some topic, interrogating someone, or resolving some problem. The notion of dialogue was introduced by the Greek philosopher Socrates as a Q&A exchange between a teacher and a pupil, designed to elicit understanding on the part of the latter. The so-called "Socratic dialogue" is still used in education in order to impart knowledge and skill to learners.

Discourse refers to a broader use of language to convey unstated or assumed beliefs, ideologies, and intents. The importance of discourse was put forward as early as the 1920s by the Russian literary scholar Mikhail Bakhtin (1981), who anticipated many key notions of current discourse theories. He was the first to use the term *discourse* to denote the particular way in which language was used by specific groups for ideological or specialized purposes. This is why we talk about "political discourse" or "sports discourse," in reference to the kinds of speech used by certain people or groups to reveal shared interests, values, worldviews, beliefs, biases, and so on. These "discourses" are typically characterized by keywords, jargon, a specific style, and coded structures (such as so-called "dog whistles") that appear frequently in speech acts (Stubbs 2008). As Scollon and Wong Scollon (2001) have amply documented, discourses invariably imply subtexts tied to a particular ideology or worldview. This is what makes them so powerful among speakers.

6.3.1 Discourse

Discourse characterizes the kinds of ingroup speech in families, schools, corporations, universities, the media, and other groups that develop specific styles of speech. So, in politics, for instance, a certain form or style of discourse is established by a leader or by an authoritative source. "Marxist discourse," for example, is a style code for sharing presuppositions and evaluations of events among those who espouse a Marxist ideology of society and politics. In instantiations of this discourse, keywords such as "capitalism," "proletariat," "superstructure," "means of production," "dialectic materialism," and the like are indexes of these presuppositions. In contrast, the same topic will be treated differently by those who espouse a capitalist ideology, marked by keywords such as "marketplace economy," "middle-class workers," "manufacturing industries," and the like. When speakers of the two ideologies clash in a communicative event, these keywords neutralize one another, leading to a blockage of understanding.

In addition to keywords, discourses are characterized by *intertextuality*, defined as the direct or indirect citation of meaningful authoritative or canonical texts for the group. For example, the Bible figures prominently in Christian discourse, whereas *Das Kapital* (a founding text of Marxism) figures noticeably in Marxist discourse. The Bible, Shakespeare, Martin Luther King's speeches, and the like are canonical for, say, religious groups, English scholars, and politicians respectively. These allow speakers to make meaningful connections to their ideas via direct or indirect citation.

In addition to ideologically motivated discourse, societies also develop *specialized* and *popular discourse* genres for specific communicative purposes. The former is characteristic, for example, of job interviews, university lectures, medical consultations, courtroom interactions, and the like, where keywords index specific notions, events, and points of background informational reference. The latter emerge in recurrent settings which induce specific speech styles in people who frequent or belong to the settings. The expressions "media discourse" or "pop culture discourse" are examples.

Box 6.3 Discourse Glossary

Common ground

the common beliefs, worldviews, etc. shared by interlocutors participating in a discourse-based event

Genres

types of discourses reflecting specific styles of delivery—speeches, interviews, and so on

Intertexuality

allusion to meaningful texts in certain groups (the Bible, Shakespeare, and so on) strengthening the common ground

As an example of keyword usages in pop culture discourse, consider again the word *cool* used to describe attractive lifestyles (Chapter 4). This comes out of jazz culture (as mentioned earlier) and is now an intrinsic part of everyday discourse, alluding to a stylish and smart mode of dressing, acting, and talking that is in synch with the times. The counterpart of *cool* is *hot* to indicate that someone is sexy (including morphemic variants such as *hottie*). A 1933 film named *Hot Pepper*, with Lupe Velez playing a sexy character, epitomized, and probably ensconced, the use of *hot* as a keyword for "sexual allure." From the 1930s to the 1960s the expression *hot pants* emerged as a slang term for sexy men and women. So, the use today of *hottie* in a sexual sense has really been a part of common pop discourse for a long time.

Movies have been particularly important in creating pop discourse trends. *Animal House* (1978) introduced colloquial expressions still used today, such as *wimp* (someone who is scared or has no courage) and *brew* (getting a beer). *Clueless* (1995) introduced the expression *whatever* to convey disinterest in what another person is saying. *Mean Girls* (2004) introduced *plastic*, meaning fake girls who look like Barbie dolls.

The term *pop language* was coined by journalist Leslie Savan in her book *Slam Dunks and No-Brainers* (2005) to refer to this type of discourse. Throughout contemporary society, Savan notes, people use a discourse style, which derives from mass entertainment events. Phrases such as "That is so last year," "Don't go there," "Get a life," "I hate it when that happens," "It doesn't get any better than this," come from television sitcoms and popular movies. Pop discourse is used by ordinary people, claims Savan, because it is perceived to be *au courant* and meaningful. The number of keywords from pop culture that have entered the communal lexicon since the 1920s is truly mind-boggling, constituting strong evidence that pop discourse informs everyday speech to a high degree.

6.3.2 Ritualistic Discourse

The term *ritualistic discourse* designates the kind of speech that characterizes some ritualistic situation, including one that is simply repeated over and over becoming part of communal understanding. Ann Gill (1994: 106) describes the power of such discourse to influence perception and belief as follows:

By portraying experience in a particular way, words work their unconscious magic on humans, making them see, for example, products as necessary for success or creating distinctions between better or worse—be it body shape, hair style, or brand of blue jeans. Words create belief in religions, governments, and art forms; they create allegiances to football teams, politicians, movie stars, and certain brands of beer. Words are the windows of our own souls and to the world beyond our fingertips. Their essential persuasive efficacy works its magic on every person in every society.

In many early cultures, knowing the name of a deity was purported to give the knower great power—for example, in Egyptian mythology, the sorceress Isis tricked the sun god Ra into revealing his name and, thus, gained power over him and all other gods. In some cultures, the ritual of bestowing an ancestral name to a newly born is perceived to weave a sort of magical protective aura on the child by the ancestor's spirit (Chapter 5). In some traditional Inuit societies, individuals will not pronounce their names randomly, fearing that this senseless act could break the magical spell of protection that the name brings with it. As Espes Brown (1992: 13) puts it: "The fact that when we create words we use our breath, and for these people and these traditions breath is associated with the principle of life; breath is life itself. And so if a word is born from this sacred principle of breath, this lends an added sacred dimension to the spoken word."

6.3.3 Critical Discourse

Critical discourse analysis (CDA) is a branch of discourse analysis that aims to describe discourses in social contexts and to offer explanations of why some forms of language can unconsciously convey emphases or biases. A common example is the difference between *this* and *that*. When a speaker says "This is true" it foregrounds the topic to a level of importance, thus empowering the speaker's ideas; contrariwise, "That is true" appears to background it, thus neutralizing what the interlocutor said and thus disempowering the speaker's ideas. CDA aims to show that differences in power alignments through speech cues are part of assumed hierarchies of social importance within institutions. The dominant critical discourses are those associated with education, the law, the government, and other authoritative agencies.

Fairclough (2003) developed a three-pronged approach to CDA, which allows sociolinguists to differentiate critical discourse from other types:

1   the analysis of specific types of texts (such as academic or political ones) in order to glean from them presuppositions and cues that signal differential power relations
2   the analysis of discourse practices themselves, such as text production, distribution, and consumption (that is, who decides which texts get out there and influence people's beliefs)
3   the analysis of events that certain discourses bring about (such as at pep rallies).

The starting point for CDA is commonly traced to the work of French philosopher Michel Foucault (1972), who described how particular types of language are used by people and institutions to manipulate the perception of reality. In this sense, discourse is a form of power that articulates and ensconces ideas that are felt as being the truth by a specific group.

6.3.4 Dialogue

Dialogue, as discussed above, involves intentional or skilled uses of Q&A sequences for various social functions, from the theatrical and narrative arts, to education and courtroom interactions. It is a purposeful (and even scripted) use of speech to achieve knowledge, understanding, or to impart sense (as in a play). It was Plato who introduced the systematic use of dialogue as a distinctive form of philosophical inquiry, after his teacher, Socrates, established the dialogue as a mode of knowledge imparting. Almost all of Plato's writings are constructed in dialogical form. After Plato, the dialogue was relegated primarily to the literary theatrical domain, although it is said that Aristotle (Plato's pupil) wrote several philosophical treatises in dialogical style, none of which, however, has survived. The dialogue was revived somewhat by early Christian writers, especially St. Augustine, Boethius, and somewhat later by Peter Abelard. However, under the powerful influence of Scholasticism, the dialogue was replaced by the more formal and concise *summa*, or synthetic treatise, of which the most famous is the one written by medieval theologian St. Thomas Aquinas.

The dialogue was reintroduced into scientific and philosophical inquiry by various intellectuals starting in the late seventeenth century. For example, in 1688, the French philosopher Nicolas Malebranche published his *Dialogues on Metaphysics and Religion*, contributing to the genre's revival. The Irish prelate George Berkeley employed it as well in his 1713 work, *Three Dialogues between Hylas and Philonous*. But perhaps the most well-known use of the dialogue was by Galileo in his *Dialogue Concerning the Two Chief World Systems* of 1632.

There are many uses of dialogue today, from education to psychotherapy. The latter involves a controlled dialogue between patient and therapist. The latter's questions are aimed at detecting some factor in the patient's life that is causing mental or emotional problems. The trained analyst uses the responses to diagnose what the problems are and to enable the patient to build an understanding of such problems. True therapeutic dialogue is nonjudgmental; it seeks to unravel hidden problems.

Contrary to this type of dialogue, courtroom interrogations are often conflictual, designed to get a witness or an accused person to reveal something, which may not even be connected to the truth of the matter, but is usable by the interrogator to argue for or against the innocence of an accused person. The goal in a cross-examination is to get the respondent to commit to a particular position. The questioner then has the option of using the answer as the basis of further argumentation. Here is a hypothetical example:

Prosecutor: Did you see the victim the day before?
Accused: No, I didn't.
Prosecutor: But then why did you say that you met often on that day?
Accused: Something happened on that day.
Prosecutor: Can you explain?

The prosecutor uses the "No" answer to connect something said previously to the present situation. At this point, the dialogue can take a different course, allowing the prosecutor to extract statements needed for subsequent interrogation. If the evidence has no bearing on the case, then the prosecutor can still use the dialogue to cast doubt on the veracity of the accused person. By arranging the content of questions strategically, damaging admissions can be obtained. These lines of questioning are used typically to get someone to commit to some situation: (1) "How do you know that?" (2) "What do you mean by that?" and (3) "Doesn't this contradict your previous statement?" Obtaining information and agreements, however, is not the sole purpose of cross-examinations. Of great importance is the impression made by the questioners and respondents on the judge or the jury. Because cross-examination is so revelatory, it can become a basis for portraying the character of the participants. Needless to say, the assessment is not always accurate, but it is always affected in some way by the cross-examination itself.

Among the dialogical strategies that characterize successful cross-examinations, the following ones stand out:

- The questioner should avoid appearing crafty or adversarial at first, so that witnesses may let down their defensive mechanisms.
- The questions should be clear and comprehensible.
- The questioner should not stray from a particular line of questioning.
- The respondent must not be allowed to take over the cross-examination. This can be done by interrupting long-winded and circuitous responses— "OK"; "Thank you"; "Let's go on."
- There may be situations in which politeness is paramount, in order to get the respondent to be compliant. This is sometimes called "playing possum," whereby the intention is to lure the respondent into admitting something they want to hide.

6.3.5 Online Discourse

Conversations, dialogues, and discourses that take place in online contexts serve the same social functions as those in offline contexts. Analysis of online conversations, such as on Twitter (Gillen and Merchant 2013), has shown that the medium does not affect the functions of discourse to any significant degree; even if they might be verbalized differently according to social medium (Foxtree, Mayer, and Betts 2011; Carr, Schrock, and Dauterman 2012).

The main difference between F2F and online conversations and discourses is that the latter may be perceived and planned as public and personal at the same; that is, they involve not only individual interlocutors but at an audience as well. This might explain why many online conversations involve some form of wordplay, perhaps as a means of deflecting attention away from the intents and Self-image of the addresser. As Reyes, Rosso, and Veale (2013) found, this type of "ludic" (playful) form of communication is common in online venues through such devices and strategies as the following: *signatures* ("you're loving person" after a bitter text); *unexpectedness*, such as throwing in a satirical comment when unexpected ("she said that she was coming, as she always does, btw"); *style* ("That is so yesterday"); and *emotivity* (such as using ! after an assertive, indicating that it was meant ironically). With a corpus of 40,000 tweets, automatically harvested from Twitter, the researchers found that users do not have a single, precise notion of irony or communicative intent; rather, they seem to possess a diffuse understanding of what it means for a text to be effective.

6.4 Nonverbal Aspects

When we converse in F2F contexts, we typically use hand gestures, facial expressions, head movements, body postures, and the like that reinforce, emphasize, and generally complement the vocal speech act. It has been found that we communicate over two-thirds of our ideas and feelings through such "body language," as it is commonly called (Morris et al. 1979). Some societies even use dual communication modalities—vocal and gestural—for special reasons. The Plainspeople of North America, for example, use a gestural language to communicate with social groups that speak different vocal languages. A detailed conversation is possible using the gestures alone (Mallery 1972). The sociolinguistic study of conversation now includes body language, either independently of vocal language or as its complement during speech acts: (1) What does a certain nonverbal sign (a gesture, a facial expression, and so on) imply? (2) What responses does it bring about? (3) Which nonverbal signs correlate with verbal ones during speech?

6.4.1 Kinesic and Proxemic Patterns

The scientific study of body language is called more technically *kinesics*. It was first developed by the American anthropologist Ray L. Birdwhistell (1952, 1970), who analyzed slow-motion films of speakers interacting during conversations, noting that specific bodily actions and reactions surfaced typically in them. He adopted notions from linguistics to characterize the patterns, believing that they were similar in function to the grammatical and lexical structures of language. He classified what he called "kinesic signs" as innate (involuntary), learned (voluntary), or a mixture of the two. Blinking, throat clearing, and facial flushing are innate (involuntary) signs, as are facial expressions of happiness, surprise, anger, disgust, and other basic emotions. Laughing, crying, and shrugging the shoulders are examples of mixed signs. They may originate as instinctive actions, but cultural rules shape their structure, timing, and uses. Winking, raising a thumb, or saluting with the hands are learned (voluntary) signs. Logically, their meanings vary from culture to culture. As Duncan and Fiske (1977: xi) observe, kinesic communication "can be construed as having a definite organization or structure."

Posture in F2F settings is a kinesic strategy that communicates information about one's sense of self, mood, motivation, and attitude. A pose can be broken down into a series of specific kinesic signs conveying various meanings, some of which are universal and others culture-specific. For example, research exists to show that the following poses and postures are unmarked culturally, that is, they tend to occur across cultures with moderate variation:

1   Slumped posture = low spirits.
2   Erect posture = high spirits, energy, and confidence.
3   Leaning forward = open and interested behavior.
4   Leaning away = defensive or disinterested behavior.
5   Crossed arms = defensive behavior.
6   Uncrossed arms = willingness to listen.

Most other poses are marked culturally. Hand gestures and touch patterns during conversations also tend to be mixed sign systems. The study of such patterns falls more specifically under the rubric of *haptics* (from Greek *haptikos*, "grasping," "touching"). Using the hands to shield oneself from an attack is an innate haptic reaction. So, too, is raising the hand to warn someone. But most other haptic signs are culture specific. These include patting someone on the arm, shoulder, or back to indicate agreement or praise, linking arms to designate companionship, putting an arm around the shoulder to indicate friendship or intimacy, holding hands to express intimacy, hugging to convey happiness, and so on.

The study of the zones people maintain between themselves during conversation comes under a different rubric, known as *proxemics*. This field was founded by the American anthropologist Edward T. Hall in the late 1950s, who developed it substantively over subsequent years (see Hall 1959; Eco 1968). As a soldier during World War II, Hall had noticed that people maintained recognizable distances between themselves during conversations, coming soon to realize that many (if not most) breakdowns in communication were attributable to infractions of these zone patterns. The unconscious differences in the ways that people of diverse cultures perceive interpersonal zones and in the ways they behave within them play a powerful role in influencing the outcomes of F2F interactions. Hall measured and assessed these critical interpersonal zones with statistical techniques. The zones can, in fact, be measured with great accuracy, varying according to age, gender, and other social variables.

Some proxemic patterns seem to be universal. For example, the immediate physical zone around a human being constitutes a sphere of privacy. The size of the zone will vary somewhat from culture to culture, but all cultures tend to perceive this zone as an intimate one. The next is within a person's reach, but falls outside the privacy zone. This is the zone in which handshaking can occur. The intimate zone (from 0–18 in.), Hall surmises, is rooted in our biological past, and is thus based on our innate sense of territoriality, which involves establishing boundaries. In the close phase (from 0–6 in.), the senses are activated and the presence of the other is unmistakable. This phase is typically reserved for lovemaking, comforting, and protecting; the far phase (from 6–18 in.) is the zone in which family members and close friends interact under normal conditions. The actual dimensions may vary somewhat, but the intimate zone and its phases seem to have a universal validity. Each of Hall's zones matches linguistic registers, corresponding more or less to Joos' typology (Chapter 4). So, in the intimate zone, the register used is also intimate, whereas in the more distant formal zones the register is also formal. In effect, vocal and body language form an integrated system of communication.

6.4.2 Gesture

When children tell a lie, they will tend to cover their mouth with one or both hands immediately afterwards. This gesture is used unwittingly later in life as well. Often the adult pulls the hand away at the last moment, touching the nose instead. The latter gesture is more sophisticated and less obvious, but it still implies mendacity.

American linguist David McNeill (1992, 2005) has shown that during conversations, gesture is an unconscious complementary sign system to vocal language. He videotaped a large number of people as they spoke, gathering a substantial amount of data on the gesture signs that accompany speech, which he termed *gesticulants*. His findings suggest that these are used in concomitance with words, exhibiting images that cannot be communicated overtly in vocal utterances. Psychologically, they are traces to what the speaker is thinking about. McNeill classified gesticulants into five main categories:

1   *Iconic* gesticulants bear a close resemblance to the referent or referential domain of an utterance: for example, when describing a scene from a story in which a character bends a tree back to the ground, a speaker observed by McNeill appeared to grip something and pull it back. His gesture was, in effect, a manual depiction of the action talked about, revealing both the speaker's memory image and point of view (the speaker could have taken the part of the tree instead).

2   *Metaphorical* gesticulants are also pictorial, but their content is abstract, rather than purely iconic. For example, McNeill observed a male speaker

announcing that what he had just seen was a cartoon, simultaneously raising up his hands as if offering his listener a kind of object. He was obviously not referring to the cartoon itself, but to the genre of the cartoon. His gesture represented this genre as if it were an object, placing it into an act of offering to the listener. This type of gesticulant typically accompanies utterances that contain metaphorical expressions such as *presenting an idea, putting forth an idea, offering advice,* and so on.

3 *Beat* gesticulants resemble the beating of musical tempo. The speaker's hand moves along with the rhythmic pulsation of speech, in the form of a simple flick of the hand or fingers up and down, or back and forth. These gesticulants mark the introduction of new themes in an utterance.

4 *Cohesive* gesticulants serve to show how separate parts of an utterance are supposed to hold together. Cohesives can take iconic, metaphorical, or beat form. They unfold through a repetition of the same gesticulant. It is the repetition itself that is meant to convey cohesiveness.

5 *Deictic* gesticulants involve some form of indication (*here, there, up, right,* etc.). They are aimed not at an existing physical place, but at an abstract concept that had occurred earlier in the conversation. These reveal that we perceive concepts as having a physical location in space.

McNeill's work gives us a good idea of how the gestural mode intersects with the vocal one in normal conversations. Gestural cues are also used in utterances to relay emotional meaning (for example, the typical hand movements that accompany happiness, surprise, fear, anger, sadness, contempt, disgust, etc.); to help monitor, maintain, or control the speech of someone else (as, for example, the hand movements indicating *Keep going, Slow down, What else happened?*, etc.); and to convey some need or mental state (for instance, scratching one's head when puzzled, rubbing one's forehead when worried, etc.) (see Ekman 1973).

6.4.3 Facial Expression

Interest in facial expression as a vehicle of emotional communication started with Charles Darwin's book *Expression of the Emotions in Man and Animals*, published in 1872. Darwin's work led, a century later, to the scientific study of facial expressions. A schematic timeline of such study is the following one:

- Anthropologist Margaret Mead's (1964) work with isolated communities suggested that facial expressions are, by and large, culture specific.
- At about the same time, psychologist Silvan Tomkins and his research associates (Tomkins and Izard 1965) argued that some expressions are cross-cultural and thus likely to be universal.
- Psychologist Gordon H. Bower (1980) linked emotional states to memory, suggesting as well that facial expressions may be shaped by environmental forces.

- The work of Paul Ekman on facial expressions has led to a deeper understanding of how these expressions are part of how we communicate emotivity in conversations (Ekman and Friesen 1975; Ekman 1976, 1980, 1982, 1985, 2003).

Of special value to sociolinguistics is, actually, Ekman's breakdown of facial expressions into units of eyebrow position, eye shape, mouth shape, nostril size, and so on. In various combinations these reinforce the meaning of a particular expression. From this, a standard set of units (which he called *microexpressions*) can be catalogued and studied for consistency and variation across cultures. So, for example, closing the eyes typically accompanies an exhortation such as "Ouch, it hurts!" Contrariwise, a smile and wide open eyes accompany an expression such as "Wow, this is great!" As obvious as these examples might seem, they still bring out the fact that verbal and nonverbal forms of expression form an integrated system of communicative competence in normal circumstances.

References and Further Reading

Austin, J. L. (1961). *How to Do Things with Words*. Cambridge, MA: Harvard University Press.

Bakhtin, M. M. (1981). *The Dialogic Imagination*. Trans. C. Emerson and M. Holquist. Austin, TX: University of Texas Press.

Birdwhistell, R. L. (1952). *Introduction to Kinesics*. Ann Arbor, MI: University of Ann Arbor.

Birdwhistell, R. L. (1970). *Kinesics and Context: Essays on Body Motion Communication*. Harmondsworth: Penguin.

Bower, G. H. (1980). *Theories of Learning*, 5th ed. Boston, MA: Pearson.

Brown, P. and Levinson, S. C. (1987). *Politeness: Some Universals in Language Usage*. Cambridge: Cambridge University Press.

Carr, C., Schrock, D. and Dauterman, P. (2012). Speech Acts Within Facebook Status Messages. *Journal of Language and Social Psychology* 31: 176–196.

Clift, R. (2016). *Conversation Analysis*. Cambridge: Cambridge University Press.

Dore, J. (1975). Holophrases, Speech Acts and Language Universals. *Journal of Child Language* 2: 21–40.

Duncan, S. and Fiske, D. W. (1977). *Face-to-Face Interaction*. Hillsdale, NJ: Erlbaum.

Eco, U. (1968). *Einführung in die Semiotik*. Munich: Fink.

Ekman, P. (1973). *Darwin and Facial Expression: A Century of Research in Review*. New York: Academic.

Ekman, P. (1976). Movements with Precise Meanings. *Journal of Communication* 26: 14–26.

Ekman, P. (1980). The Classes of Nonverbal Behavior. In: W. Raffler-Engel (ed.), *Aspects of Nonverbal Communication*, pp. 89–102. Lisse: Swets & Zeitlinger.

Ekman, P. (1982). Methods for Measuring Facial Action. In: K. R. Scherer and P. Ekman (eds.), *Handbook of Methods in Nonverbal Behavior*, pp. 45–90. Cambridge: Cambridge University Press.

Ekman, P. (1985). *Telling Lies*. New York: Norton.

Ekman, P. (2003). *Emotions Revealed*. New York: Holt.

Ekman, P. and Friesen, W. (1975). *Unmasking the Face*. Englewood Cliffs, NJ: Prentice-Hall.

Espes Brown, J. (1992). Becoming Part of It. In: D. M. Dooling and P. Jordan-Smith (eds.), *I Become Part of It: Sacred Dimensions in Native American Life*, pp. 1–15. New York: HarperCollins.

Fairclough, N. (2003). *Analysing Discourse*. London: Routledge.

Foucault, M. (1972). *The Archeology of Knowledge*. New York: Pantheon.

Foxtree, J., Mayer, S. and Betts, T. (2011). Grounding in Instant-Messaging. *Journal of Educational Computing Research* 45: 455–475.

Gill, A. (1994). *Rhetoric and Human Understanding*. Prospect Heights, IL: Waveland.

Gillen, J. and Merchant, G. (2013). Contact Calls: Twitter as a Dialogic Social and Linguistic Practice. *Language Science* 35: 47–58.

Goffman, E. (1955). On Face-Work: An Analysis of Ritual Elements in Social Interaction. *Psychiatry: Journal for the Study of International Processes* 18: 213–231.

Goffman, E. (1978). Response Cries. *Language* 54: 787–815.

Goodwin, C. and Goodwin, M. H. (1992). Assessments and the Construction of Context. In: A. Duranti and C. Goodwin (eds.), *Rethinking Context: Language as an Interactive Phenomenon*. Cambridge: Cambridge University Press.

Grice, H. P. (1975). Logic and Conversation. In: P. Cole and J. Morgan (eds.), *Syntax and Semantics*, Vol. 3, pp. 41–58. New York: Academic.

Grice, H. P. (1989). *Studies in the Way of Words*. Cambridge, MA: Harvard University Press.

Hall, E. T. (1959). *The Silent Language*. Greenwich: Fawcett.

Hall, E. T. (1966). *The Hidden Dimension*. Garden City, NJ: Anchor.

Halliday, M.A.K. (1985). *Introduction to Functional Grammar*. London: Arnold.

Hutchby, I. and Wooffitt, R. (1998). *Conversation Analysis*. Cambridge: Polity Press.

Hymes, D. (1971). *On Communicative Competence*. Philadelphia: University of Pennsylvania Press.

Ide, S. (1989) Formal Forms and Discernment: Two Neglected Aspects of Universals of Linguistic Politeness. *Multilingua* 8: 223–248.

Jakobson, R. (1960). Linguistics and Poetics. In: T. Sebeok (ed.), *Style and Language*. Cambridge, MA: MIT Press.

Lakoff, R. (1975). *Language and Woman's Place*. New York: Harper & Row.

Leech, G. (2014). *The Pragmatics of Politeness*. Oxford: Oxford University Press.

Malinowski, B. (1922). *Argonauts of the Western Pacific*. New York: Dutton.

Mallery, G. (1972). *Sign Language Among North American Indians Compared with That Among Other Peoples and Deaf-Mutes*. The Hague: Mouton.

Matsumoto, Y. (1988) Reexamination of the Universality of Face: Politeness Phenomena in Japanese. *Journal of Pragmatics* 12: 403–426.

McNeill, D. (1992). *Hand and Mind: What Gestures Reveal About Thought*. Chicago: University of Chicago Press.

McNeill, D. (2005). *Gesture & Thought*. Chicago: University of Chicago Press.

Mead, M. (1964). *Continuities in Cultural Evolution*. New Haven, CT: Yale University Press.

Meyerhoff, M. (2006). *Introducing Sociolinguistics*. London: Routledge.

Morris, C. W. (1938). *Foundations of the Theory of Signs*. Chicago: University of Chicago Press.

Morris, D., Collett, P., Marsh, P., O'Shaghnessy, M. (1979). *Gestures: Their Origins and Distributions*. London: Cape.

Nastri, J., Pena, J., and Hancock, J. T. (2006). The Construction of Away Messages: A Speech Act Analysis. *Journal of Computer-Mediated Communication* 11: 1025–1045.

Peirce, C. S. (1931–1958). *Collected Papers*. Cambridge, MA: Harvard University Press.

Reyes, A., Rosso, P., and Veale, T. (2013). A Multidimensional Approach for Detecting Irony on Twitter. *Language Resources & Evaluation* 47: 239–268.

Sacks, H., Jefferson, G., and Schegloff, E. A. (1995). *Lectures on Conversation*. Oxford: Wiley-Blackwell.

Savan, L. (2005). *Slam Dunks and No-Brainers: Language in Your Life, the Media, Business, Politics, and, Like, Whatever*. New York: Alfred A. Knopf.

Scollon, R. and Wong Scollon, S. (2001). *Intercultural Communication*, 2nd ed. Oxford: Wiley-Blackwell.

Searle, J. R. (1969). *Speech Acts: An Essay in the Philosophy of Language*. Cambridge: Cambridge University Press.

Sidnell, J. (2010). *Conversation Analysis: An Introduction*. Oxford: Wiley-Blackwell.

Sidnell, J. and Stivers, S. (eds.) (2014). *The Handbook of Conversation Analysis*. Oxford: Wiley-Blackwell.

Stubbs, M. (2008). Three Concepts of Keywords. Paper presented to the conference on Keyness in Text, University of Siena.

Tomkins, S. and Izard, C. E. (1965). *Affect, Cognition, and Personality: Empirical Studies*. New York: Springer.

Watts, R. (2003). *Politeness*. Cambridge: Cambridge University Press.

Whorf, B. L. (1956). *Language, Thought, and Reality*, J. B. Carroll (ed.). Cambridge, MA: MIT Press.

Wooffitt, R. (2005). *Conversation Analysis and Discourse Analysis: A Comparative and Critical Introduction*. London: Sage.

7 Writing and Society

The language–society nexus comes out not only in oral conversations, but also in practices and traditions of writing (Sebba 2009). Before the advent of alphabets, people communicated and passed on knowledge mainly through the spoken word. But even in oral cultures, tools had been invented for recording and preserving ideas in pictographic form, inscribed on walls, artifacts, and earthen structures. So instinctive is pictography, which is essentially writing in pictures, that it comes as little surprise to find that it has not disappeared from the modern world. The signs in public buildings (such as the "No Smoking" one), the emoji figures used in text messages and tweets, among many others, are modern-day manifestations of pictography.

Writing serves a host of social and cultural functions, from education to recreation. Some written texts, such as sacred, philosophical, and literary ones, are preserved by official institutions and studied in school, attesting to the investment of meaning put into them in a culture's history. The purpose of this chapter is to take a look at some of the main modalities and functions of writing in society. As mentioned in Chapter 3, Marshall McLuhan (1962) claimed that the medium of communication that becomes dominant in a particular society in a certain era of time affects people's ways of thinking as well as how they will evolve socially and intellectually. In a phrase, each major period in history takes its character from the medium of communication used most widely at the time. McLuhan called the period from 1700 to the mid-1900s the "age of print," because print artifacts, such as books, were the primary means by which people gained and shared knowledge. So, literacy became a major social value. With the advent of the electronic age, starting in the twentieth century, this value has not receded; it has been revised in terms of a broader view of literacy based in multimodal forms of writing on the Internet. As McLuhan anticipated, these have led to cultural paradigm shifts that parallel the rise of print literacy in the past— shifts that will be discussed in this chapter as well.

7.1 Writing Systems

The earliest pictographs were essentially picture signs representing objects and events that were of some importance to the users, given the effort to make them and inscribe them onto some surface. One of the first civilizations to utilize pictography as a means of keeping track of transactions and transmitting knowledge was ancient China. According to some archeological estimates, Chinese writing may date as far back as the fifteenth century BCE. As Figure 7.1 shows, pictographs start out as imitative sketches of something—for example, the sun and the moon. These then undergo stylization over time, so as to make the drawings easier to reproduce quickly and with less effort. The end result is a set of symbols, which are outlines of the original picture signs; these symbols form the basis of a writing system.

Pictographs are typically drawings that stand for concrete objects and ideas through resemblance. Drawing abstract or complex referents requires a more suggestive approach; one such approach is called *ideography* (Billeter 1990). An example of a contemporary sign constructed ideographically is the common "No Smoking" one, where a cigarette is crossed out to indicate that the action of smoking is not permitted. Increasingly abstract ideographs are known as *logographs*. These are signs replacing words or phrases, such as the following ones found commonly on keyboards: $, £, §, &, @, %, +.

7.1.1 Pictography and Alphabets

One of the earliest pictographic-ideographic writing systems was the one used in the ancient Sumerian civilization around 5,000 years ago, called *cuneiform*. It consisted of wedge-shaped characters, which the Sumerians inscribed on clay tablets, making writing expensive and effortful (Walker 1987; Goldwasser 1995). It was thus, at first, the privilege of the few, generally the wealthy and those in positions of authority. Nonetheless, literacy was considered an important value and imparted in Sumerian schools. To facilitate the speed of writing, the original cuneiform characters were streamlined and rendered more easily reproducible, as Figure 7.2 shows.

By about 3000 BCE, the Egyptians developed their own writing script—known as *hieroglyphics*—which they used to record hymns and prayers, to register the names and titles of individuals and deities, to annotate various community activities, to record historically significant events, for education purposes, and for other socially important functions. The script eventually

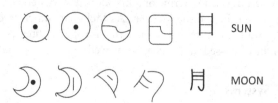

Figure 7.1 Pictographs

MEANING		OUTLINE CHARACTER, B. C. 3500	ARCHAIC CUNEIFORM, B. C. 2500	ASSYRIAN, B. C. 700	LATE BABYLONIAN, B. C. 500
1.	The sun				
2.	God, heaven				
3.	Mountain				
4.	Man				
5.	Ox				
6.	Fish				

Figure 7.2 Cuneiform Writing

developed *phonographic* elements within it—*phonographs* are signs standing for syllables or phonemes. In the case of the former, the system is known more accurately as a *syllabary* and in the case of the latter it is called *alphabetic*. Some of the first syllabaries were developed during the last half of the second millennium BCE. They are still used in some societies. Japanese, for example, is written with two complete syllabaries—the *hiragana* and the *katakana*—devised to supplement the characters originally taken over from Chinese.

A complete phonographic system for representing phonemes is called alphabetic. The first one emerged in the Middle East, and was transported by the Phoenicians (a people from a territory on the eastern coast of the Mediterranean, located largely in modern-day Lebanon) to Greece. It contained signs for consonant phonemes only. The Greeks added signs for vowel phonemes to complete it.

The transition from pictography to alphabetic writing was evolutionary, not revolutionary. The transition is explained in terms of the *rebus principle*, which implies that an alphabet character is the result of a stylistic alteration to some pictograph. Take, for example, the alphabet character A. It started out as a pictograph of the head of an ox in parts of the Middle East. The full head was drawn at some point only in outline form, standing for the word for "ox" (*aleph*). Around 1000 BCE, Phoenician scribes, who wrote from right to left, drew the ox outline sideways (probably because it was quicker to do so). The slanted Phoenician figure came to stand just for the first phoneme in the word *aleph*, which was pronounced as a consonant. At that point, the same sign could be used for the same phoneme, no matter what word contained it. The Greeks, who wrote from left to right, stylized the Phoenician letter further, and

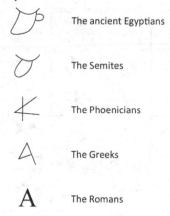

The ancient Egyptians

The Semites

The Phoenicians

The Greeks

The Romans

Figure 7.3 The Evolution of "A"

used it to represent a vowel phoneme. Around 500 BCE, alphabetic writing spread broadly. The A assumed the upright position it has today in Roman script, from which English has derived its alphabet. The "history of A," as it can be called, is shown schematically in Figure 7.3.

The Greeks started the practice of naming each letter with words, such as *alpha, beta, gamma,* and so on, which were imitations of Phoenician words (*aleph,* "ox," *beth,* "house," *gimel,* "camel"). They also introduced the idea of an alphabetic order, using the letters as well to stand for numbers in order—alpha stood for 1, beta for 2, gamma for 3, and so on.

It is interesting to note that alphabetic symbols, like any human symbol, have over time acquired social values. For instance, in American society, A is today a sign of high achievement, perhaps because it is the first letter in the alphabet. In a fascinating book titled *Sign after the* X (2000), Marina Roy has traced the history of the X sign, showing that it has had very little to do with phonetics at any period of its history, but everything to do with symbolism. Here are a few of its uses:

- any unknown or unnamed factor, thing, or person
- the sign for mistake
- cancellation
- the unknown, especially in mathematics
- the multiplication symbol
- a location on a map
- choice on a ballot
- the symbol for a kiss
- the symbol for Chronos, the Greek god of Time
- the symbol for planet Saturn in Greek and Roman mythology.

As this shows, whenever symbols gain social currency they quickly accrue connotative values. It is relevant to note that alphabets have been used to facilitate classification—for example, we might arrange books in a section of a library according to the names of the authors in alphabetical order. The transfer of databases onto the Internet has made classification more efficient and broader. Hyperlinks and search engine indexing systems now collect, parse, and store data to facilitate rapid information retrieval.

7.1.2 Writing and Society

As discussed briefly in Chapter 3, literacy and social power have been intertwined since antiquity. Those who gained high levels of literacy tended to be those who wielded authority and influence. Illiterate people relied on them to read and write for them; illiteracy has always implied power-lessness, socially and intellectually.

Literacy became a common social value after the invention of the printing press in the 1400s (Chapter 2). Although a Chinese printer named Bi Sheng invented movable type in the 1000s CE, it was not until the late 1430s that German printer Johannes Gutenberg perfected movable metal type technology, developing the first mechanical printing press capable of producing numerous copies of paper documents quickly and cheaply. The event was a paradigmatic one in the history of civilization. Printing shops sprung up all over Europe, publishing books, newspapers, pamphlets, and many other kinds of paper documents inexpensively. As more print materials became available, more and more people desired to gain literacy because it became an increasingly useful and necessary skill. Ideas could now be spread more broadly than ever before. This situation is cited by historians as the basis for the revolutions of an educational, religious, political, social, and scientific nature that led eventually to the Renaissance, the period marking the transition from medieval to modern times. Standardized ways of doing things in the scientific, education, and business worlds emerged, bringing people of different countries more and more into contact with each other, leading to the desire to learn each other's language. In a phrase, the invention of the printing press was an event that paved the way to the establishment of a global civilization. Marshall McLuhan (1962) called this new world order the "Gutenberg Galaxy," as mentioned briefly in Chapter 3.

With the Industrial Revolution during the eighteenth and nineteenth centuries, literacy became increasingly a society-wide necessity, as large numbers of people required even a minimal level of literacy to be able to work in the new urban centers. Governments began to understand the importance of literacy for everyone, not just for privileged classes, creating legislation to make elementary schooling obligatory. As a result, the literacy rate rose rapidly. Literacy has psychological and social consequences. It correlates with better health and social mobility. Public health research has shown that access to healthcare and improvements in health are connected with levels of literacy (Levine and Rowe 2009). For such reasons, literacy is now seen as a basic human right in many countries.

As discussed in Chapter 3, traditional print literacy is divided into two levels—pure and functional. The former refers to the ability to comprehend and produce writing; the latter refers instead to the ability to extract meaning from writing and to use it for intellectual and various social purposes (Gee 1996). Functional literacies have shaped knowledge practices throughout history (Schuster 1990; Lillis 2013). Illiteracy assigns people to marginalized communities. However, as we have seen, in the Internet age, the concept of literacy is morphing on a daily basis. Cynthia Selfe (1999) argues that the traditional notions of literacy, based on printed texts, must now include different kinds of literacies related to the new technologies. The range of literacy in the post-print era, therefore, includes not only the ability to read and write written text functionally, but also numeracy (mathematical literacy), and technological literacy itself, as well as the ability to access and use information technologies effectively and meaningfully. Nevertheless, the ability to read and write language remains a fundamental skill today. Even multimodal writing involves the amalgamation of print literacy with other literacies, especially visual literacy (Chapter 2), as will be discussed subsequently in this chapter.

7.1.3 Stylometry

The way people write can be used to identify them, since it constitutes an idiolect in the area of writing. It too is part of our linguistic identity (Chapter 5).

A branch of sociolinguistics called *stylometry* studies writing as a means to identify individuals. This has become a useful branch in areas such as authorship identification in literary criticism and in forensic science. It started with the work of Polish philosopher Wincenty Lutosławski in 1890 and is now based on the analysis of the relative frequencies of words and syntactic constructions that can be associated with a literary genre or a specific author. The data are collected and analyzed statistically to determine specific stylistic features, the sources of a text, the historical meaning of a text, etc. in order to determine who a writer of a text might be, or else what category of writing the text illustrates.

We all habitually use certain words, phrases, and other linguistic structures as part of our idiolect and communication style, even though we are hardly conscious of doing so. The stylometrist uses a statistical analysis of idiolectal habits as a means of establishing the identity of an unknown author of a text. But the method is not foolproof, because idiolects are always susceptible to variation from external influences, including contact with other speakers, the media, and changes in a language itself. Nevertheless, stylometric research has shown that grammatical and vocabulary styles tend to be fairly stable in individuals and largely impervious to outside influences even as people age. A written text can thus be examined for idiolectal patterns within it, measuring them statistically against known style features of the author. The analysis may at the very least be sufficient to eliminate an individual as an author or narrow down an author from a group of subjects.

A precursor example of stylometry is Lorenzo Valla's 1439 proof that the fourth-century document *Donation of Constantine* was a forgery. Valla based his argument in part on the fact that the Latin used in the text was not consistent with the language as it was written in fourth-century documents. One of the features that suggested forgery to Valla was the fact that some of the words could not have been written in that century. For example, Valla remarked, correctly, that the term *fief*, meaning "an estate of land associated with the feudal system," emerged much later.

Much scientific suspicion about the validity of stylometry existed until Donald Foster's study that correctly identified the author of the pseudonymously authored book *Primary Colors* as Joe Klein (Foster 2001). After that, its use spread broadly among linguists and forensic scientists, who use it to identify the author of some criminal text (Arntfield and Danesi 2017). The main technique (called *lexicometry*) involves identifying the most common lexemes that a particular person tends to use and then plotting them against their frequency distribution in a given text.

Stylometry is now a branch of *corpus linguistics*, or the quantitative study of language samples known as *corpora*. The objective is to derive a set of general principles of language design and usage, by extrapolating them from a statistical analysis of (primarily) written texts. For example, Quirk's 1960 survey of English usage and Kucera and Francis's 1967 quantitative analysis of a carefully chosen corpus of American English, consisting of nearly 1 million words, are early examples of corpus linguistic analysis. One of the offshoots of this type of work has been the preparation of dictionaries combining prescriptive information (how language should be used) and descriptive information (how it is actually used). Examples of the prescriptive versus descriptive dichotomy are included in Table 7.1. (Note that the term "descriptive" here refers to the actual form as it is used.)

7.2 Compressive Writing

The more a word or expression is written the more likely it will be replaced by a shorter equivalent, thus minimizing the effort expended to write it. This is

Table 7.1 Descriptive and Prescriptive

Actual form (descriptive)	Prescribed form
ain't	am not, is not, are not
gonna	going to
yeah	yes
outta here	out of here
goin'	going

why we abbreviate the names of friends and family members (*Alex* for *Alexander*, *Bob* for *Robert*, *Cathy* for *Catharine*, *Debbie* for *Deborah*), of common phrases (*TGIF* for *Thank God it's Friday*), and of anything else that refers to something common or familiar. Compression also takes the form of acronymy, that is, the abbreviation of phrases by using the first letters of their separate words (see Box 7.1).

Box 7.1 Common Compressive Forms

English

- 24/7 (24 hours a day, seven days a week)
- aka (also known as)
- ad (advertisement)
- ATM (automated teller machine)
- CD (compact disc)
- CEO (chief executive officer)
- DIY (do it yourself)
- DNA (deoxyribonucleic acid)
- ETA (estimated time of arrival)
- GNP (gross national product)
- IQ (intelligence quotient)
- PC (personal computer)
- PIN (personal identification number)
- TGIF (Thank God it's Friday)
- VIP (very important person)

French

- BP (*boîte postale* = post office box)
- H (*heure* = o'clock)
- HS (*hors service* = out of order)
- PDG (*président-directeur general* = CEO)
- RN (*revenu national* = GNP)

Spanish

- CÍA (*compañía* = company)
- LIC (*licenciado* = attorney)
- SL (*sociedad anónima* = Ltd)
- WC (*water closet* = bathroom)
- TEL (*teléfono* = telephone)
- UD (*usted* = you)

Whatever undergoes compression is either common or important. This is perhaps why (in the case of the latter) many institutions use abbreviations to represent themselves. These impart an implied symbolic status to them: AMA (American Medical Association), AP (Associated Press), CIA (Central Intelligence Agency), EPA (Environmental Protection Agency), EU (European Union), FBI (Federal Bureau of Investigation), IBM (International Business Machines Corporation), NATO (North Atlantic Treaty Organization), PBS (Public Broadcasting System), UN (United Nations), and so on.

7.2.1 Implications

As the foregoing discussion implies, compressive writing is used not only for the sake of expedience but also for symbolic reasons, conveying a kind of implicit expertise or savvy. It continues to be used commonly in this way in technical and scientific writing practices (in indexes, in footnotes, in bibliographies) (Nida 1992):

- ad lib (*ad libitum*) = as one pleases
- e.g. (*exempli gratia*) = for example
- et al. (*et alibi*) = and others
- etc. (*et cetera*) = and so forth
- ibid. (*ibidem*) = in the same place
- id. (*idem*) = the same
- loc. cit. (*loco citato*) = in the place cited
- NB (*nota bene*) = note well
- op. cit. (*opus citatum*) = the work cited
- QED (*quod erat demonstrandum*) = which was to be shown or proved
- q.v. (*quod vide*) = which see
- i.e. (*id est*) = that is
- v. (*vide*) = see
- vs. (*versus*) = against.

For everyday intents and purposes, compressed writing is used to make writing rapid and efficient. This is the case of frequently used words such as *laser* and *radio*, which are compressions (*laser* = light amplification by stimulated emission of radiation; *radio* = radiotelegraphy). It is also evident in the contraction of separate words into single forms to describe notions that have arisen for which no single word existed, such as *motel* (*motor + hotel*), *brunch* (*breakfast + lunch*), and *guestimate* (*guess + estimate*). It is also a central feature of netlingo, because it makes communication in cyberspace rapid (Box 7.2).

Netlingo, also called *textspeak*, is an ever expanding form of digital literacy. It now also involves word creations, such as those that result from blending separate morphemes, to make new ones in order to refer to digital culture more appropriately: *webonomics, netlag, netizen, hackitude,*

Box 7.2 Common English Netlingo Forms

2moro	tomorrow
2nite	tonight
brb	be right back
btw	by the way
fwiw	for what it's worth
gr8	great
ilu/ily	I love you
l8r	later
lmk	let me know
lol	laughing out loud
NVM	never mind
omg	oh my god
pov	point of view
ROFL	rolling on floor laughing
smh	shaking my head
swak	sealed with a kiss
YOLO	you only live once
xoxo	hugs and kisses

geekitude. Interestingly, as for all linguistic codes, variation now characterizes netlingo, so that it is no longer a singular form of online literacy, but rather one that differs according to users and Internet venue. For this reason, there are now Internet style guides that are aimed specifically at promoting general forms of netlingo. But, variation cannot be avoided—a fundamental principle of sociolinguistics. The linguistic diversity that is unfolding online may be different in detail from the one in offline contexts, but it nonetheless reveals how variation is part of language, no matter what medium is involved.

Netlingo developed originally in bulletin board systems and chatrooms so that users could type more quickly, relying on the redundancy features built into language: vowels, for example, are largely predictable in written words and thus can be eliminated with a minimal loss of meaning. Netlingo occurs across languages. In Mandarin Chinese, for example, numbers that sound like words are used in place of the words. There is now software that attempts to infer what words are being typed so that it can occur even more quickly. Websites such as *transl8it* (translate it) provide updates on netlingo so that it can be used more systematically and broadly for communication, like the Morse code and other telegraphic writing systems before it. As a consequence, there are now standard dictionaries and glossaries of textspeak available online.

The basic pattern in constructing textspeak words involves shortening a word in some linguistically logical way. For example, *I love you*, is shortened to *i luv u* or *ilu/ily*. Deciphering the form is dependent on user familiarity. Words and expressions that are used frequently in digital communications get shortened systematically. People use textspeak not to generate thoughtful and sophisticated communication, but to keep in contact and to facilitate communication quickly. In no way does this imply that people have lost the desire to read and reflect on the world. It is relevant to note that no less an authority on language trends than the Oxford English Dictionary has introduced many items from textspeak into its dictionary. This is an affirmation of the plasticity and adaptiveness of language.

7.2.2 Zipf's Law

Compressive writing brings out a communication principle—the reason why speakers minimize articulatory effort by shortening the length of words and utterances is to save on effort. As Harvard linguist George Kingsley Zipf (1932, 1935) demonstrated statistically, there exists an intrinsic correlation between the length of a specific word (in number of phonemes) and its rank order in the language (its position in order of its frequency of occurrence in texts of all kinds). This is known as Zipf's Law. It states that the higher the rank order of a word (the more frequent it is in actual usage), the shorter it tends to be (made up with fewer phonemes). For example, articles (*a*, *the*), conjunctions (*and*, *or*), and other grammatical morphemes (*to*, *it*), which have a high rank order in English (and in any other language for that matter), are typically monosyllabic, consisting of one to three phonemes. This law manifests itself commonly in the tendency for expressions that come into popular use to become abbreviated (*FYO*, *24/7*, and so on).

In 1958, psycholinguist Roger Brown claimed that compression tendencies correlate with meaning patterns, reflecting a broader principle, namely that language users will encode the concepts that they regularly need. And this determines the size of their lexemes. If speakers of a language need color terms to encode their experiences, then they will develop more words for color concepts than do other languages; and these words will be shorter than others: *red* (three letters), *green* (five letters), *blue* (four letters), and so on. Brown (1958: 235) puts it as follows:

> Suppose we generalize the finding beyond Zipf's formulation and propose that the length of a verbal expression (*codability*) provides an index of its frequency in speech, and that this, in turn, is an index of the frequency with which the relevant judgments of difference and equivalence are made ... Such conclusions are, of course, supported by extralinguistic cultural analysis, which reveals the importance of ... cattle to the Wintu, and automobiles to the American.

This interpretation of compression is not without its critics. The linguist George Miller (1981: 107) dismisses it as follows: "Zipf's Law was once thought to reflect some deep psychobiological principle peculiar to the human mind. It has since been proved, however, that completely random processes can also show this statistical regularity." But a resurgence of interest in Zipf's Law in the Internet age suggests something different— namely, that the relation between form and meaning is not arbitrary and that it evolves in specific contexts. In compression strategies there are two forces at work: a social force (the need to be understood) and the desire to be brief and relevant (which is one of Grice's maxims).

7.3 Literacy Practices

The topic of writing invariably leads to the social roles of literature traditions and literacy practices. All forms of literature, from poetry to fictional novels, constitute literacy and social practices at once. Myths, for example, are not just imaginative or fanciful stories, but also founding narrative theories about how cultural, ethical, and moral systems emerged in human life.

As Michel Foucault (1971) has argued, narratives are thus more than stories; they are tools of knowledge and of socialization, because literature "from high to low, from epic poems to Sunday-school prize books, [have] played a key role in shaping and effecting transformations in schooling and in the social function of reading" (Foucault 1971: xiv); and "literary texts help constitute the educational discourses and practices of their time as well as critically addressing them" (Foucault 1971: 32). Whether stimulating the childhood imagination, endorsing innovative educational methods, or appealing to specific reading publics, literature has always been crucial to social systems.

7.3.1 Myth and Narrative

In early societies, myths and sacred writing were linked. The word *myth* derives from the Greek *mythos*, "word," "speech," "divine tale." A founding myth (called *cosmogonic*) is a narrative in which the main characters are gods, superhuman heroes, mystical beings, and various supernatural creatures who interact with mortal and weak humans; the plots revolve around the origin of the world; and the setting juxtaposes the real world against a metaphysical backdrop. In the early writing systems, such as the cuneiform and hieroglyphic ones, myths were a primary form of narration. They recounted the imagined histories of early cultures.

Myth and language evolved in tandem. The Zuñi people of North America claim to have emerged from a hole in the earth, thus establishing their kinship with the land. From this founding story, the Zuñi language has a core vocabulary that involves metaphorical reference to the earth, farming, and the power of nature to bless and destroy human life. The Romans wrote down their early myths, such as the one of Romulus, who as an infant had to be suckled by a wolf, thus alluding to a supposed fierceness of the Roman people. The abundant vocabulary regarding war in Latin attests to the significance of this origin myth in Roman culture. English words such as *bellicose, battle, assault, antebellum, ally*, and others derive from this ancient core vocabulary.

Myths explain natural processes or events perceived to be crucial to the origins of a society through metaphorical language. The people of the Trobriand Islands in the Pacific Ocean believed that humans were immortal when the world originated. When they began to age, they swam in a certain lagoon and shed their skin. They quickly grew new skin, renewing their youth. One day, a mother returned from the lagoon with her new skin. But her unexpected youthful appearance frightened her little daughter. To calm the child, the mother returned to the lagoon, found her old skin, and put it back on. From then on, according to this myth, death could not be avoided. The lexicon of the Trobriand language is replete with metaphors relating age and mortality to physical appearance. The same metaphors are used to evaluate everyday occurrences in that language to this day.

Mythic metaphors leave their residues in all languages. We get the concept that "up" is where good resides and "down" where bad dwells from ancient myths. Many of the sacred places in antiquity were thought to be in the sky, on top of mountains; and the evil ones below the earth. The most sacred place in Japanese mythology is Mount Fuji, the tallest mountain in Japan. During part of their history, the Greeks believed that their divinities lived on Mount Olympus in northern Greece. The Greeks also believed in a mythical place beneath the ground, called Hades, where the souls of the dead lived. The Norse similarly believed in an underground place for the souls of dead persons, called Hel (the source of English *hell*), except for slain warriors, who went to Valhalla, a great hall in the sky.

The Greeks symbolized the sun as the god Helios driving a flaming chariot across the sky. The scientific word *helium* is a residue of this metaphorical symbol. Words for natural phenomena are typically derived from mythology. From the Germanic and Roman myths, we have inherited the names of the days of the week and months of the year: *Tuesday* is the day dedicated to the Germanic war god Tiu, *Wednesday* to the chief god Wotan, *Thursday* to Thor, *Friday* to the goddess of beauty Frigga, *Saturday* to the Roman god Saturn, *January* to Janus, and so on. Our planets bear a similar mythological nomenclature: *Mars* is named after the Roman god of war, *Venus* after the Roman goddess of love, and so on. This kind of analysis led anthropologist Claude Lévi-Strauss (1978) to claim that mythic language was the primordial mode of understanding, and that it continues to reverberate below the threshold of awareness in the words themselves.

Narrative traditions are derived from the early myths (Hodges and Davies 2013). To this day, we tell stories to children not only for entertainment and engagement, but also to impart knowledge, ethics, and the values that are significant to the culture in which they are reared. Children are never taught what a story is; they respond to it naturally, implying that narrative structure may be part of an innate competence. The term *emergent literacy*, introduced by Marie Clay in 1966, is used to refer to children's instinctive knowledge of what reading and stories imply before they gain formal literacy. It can be seen in the following typical childhood behaviors:

- Children are spontaneously interested in stories and storybooks, with no particular prompting.
- Children become aware early on of what storytelling and what reading entail; that is, they learn how to handle books (turn pages, for example) and how to follow words on a page.
- As children follow along when someone reads to them, they become aware of the connection between narrative and life.
- Narratives allow children to understand the function of words in describing events in the world.
- The child can easily reiterate plot lines and character descriptions meaningfully, connecting them to the words.

The Russian scholar Vladimir Propp (1928) argued that ordinary discourse was implanted in narrative traditions. The themes, concepts, and turns of phrase that become standardized in discourse practices derive typically from culturally significant narratives. For example, a concept such as *doublespeak* comes from the novel by George Orwell, *Nineteen Eighty-Four*. The actual term is not used in the novel—it is a blend of two words in it—*doublethink* and *Newspeak*. But the word has resonance beyond the narrative, because it is a semantic template for understanding aspects of contemporary society and discourse.

7.3.2 New Literacies

As Pérez-Sabater (2012) found in her study of writing practices on Facebook, new forms of literacy have evolved online, spreading to offline venues as well. In schools, it is not uncommon today for educators and students to move back and forth between online and offline literacies depending on writing tasks and functions (Crystal 2011). This bears significant implications for the future of functional literacy practices. Naomi Baron (2008) has claimed, however, that online literacy practices have little effect on offline ones, because they now exist as a dichotomy, with each one contextualized according to medium and social function. Others claim instead that online writing is strongly influencing how we view writing and even functional literacy.

Online writing practices may have actually increased sensitivity to the significance of writing itself, producing a kind of expanded literacy competence, which involves:

1   knowing when and how to use online literacy practices versus traditional forms of writing
2   knowing how to communicate effectively in both online and offline situations

3 recognizing differences between print and electronic literacies
4 understanding how traditional forms of writing can be enhanced via multimodality (photos, videos, and audio)
5 knowing how to communicate in virtual spaces according to online community
6 knowing how different slangs or jargons now interact in online and offline contexts
7 knowing how to mine information from the Internet and use it for both online and offline communications.

Today, "looking up something" means either consulting a wiki or Google, rather than a print dictionary or encyclopedia. The term *wiki* refers to any website that provides information of a specific kind—*Wikipedia* (encyclopedic), *Wiktionary* (dictionary), and so on. The difference between these information sources and the print ones is that they can be updated and edited routinely. Wikipedia is arguably the most influential of all the wikis. It was launched on January 15, 2002, by Larry Sanger and Ben Kovitz, who wanted, at first, to create an English-language encyclopedia project called Nupedia, to be written by expert contributors, in line with the Internet-based encyclopedia project called the Interpedia (launched in 1993). But they soon made the decision to have it written and edited collaboratively by volunteers and visitors to the site.

Needless to say, there has been controversy over Wikipedia's accuracy and overall reliability, because it is susceptible to the whims of users. The encyclopedia has remedied this situation somewhat (especially with "warning" annotations), but it still remains a kind of marketplace reference source, where knowledge can be negotiated, tailored, and discarded as the values of that marketplace change. The main idea behind Wikipedia is to bring the domain of knowledge within everyone's reach. The founders described it as "an effort to create and distribute a multilingual free encyclopedia of the highest quality to every single person on the planet in his or her own language." It makes further information gathering efficient by providing hyperlinks and other cross-referencing tools. The wiki entries are also linked to other digital forms (such as dictionaries provided by computer programs). Wikipedia allows anyone to be involved in a continuing process of creation, reconstruction, and collaboration in coding information and knowledge that is of relevance to a society (and even the world). Critiques of Wikipedia are that it is inaccurate and poorly edited. This may have been true at the start, but the Wikipedians have actually turned it more and more into a traditional, quality-controlled reference tool. Moreover, its infelicities soon get noticed and eliminated. Google has also changed many traditional literacy and literary practices and concepts, including copyright, authorship, and publication. When works fall into the public domain, anyone can use them as they wish without having to pay royalties and without being subject to any liability. This has led to a reevaluation of what constitutes copyright and how to enforce it. Millions of books are now available online. The noble idea of opening up all texts to everyone is highly idealistic, but it is problematic for the authors of books. In the US, copyright was included in the Constitution (Article 1, Section 8) for "limited times" and only to promote "the progress of science and useful arts." The Constitution put the public's right to access information before private profit. Google sees its mission as putting library collections online as a means of encouraging universal literacy—the ultimate goal of enlightened democracies as it has constantly asserted.

But, in actual practice, it is not the attainment of universal literacy that drives Google; statistics and popularity rule the Google universe (Carr 2008; Auletta 2009). Using algorithms, Google can easily determine the relevancy of sites via the number of clicks on the site, as well as the number of "Likes," and thus, by implication, the value of the site's content. As Carr (2008) argues, this meaning of value and relevancy is based on a science of measurement, not around any assessment of the intrinsic value of texts. As a result, Carr believes, Google has conditioned us to process information efficiently and statistically, not in terms of understanding. So, rather than encourage reading in the reflective sense of the word, Carr asserts, Google is leading to selective and superficial browsing, guided by the criterion of popularity. As Vaidhyanathan (2011: 89) has similarly put it: "We are not Google's customers: we are its product. We—our fancies, fetishes, predilections, and preferences—are what Google sells to advertisers." The questions raised by Google are the substance of ongoing debates across the social sciences and philosophy.

7.3.3 *Digital Literacy*

The study of the different literacies that have emerged in online contexts is sometimes included under the general rubric of *digital literacy* (Gilster 1998; Hobbs 2017). This can be defined as the ability to decipher, create, understand, and interpret digital texts (websites), platforms and venues (social media), and other aspects of digital culture correctly or meaningfully. Digital literacy implies the development of various subliteracies, such as the following (see also Chapter 9):

1   *mobile literacy*, which involves the ability to create and understand texts on mobile devices
2   *blog literacy*, which is similar to parallel offline literacy practices, such as the newspaper editorial
3   *virtual worlds literacy*, which implies gaining the capacity to function in virtual communities, which have developed new forms of language within them
4   *email literacy*, which is the closest to traditional print literacy, as used by businesses, schools, and other institutions; it is thus more sensitive to formal registers than other types of digital literacies

5   *instant messaging (netlingo) literacy*, which has developed its own informal language style, although corrective devices on mobile devices make spelling more complete.

Many features of digital writing parallel F2F communication. The term used in reference to this is *digital orality*, which implies that today's electronic media are retrieving a form of orality that harkens back to pre-alphabetic cultures. For instance, digital communications now typically entail real-time responses, whereas traditional written communications involve a time lag in receiving responses. As Walter Ong argued in *Orality and Literacy* (1982), the orality mode of early cultures can be called "primary"; the orality that has surfaced today through electronic communications can instead be called "secondary." So, paradoxically, even though we communicate by writing (emails, text messages, and so on), our expectations from the act of communication are similar to those of oral communication—that is, we expect an immediate or quasi-immediate response.

Written communication in social media also has the following features of orality:

1   It is elliptical and compressed in ways that parallel common oral speech.
2   It is synchronous (occurring in real time) like vocal speech, while it is also editable, like writing.
3   It is typically informal and highly conversational in style and mode of delivery.
4   It encourages immediate replies from one's interlocutor, as in oral communication.

7.4 International Writing Systems

In 2015 The Oxford Dictionary's "Word of the Year" was an emoji—the "face with tears emoji" (see Figure 7.4). The rationale for this selection was, simply, that the emoji was one of the most used new "words," and thus deserving of its word-of-the-year status.

This event signaled that a change in how we view writing in a globalized world of international digital communications had occurred. A word written with alphabet characters is designed to represent its phonemic structure, as discussed in this chapter. By the same token, an emoji is a pictograph that stands for a referent directly. It is a "picture word" that can be, in principle, used by anyone, regardless of native language, with the same (approximate) meaning. The original objective was in fact to allow people all over the world who wrote with different scripts to be able to communicate via this new form of pictography. Since 2010, Unicode has made a large repertory of emoji signs available for installation on mobile device keyboards and on apps, making emoji use a matter of routine—Unicode is an international encoding standard for use with different scripts.

Figure 7.4 Face-with-Tears Emoji

But the emoji phenomenon is not the first attempt to develop an international writing system—a kind of lingua franca script that would facilitate global communications. There have been previous attempts to unify people of the world through a common writing system—a fact that brings out, at the very least, the importance of writing in human civilization.

7.4.1 Artificial Systems

Several hundred artificial language systems had been proposed long before the advent of emoji. The term "artificial" is used to designate a language or writing system constructed for specific purposes. Today, only Esperanto is used somewhat regularly as an artificial language. It was devised by Ludwik Lejzer Zamenhof, a Polish physician, in 1887. It has a simple, uniform grammar—for example, adjectives end in /-a/, adverbs end in /-e/, nouns end in /-o/, /-n/ is added at the end of a noun used as an object, and plural forms end in /-j/. Its core vocabulary consists mainly of root morphemes common to the Indo-European languages. Its affinity to Romance languages, such as Spanish, would make it easily understandable to speakers of those languages; but not so much to speakers of other languages, thus decreasing its universality. Esperanto was supposed to be immune from outside interferences and to the typical dialectal and sociolectal variation of natural languages. However, as Benjamin Bergen (2001) discovered, even in the first generation of Esperanto speakers, the language underwent fragmentation and diversification, leading to Esperanto dialects.

Before Esperanto, the seventeenth-century philosopher and mathematician Gottfried Wilhelm Leibniz proposed a *characteristica universalis* as a set of symbols that he believed could be used universally to communicate philosophical, mathematical, and scientific concepts unambiguously. The international expansion of economic, scientific, and political relations in Leibniz's era made his project an attractive and significant one for many. But, as it turned out, the existing mathematical and logical symbol systems in use made Leibniz's *characteristica universalis* virtually superfluous.

Another well-known project for creating an artificial writing system is the one by Charles Bliss (1949, 1955). While living in China, Bliss became fascinated by the writing on shop signs. He quickly taught himself how to read them, with backup training, coming to the realization that he had been reading them not in Chinese, but through the conceptual lens of his own native language of German. From this experience, he set himself the mission of creating a system of written communication that could be used universally through symbols and that could be easily comprehended and used uniformly by anyone.

The script he developed, called Blissymbolics, consists of over 2,000 symbols, made up of basic shapes that can be combined to compose new symbols and even entire sentences and texts. The sequence in Figure 7.5 corresponds to the English sentence "I want to go to the movies."

The pronoun "I" is represented by the symbol for person (an upright stick on a platform) and the number "1," standing for "first person." The heart symbol stands for desire or wanting, and the curvy sign ("fire") emphasizes this meaning. The inverted cone figure on top identifies the symbol as a verb. The third figure stands for "to go" and is composed of the symbol for "leg" and the cone symbol for verb. The last symbol, which stands for "movies," is constructed with a house figure followed by the symbol for film ("camera") with the arrow indicating movement.

Clearly, Blissymbolics has qualities that could potentially bridge different systems of writing. However, outside of educational circles, where Blissymbolics has been found to help children with learning challenges acquire the ability to read and write effectively, Bliss's dream of an international writing system has never been realized.

7.4.2 Emoji Writing

Bliss's objective has been achieved somewhat by emoji writing, because of its spread through digital media, constituting a component of digital literacy (Danesi 2016). Text messages, tweets, Instagram notations, and even emails now are constructed typically with a blend of alphabetic and emoji writing.

Emoji are picture words, standing for both concrete and abstract referents. For example, a cloud emoji is a concrete sign that suggests the outline

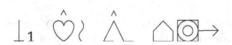

Figure 7.5 A Sentence in Blissymbols

Figure 7.6 Cloud and Sunrise Emojis

of a cloud. A sunrise emoji, however, is an abstract sign, showing the shape of a sun as it rises up from a background (see Figure 7.6).

Emoji surfaced as a means to enhance a broader comprehension of written texts in an age of global communications. But the diversity principle enunciated several times in this book has attenuated this laudable objective. Today, culturally based variation in emoji semantics and usage has emerged. Even facial emoji (or smileys) have undergone modification due to culture-specific needs. The smiley was presumed to be as culturally neutral as possible, with its yellow color that, ostensibly, would remove recognizable facial features associated with race or ethnicity, and with its round shape, again to attenuate specific details of facial structure that would otherwise suggest specific identity. But, almost right after the emoji gained international currency, new smileys were constructed to respond to the demand of users to make them more culturally sensitive or appropriate. So, different colors and shapes for the smiley emerged.

The ever broadening research on emoji use suggests that it has gone beyond a simple pictographic-ideographic script. It has assumed common discourse functions. For example, a smiley used at the beginning of a text message is an opening protocol, providing (usually) a positive tone that aims to ensure a phatic bond between interlocutors. Emoji usage also entails a considerable level of emotivity. In F2F communication, interjections, intonation, and other prosodic strategies are employed, alongside specific keywords and phrases, to convey feelings, explicitly or implicitly. In digital communications, these are typically rendered by emoji signs. Corroborating that the emoji code is, arguably, more a language than a script is the practice of writing texts completely with emoji. A famous example was PETA's (People for the Ethical Treatment of Animals) 2014 mobile-based campaign calling for social action against the mistreatment of animals. The campaign was known, significantly, as "Beyond Words." One of the original messages in the campaign can be seen in Figure 7.7.

The message implores a young woman (the leftmost emoji) to reconsider (shown by the thought bubble above her) that the items she might wish to buy (dress, shoes, purse, lipstick, boots), laid out in that order to become a "princess" (the rightmost emoji), are all animal products and thus destructive of animal life for purely casual lifestyle reasons. Interpreting the message requires more than just knowledge of the semantic possibilities of the emoji. It also requires knowledge of how they are combined

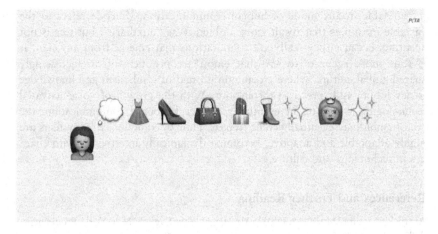

Figure 7.7 PETA Emoji Campaign

and laid out and, thus, how these are connected to each other sequentially and conceptually. Emoji texts of this kind require what can be called "emoji competence." Not everyone who sees the text will, in fact, make the association between the products and animals. In other words, like any mode of language use, the meaning of the message is implanted in modalities of contextualization.

The failure to eliminate variation and semantic ambiguity in emoji usage brings out the fact that all human systems are variable. The thumbs-up emoji is a case-in-point. In English culture, it is a sign of approval (see Figure 7.8).

This same emoji is offensive in various other parts of the world, where it is the equivalent of using the middle finger in America. The list of such culturally coded emoji is an extensive one, and need not concern us here. The point is that ambiguity, misinterpretations, and cultural coding are

Figure 7.8 The Thumbs-Up Emoji

unavoidable in any mode of human communication. Unicode refers to the variable meanings that result from ambiguity as "auxiliary"; but this is not accurate, because they really are connotations that emerge from any sign. It is thus more accurate to say that emoji are products of an increasingly shared global culture, where a common ground of symbolism and knowledge is developing and spreading throughout. With the growth of voice-activated technologies, which might eventually replace keyboard communication, the era of emoji may eventually come to pass. Human communicative systems are highly adaptable and adaptive, becoming dynamically intertwined with changes in technology and culture.

References and Further Reading

Arntfield, M. and Danesi, M. (2017). *Murder in Plain English*. New York: Prometheus.
Auletta, K. (2009). *Googled: The End of the World as We Know It*. New York: Penguin.
Baron, N. S. (2008). *Always On*. Oxford: Oxford University Press.
Bergen, B. (2001). Nativization Processes in L1 Esperanto. *Journal of Child Language* 28: 575–595.
Billeter, J. F. (1990). *The Chinese Art of Writing*. New York: Rizzoli.
Bliss, C. K. (1949). *International Semantography: A Non-Alphabetical Symbol Writing Readable in All Languages. A Practical Tool for General International Communication, Especially in Science, Industry, Commerce, Traffic, etc. and for Semantical Education, Based on the Principles of Ideographic Writing and Chemical Symbolism*. Sydney: Institute of Semantography.
Bliss, C. K. (1955). *Semantography and the Ultimate Meanings of Mankind: Report and Reflections on a Meeting of the Author with Julian Huxley. A Selection of the Semantography Series; with "What Scientists Think of C.K. Bliss' Semantography."* Sydney: Institute of Semantography.
Brown, R. (1958). *Words and Things: An Introduction to Language*. New York: Free Press.
Carr, N. (2008). *The Shallows: What the Internet Is Doing to Our Brains*. New York: Norton.
Clay, M. (1966). *Reading: The Patterning of Complex Behavior*. Auckland: Heinemann.
Coulmas, F. (1989). *The Writing Systems of the World*. Oxford: Wiley-Blackwell.
Crystal, D. (2011). *Internet Linguistics: A Student Guide*. New York: Routledge.
Danesi, M. (2016). *The Semiotics of Emoji: The Rise of Visual Language in the Age of the Internet*. London: Bloomsbury.
Foster, D. (2001). *Author Unknown: Tales of a Literary Detective*. New York: Holt.
Foucault, M. (1971). *The Archeology of Knowledge*. Trans. A. M. Sheridan Smith. New York: Pantheon.
Gee, J. P. (1996). *Social Linguistics and Literacies: Ideology in Discourses*. London: Taylor & Francis.
Gilster, P. (1998). *Digital Literacy*. New York: John Wiley.
Goldwasser, O. (1995). *From Icon to Metaphor: Studies in the Semiotics of the Hieroglyphs*. Freiburg: Universitätsverlag.
Hobbs, R. (2017). *Create to Learn: Introduction to Digital Literacy*. London: Wiley-Blackwell.

Hodges, G. and Davies, B. (eds.) (2013). *Narrative and Literacy*. Special Issue of *Literacy*, 47, April 2013.

Kucera, H. and Nelson Francis, W. (1967). *Computational Analysis of Present-day American English*. Providence, RI: Brown University Press.

Levine, R. A. and Rowe, M. (2009). Maternal Literacy and Child Health in Less-Developed Countries: Evidence, Processes, and Limitations. *Journal of Developmental & Behavioral Pediatrics* 30: 340–349.

Lévi-Strauss, C. (1978). *Myth and Meaning: Cracking the Code of Culture*. Toronto: University of Toronto Press.

Lillis, T. (2013). *The Sociolinguistics of Writing*. Edinburgh: Edinburgh University Press.

McLuhan, M. (1962). *The Gutenberg Galaxy: The Making of Typographic Man*. Toronto: University of Toronto Press.

McLuhan, M. (1964). *Understanding Media: The Extensions of Man*. London: Routledge.

Miller, G. A. (1981). *Language and Speech*. New York: W. H. Freeman.

Nida, E. A. (1992). Sociolinguistic Implications of Academic Writing. *Language in Society* 21: 477–485.

Ong, W. (1982). *Orality and Literacy*. New York: Methuen.

Pérez-Sabater, C. (2012). The Linguistics of Social Networking: A Study of Writing Conventions on Facebook. *Linguistik Online*56. www.linguistik-online.de/56_12/perez-sabater.html.

Propp, V. J. (1928). *Morphology of the Folktale*. Austin, TX: University of Texas Press.

Quirk, R. (1960). Towards a Description of English Usage. *Transactions of the Philological Society*:40–61.

Roy, M. (2000). *Sign After the X*. Vancouver: Advance Artspeak.

Schuster, C. (1990). The Ideology of Literacy: A Bakhtinian Perspective. In: E. A. Lunsford, H. Moglen, and J. Slevin (eds.), *The Right to Literacy*. New York: Modern Language Association.

Sebba, M. (2009). Sociolinguistic Approaches to Writing Systems Research. *Writing Systems Research* 1: 35–49.

Selfe, C. (1999). *Technology and Literacy in the Twenty-First Century: The Importance of Paying Attention*. Carbondale, IL: Southern Illinois University Press.

Vaidhyanathan, S. (2011). *The Googlization of Everything (and Why We Should Worry)*. Berkeley: University of California Press.

Walker, C. B. F. (1987). *Cuneiform*. Berkeley: University of California Press.

Zipf, G. K. (1932). *Selected Studies of the Principle of Relative Frequency in Language*. Cambridge, MA: Harvard University Press.

Zipf, G. K. (1935). *Psycho-Biology of Languages*. Boston, MA: Houghton-Mifflin.

8 Language, Mind, and Culture

As discussed in the opening chapter, linguistic anthropology and socio-linguistics share a large territory of research, theoretical interests, and overall objectives. The difference is one of emphasis. Linguistic anthropology focuses on the relation between language, mind, and culture; sociolinguistics on the social structures mirrored in, and shaped by, language and verbal interaction, as well as on the nature of variation in language usage. The dividing line between the two is a thin one indeed.

What connects the two branches in particular is a focus on how a language reflects the categories that are important to a culture and how these manifest themselves in vocabulary, grammar, and pragmatic strategies. As Edward Sapir (1921: 75), a founder of linguistic anthropology, wrote, the specific linguistic categories that speakers acquire in cultural context shapes how they understand the real world:

> Human beings do not live in the object world alone, nor alone in the world of social activity as ordinarily understood, but are very much at the mercy of the particular language system which has become the medium of expression for their society. It is quite an illusion to imagine that one adjusts to reality essentially without the use of language and that language is merely an incidental means of solving specific problems of communication or reflection. The fact of the matter is that the "real world" is to a large extent unconsciously built up on the language habits of the group.

This means that studying the linguistic categories of a people or a group will reveal cultural realities and needs and how these categories will double back on the mind, influencing perception and memory. John Lucy (1996) reviewed the effect of grammatical differentiation on memory tasks in English and Yucatec (a Mayan language) speakers, focusing on the presence of a dichotomy between the two languages: English requires a plural morpheme (/-s/) for count nouns, whether or not they refer to animate or inanimate things; Yucatec marks the plural only of nouns referring to animate things. Lucy presented pictures of Yucatec village scenes to both English and

Yucatec speakers, asking them to perform a recall task on the number of specific referents in the scenes. He found that English speakers were able to recall the number of both animate beings and objects; Yucatec speakers recalled instead the number of animate beings. Although this is a highly reductive paraphrase of the experiment, the point is that it brings out how the specific categories of a language might influence some aspect of mind, such as memory. This chapter will look at the synergy between language, mind, and culture.

8.1 Classification

In his study of American indigenous languages, Franz Boas (1940) discovered features that suggested to him that languages served people, above all else, as classificatory strategies for coming to grips with their particular environmental and social realities. For example, he noted that the Inuit language had devised various terms for the animal we call simply a *seal* in English:

- one is the general term for "seal"
- another refers to a "hair seal"
- a third refers to a "bearded seal."

This *specialized vocabulary* for referring to this particular animal is necessitated by the vital role that seals play (or have historically played) in Inuit life. In other words, the Inuit lexicon is reflective of Inuit reality—it allows speakers of the language to refer to and interpret those referents that are of significance to their everyday life in specific ways. The lexicon is thus much more than an arbitrary source of information about the things of the world; it is also a means to interpret them meaningfully and socially. In English, we use descriptive terms (usually adjectives, metaphors, and the like) for referring to seals: for example, *bull seal* and *elephant seal*, which are analogies to other animals that the seals appear to resemble. As this example shows, the study of the relation between language, mind, and culture starts with a study of the lexicon—the domain where sociolinguistics and linguistic anthropology intersect considerably.

8.1.1 The Lexicon

Words serve classificatory functions across societies, encoding realities that are perceived to be critical, useful, or common ones by particular peoples. In contemporary technological culture, specialized terms to name new devices and practices (*tablet, selfie, Snapchat,* and so on) are being devised on a regular basis, bearing witness to the importance of technology to modern society. Not too long ago, we possessed a sophisticated lexicon for referring to typewriters. Most of the terms have disappeared for the simple reason that we no longer need them, unless, of course, we are an antique collector of typewriters. In a phrase, changes in the lexicon mirror changes in society. The words we use for daily communication also have a "doubling-back" effect on us—they act as mental guides for both performing and interpreting everyday tasks. This does not block understanding beyond the words themselves. The paraphrases used above to convey the various meanings of the terms used by the Inuit language to refer to seals show that there are always ways in which the resources of any language can be used for the purpose of cross-cultural communication and understanding.

Naming the objects, events, plants, flowers, animals, beings, ideas, and so on that make up human experience allows people to organize the world conceptually. Words allow us to remember those parts of the world that are considered meaningful in the culture in which we are reared. Without them, the world would not have parts to it that can be recalled at will; it would remain a flux of impressions filtered through our senses and instincts.

Box 8.1 Inuit Vocabulary (Ottenheimer 2013: 18)

Seals

> *natchiq* (hair seal)
> *kiieaqq* (male seal in mating season)
> *tiggafniq* (strong-smelling bull seal)
> *quaibutlik* (ringed seal)
> *ugruk* (bearded seal)

Snow

> *aniu* (packed snow)
> *mixik* (very soft snow)
> *natibvik* (snowdrift)
> *nutabaq* (fresh snow)
> *pukak* (sugar snow)

Some of the detailed ways in which *seals* and *snow* are named by Inuit speakers of central Canada imply that these two referents have always played a crucial role in their society. The elaborate vocabulary they have created in this area of knowledge allows them to refer to seals and snow in ways that bring out their importance to daily life; and this leads to the emergence of specific detailed conceptual categories—categories that people who lived where, for instance, seals are not prominent in everyday life would not have needed to develop. When a word is coined for a specific reason, it automatically puts its referent into a category, projecting it into mental awareness.

Consider the word *cat*. By naming this particular animal, we have, *ipso facto*, differentiated it conceptually from other animals. Now, by having the word in our lexicon we are predisposed to attend to the presence of this creature in the world as real and distinctive. When a cat comes into view, we recognize it as such. However, since cats vary in appearance, size, etc. we might want to expand the category to include different types, naming them *Siamese*, *Persian*, etc. based on various historical reasons (which need not concern us here). This suggests a larger category that entails "catness." In English, we have devised a name for it—*feline*. Armed with this broad category, can now devise further differentiations of felines, naming them *lions, tigers, cougars, jaguars*, etc. At that point, we might stop the classification because we may no longer see lexical differentiations as useful or necessary.

Classifying felines in the way just described is just that—one way. We could easily have classified them into the some other category, along with *dogs* and *horses*, given that they are all four-legged creatures. Classification systems are not universal; they are products of historical needs and specific situational practices.

Because of the inbuilt relativity of specialized vocabularies, biologists decided early on to establish universal criteria for the classification of species, so that they could communicate with each other in a conventional way. The result has been a conventionalized lexicon that biologists use typically for their specific scientific purposes. But deciding what criteria are critical in science has always been a difficult problem. The classification of animals depends largely on the features animals are perceived to share. In general, the more features they share, the more closely they are seen to be related. The largest group is the kingdom *Animalia* itself, which includes all animals. Next, each animal is placed in a group called a *phylum*. Each phylum is divided into groups called *classes*. The classes are broken down into *orders*, and the orders into *families*. The families are split into *genera*, and the genera into *species*.

Such schemas are called *taxonomies* (from the Greek for "naming arrangements"). Taxonomies have always existed, even in prescientific eras. Early human beings divided organisms into two groups—useful and harmful, as archeological research has suggested. As people began to perceive important differences within these two broad categories, they developed new detailed ways to classify animals. One of the first generic taxonomies was put forward by Aristotle, who classified animals into those with red blood (animals with backbones) and those without it (animals without backbones). He divided plants by size and appearance into herbs, shrubs, and trees. Aristotle's scheme served as the basis for classification for almost 2,000 subsequent years. During the seventeenth century, the English biologist John Ray suggested the idea of *species* in classification, leading to the taxonomy system devised by the Swedish naturalist Carolus Linnaeus in the eighteenth century. Linnaeus classified organisms according to their physical structure, assigning distinctive names to each species. Modern classifications are based on microscopic structural and biochemical characteristics, as well as on presumed evolutionary relationships among organisms. The point here is that naming and classification are intertwined, and these two are always subject to modification according to need and social progress.

8.1.2 Concepts

Conceptual knowledge is not an innate feature of the mind; it is acquired through context. Like other animals, human infants come to understand the world at first with their senses. When they grasp objects, for instance, they are discovering the tactile properties of things; when they put objects in their mouths, they are probing their gustatory properties; and so on. In a remarkably short period of time, they start replacing sensory knowledge with conceptual knowledge, made possible by the names for things they acquire in rearing contexts. This event is extraordinary—all children require is simple exposure to words in social context for concepts to form in their minds. From that point on, they require their sensory apparatus less and less to gain knowledge, becoming more and more dependent on language to learn about the world.

Once a concept is lexicalized, then connotative processes expand its meaning considerably. Take the word *blue* in English. As a concrete concept, *blue* was probably motivated from observing a pattern of hue found in natural phenomena such as the sky and the sea, and by then noting the occurrence of the same hue in other things. At that point it became a color concept. The specific image that *blue* elicits in the mind will, of course, be different from individual to individual. But all variants will fall within a certain hue range. But that is not all there is to the meaning of *blue*. Speakers use the very same word to characterize emotions, morals, and other abstractions. Consider, for instance, these two sentences:

1   Today I've got the *blues*.
2   That piece of information hit me right out of the *blue*.

The use of *blue* in (1) to mean "sad" or "gloomy" is the result of a culture-specific emotional reaction to the color, reinforced by the tradition of "blues" music, which is perceived typically to evoke sadness or melancholy. The use of *blue* in (2) to render the concept of "unexpectedness" comes, instead, out of the mythic tradition of ascribing portentous meanings to the weather. This expansion of meaning is indirect evidence that the brain is an association-making organ, allowing us to connect referents in the world through words. In the nineteenth century, the early psychologists, guided by the principles enunciated by James Mill in his *Analysis of the Phenomena of the Human Mind* (1878), studied how subjects made such associations. They found that factors such as intensity, inseparability, and repetition played a role in associative processes: for example, arms are associated with bodies because they are inseparable from them; rainbows are associated with rain because of repeated observations of the two as co-occurring phenomena; and so on. Mill's analysis remains valid to this day—association and analogy are unconscious cognitive processes behind connotative tendencies in semantic systems.

8.2 The Whorfian Hypothesis

The view that a specific language affects perception, memory, and even world-view is commonly called the Whorfian Hypothesis (WH) (Chapter 1). The synergy between language and mind is generally unconscious, manifesting itself in various lexical and grammatical ways. For example, in English, we say that we read something *in a newspaper*, implying through that preposition (*in*) that we perceive the newspaper as a container of information "into which" we must go to seek it out. That is why we also say that *we got a lot out of the newspaper*, or that there *was nothing in it*. By way of contrast, Italian speakers use the preposition *su* ("on"), implying that the information is impressed on the surface of the pages through its words. In Italian, therefore, there are no expressions similar to *we got a lot out of the newspaper* and *there was nothing in it*. The difference in prepositional usage signals a difference in perception. This example encapsulates the essence of the WH. And, as discussed, this in no way implies blockage of understanding cross-culturally. It simply asserts that the way we perceive the world is reflected in our language categories. If cross-cultural communication is required, then we can always translate, paraphrase, and use other strategies to do so.

It must be mentioned that not every linguist accepts the WH for discussing the language–mind–culture nexus. Some have even called it a hoax (Pullum 1991; McWhorter 2016). The main critique is aimed at the so-called "strong version" of the WH, called *linguistic determinism*—namely that there is no thought without language, just feelings and instincts. This is a valid critique. The strong version is certainly not the one adopted here, neither is it the one that most anthropological linguists adopt. The so-called "weak version," or *linguistic relativity*, is much harder to debunk, for the reasons discussed already in the foregoing sections of this chapter.

Laura Martin (1986) has argued that the WH makes a specious claim, because it depends on what we mean by lexeme. In the Inuit language, it is obvious that there are different lexemic resources than there are in English for referring to snow. So, Inuit simply prefers individual lexemes, English prefers phrases and expressions instead. But the results are the same, with no influence on perception. Geoffrey Pullum (1991) concurs—morphemes such as *qani-* for "snowflake" and *apu-* for "snow lying on the ground or covering things up" are similar to English *slush*; the perceptual mechanisms are the same, the lexical ones are different (as would be expected). But this line of critique misses the point that different lexicalizations involve different needs and thus emphases. And this no doubt predisposes users of the words to pay attention to what they encode. Snow is a critical concept in Inuit culture and thus it comes as no surprise that it has salience lexically and grammatically, and that this salience doubles back on how snow is perceived by speakers of the language.

In sum, the WH claims that language and thought are intertwined and cannot be disconnected. It even finds some anecdotal validation in writing differences (Chapter 7). For example, those who are accustomed to writing from left to write tend to perceive past time as a "left-oriented" phenomenon and future time as a "right-oriented" one. To grasp what this means, consider a line which has a point on it labeled "Now."

Where would we put the labels "Before" and "After" on that line? We would tend to put "Before" to the left and "After" to the right, because we have become accustomed to seeing what is written to the left on a page as something that has been written "before," and what will be written to the right as something that will be written "after."

Those who are accustomed to writing from right to left will tend to reverse the order of the labels, for the same kind of reason.

Even before Whorf, the writings of eighteenth-century scholars such as Johann Herder (1744–1803) and Wilhelm von Humboldt (1767–1835), posited that language structures predispose native speakers to attend to certain concepts as being necessary, and others as not, even though they may exist and labeled differentially in other languages. This does not imply, however, that people cannot understand each other. The WH is a useful framework for studying languages in cultural context and how the specific categories of a language reveal what a culture considers important. Consider the way in which the device that marks the passage of time is named in English and Italian. In the former language, it is called *watch* if it is a portable object or worn on the human body, usually on the wrist, but a *clock* if it is to be put somewhere—for example, on a table or on a wall. In Italian, no such distinction has been encoded lexically. The word *orologio* refers to any device for keeping track of time, with no regard to its "portability." This does not mean that Italian does not have the linguistic resources for making the distinction, if needed. Indeed, the phrase *da* + place allows speakers to provide exactly this kind of information: *orologio da polso* ("wrist watch"); *orologio da muro* ("wall clock"); etc.

In effect, Italians did not find it necessary historically to distinguish between *watches* and *clocks*. They can refer to the portability of the device in other ways, if the situation requires them to do so. Speakers of English, contrariwise, refer to the portability distinction as necessary conceptually, attending to it on a regular basis, as witnessed by the two words in the lexicon. Historically speaking, the word *watch* originated when people started strapping time-keeping devices around their wrists. As the psychologist Robert Levine (1997) argues, this introduced a fixation with time that has been incorporated into English vocabulary and which affects how we have come to perceive time ever since.

8.2.1 Language and Thought

The idea that language shapes people's thoughts and memory recall caught the attention of the Gestalt psychologists in the 1930s. Carmichael, Hogan, and Walter, for instance, conducted a truly remarkable experiment to test this idea in 1932. The researchers found that when they showed subjects a picture and then asked them later to reproduce it, the reproductions were influenced by the verbal label assigned to the picture. The same drawing was shown to two groups of subjects (A and B)—two circles joined by a straight line. However, to group A the figure was labeled *Eyeglasses*, and to group, B, *Dumbbells*. Group A tended to draw an eyeglass figure in the recall task, and B a dumbbells one. Clearly, the name given to the figure influenced recall of the figure. There is no other way to explain the results, other than to say that the language labels influenced the way the subjects recalled the figures (see Figure 8.1).

Studies of the Navajo language of Arizona in relation to English have produced relevant insights into the nature of the WH. For example, the Navajo lexicon is rich with words referring to lines, shapes, and configurations. The language has around 100 words for this purpose, including the following three (Trask 1999: 47):

1 *dziisgai*, a word referring to "parallel white line running off into the distance"
2 *ahééhesgai*, a word referring to "more than two white lines forming concentric circles"
3 *álhch'inidzigai*, a word designating "two white lines coming together at a point."

Although the word *angle* is used in English for (3), it refers to the space between the lines, not the lines themselves. In effect, there are no equivalent words for these concepts in English. Navajo speakers have developed a sophisticated vocabulary for discussing spatial arrangements. Nevertheless, English speakers (or speakers of any other language) can come up with ways of grasping the Navajo words. The Navajo classificatory system suggests that the geometry of basic shapes has great cultural value. It thus comes as little surprise that Navajo toponyms (place names) are geometrical metaphors. Once classified, the world is passed on through language forms to subsequent

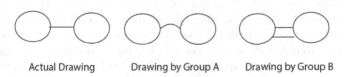

Actual Drawing　　　Drawing by Group A　　　Drawing by Group B

Figure 8.1 Recall Task (Carmichael, Hogan, and Walter 1932)

generations who acquire knowledge of the world through those very forms. Of course, subsequent generations can change their lexical filters any time they want, by simply inventing new words, discarding older ones, or modifying their meanings.

A classic study of Navajo children also dramatically showed how the connection between language and thought manifests itself (Kramsch 1998: 13–14). Navajo vocabulary lexicalizes the actions of "picking up a round object," such as a ball, and "picking up a long, thin flexible object," such as a rope, as obligatory categories. When presented with a blue rope, a yellow rope, and a blue stick, and asked to choose which object goes best with the blue rope, Navajo children tended to choose the yellow rope, associating the objects on the basis of their shapes, whereas English-speaking children almost always chose the blue stick, associating the objects on the basis of color, even though both groups of children were perfectly able to distinguish colors and shapes. In effect, the children tended to sort out and distinguish things according to the categories provided by their languages. Interestingly, Navajo children who had studied English chose the blue stick and yellow rope in a fairly equal way.

Many Navajo verbs designate specific aspects of motion and of objects affected by motion. For this reason, Navajo uses metaphors of motion, which manifest a specific kind of understanding and experience of the world that contrasts with English, as the examples in Table 2.6 of Chapter 2 show.

To reiterate here, to say "one dresses," Navajo speakers would say "one moves into clothing;" to say "one lives," Navajo speakers would say "one moves about here and there;" and so on.

Examples of differences such as those between Navajo and English abound. In English, when we say that something is *in front of us* or *ahead*, we imply that it will occur in the future; whereas something which is *behind us* is perceived as having occurred in the past:

1   Your whole life lies *in front* of you.
2   Do you know what lies *ahead*?
3   Just put all that *behind* you. It's ancient history.
4   I have fallen *behind* in my work.

These expressions seem so natural to us that we rarely stop to consider what they imply perceptually. We tend to imagine time as standing still while people travel through it, from left to right, influenced by our writing mode (above). The lexicon of the English language presents us with ways to articulate this. Greek speakers, however, perceive people as standing still while time overtakes them from behind. The future is still behind, and not yet visible, whereas the past is already in front, and thus visible. The Greek lexicon presents comparable ways to articulate this.

The language with which Whorf became fascinated was Hopi, an American indigenous language spoken in the southwest region of the United States (Whorf 1956). Today there are fewer than 11,000 Hopi people, half of whom live on a reservation in Arizona, in 11 villages on or near three high mesas (tablelands). Oraibi is one of the oldest continuously inhabited villages in America. It was founded about 800 years ago. Two things in particular about the language spoken by the Hopi caught Whorf's attention (SAE = Standard Average European):

1   *Plurality and numeration.* SAE languages form both real and ima-
    ginary plurals—"four people," "10 days." The latter is considered
    to be imaginary because it cannot be objectively experienced as an
    aggregate. SAE tends to objectify time, treating it as a measurable
    object ("two days, four months," etc.). Hopi, in contrast, does not
    have imaginary plurals, because only real aggregates can be
    counted. Moreover, it treats units of time as cyclic events, not as
    linear ones.
2   *Verb tense.* SAE languages have three basic tense categories that
    predispose speakers to view time sequences as occurring in the pre-
    sent, in the past, and in the future. Hopi verbs, however, are
    marked by validity morphemes, which indicate whether the speaker
    reports, anticipates, or speaks from previous experience, and by
    aspectual forms, which indicate duration and other characteristics of
    an action.

These two aspects of Hopi grammar, Whorf claimed, mirror their worldview and, thus, how they perceive reality and organize their societies. By not seeing time as an objectifiable phenomenon, the traditional Hopi people are less dependent on devices such as watches, timetables, and the like to carry out their daily affairs.

As American linguist Ronald Langacker (1987, 1990, 1999) maintains, phenomena such as those identified by Whorf imply that language forms are actually thought forms. Nouns, he claims, elicit images of referents that appear to trace a "region" in mind–space—for example, a count noun is imagined as referring to something that encircles a bounded region, whereas a mass noun is visualized as designating a non-bounded region. The noun *water* elicits an image of a non-bounded region, whereas the noun *leaf* evokes an image of a bounded region. This dichotomy produces specific grammatical structures—*leaves* can be counted, *water* cannot; *leaf* has a plural form (*leaves*), *water* does not (unless the referential domain is metaphorical); *leaf* can be preceded by an indefinite article (*a leaf*), *water* cannot; and so on.

Box 8.2 Nouns

Mass (noncount) noun

- a noun referring to something that cannot be counted, such as a substance or quality; in English a mass noun lacks a plural in ordinary usage: *rice, baggage, information*
- some mass nouns have a plural form when used in reference to different types: *coffees, breads, meats*

Count noun

- a noun referring to something that can be counted: *book, leaf*
- it will thus have a plural form and, in the singular, can be used with the indefinite article: *books, a book, leaves, a leaf*

8.2.2 Specialized Vocabularies

In Shinzwani (a language spoken in the Comoro Islands of the Western Indian Ocean), the word *mama* refers to both *mother* and *aunt*. The reason for this is that the two individuals perform similar kinship duties. As this example shows, naming kinship members mirrors cultural realities. In English, the primary kinship relations are lexicalized by the words *mother, father, brother, sister, grandmother, grandfather, grandson, granddaughter, niece, nephew, mother-in-law, father-in-law, sister-in-law,* and *brother-in-law.* English vocabulary also distinguishes between *first* and *second cousins* and *great-aunts, great-uncles,* and so on. However, it does not distinguish lexically between younger and older siblings. Moreover, English distinguishes a *nephew/niece* from a *grandchild.* But the latter distinction is not encoded in other languages. In Italian, for example, *nipote* refers to both "nephew/niece" and "grandchild." Amplifications to this area of a core lexicon occur whenever the need arises pursuant to social change—hence terms such as *stepmother, stepfather,* and so on.

Kinship terms reveal, in sum, how kinship is perceived, what relationships are considered to be especially important, and what attitudes towards specific kin may exist. Take, as an example, the Hawaiian kinship system, where relatives of the same generation and sex are referred to with a similar or identical term—the term used to refer to *father* is used as well for the father's brother and the mother's brother (for which we use *uncle*). Similarly, the mother, her sister, and the father's sister (for which we use *aunt*) are all classified under a single term. Essentially, kinship reckoning in Hawaiian culture involves putting relatives of the same sex and age into the same category. In the Sudanese system, the mother's brother is distinguished from the father's brother, and the mother's sister is distinguished from the father's sister. Each cousin is also named differentially. This system is one of the most precise ones in existence. In few societies are all aunts, uncles, cousins, and siblings named and treated as precisely.

Color terminologies are similarly specialized, as already discussed (Chapter 2). Potentially, we can perceive perhaps as many as 10 million hues. Our names for these are, thus, far too limited to cover them all. As a result, we often have difficulty trying to describe or match a certain color. A classic study of color terminology is the 1953 one by linguist Verne Ray. Ray interviewed the speakers of 60 different languages spoken in the southwestern part of the US. He showed them colored cards under uniform conditions of lighting, asking the speakers to name them. The colors denoted by *black, white,* and *gray* were not included in the study. Ray discovered that the terms overlapped, contrasted, and coincided. In Tenino and Chilcotin, for example, a part of the range of English *green* is covered by a term that includes *yellow*. In Wishram and Takelma, by way of contrast, there are as many terms as in English, but the hue boundaries are different. In still other cases, there are more distinctions than in English. Ray (1953: 59) concluded as follows: "Color systems serve to bring the world of color sensation into order so that perception may be relatively simple and behavioral response, particularly verbal response and communication, may be meaningful."

Shortly after, in 1955, Harold Conklin examined the four-term color system of the Hanunóo of the Philippines. He found that the four categories into which the Hanunóo grouped colors were associated with light and the plant world (the prefix *ma-* means "having" or "exhibiting"):

- *ma-biru* ("darkness, blackness")
- *ma-lagti* ("lightness, whiteness")
- *ma-rara* ("redness, presence of red")
- *ma-latuy* ("greenness, presence of green").

The *ma-biru* category implies absence of light, and thus includes not only English *black* but also many deep shades that English has named *blue, violet, green, gray,* and so on. The *ma-lagti* category implies instead the presence of light, and thus includes *white* and many lightly pigmented shades. The other two terms derive from an opposition of freshness and dryness in plants—*ma-rara* includes *red, orange,* and *yellow,* and *ma-latuy* includes *green* and *brown*. The Hanunóo language can, of course, refer to color gradations more specifically than this, if the need should arise.

In sum, specialized vocabularies serve specific cultural needs. Consider bodies of water. In English, we classify them as *lakes, oceans, rivers, streams, seas, creeks,* and so on. Because of their importance, criteria such as size enter the classificatory picture—*ocean* versus *lake*—as does width and length—*river* versus *stream*—among other features. Now, this rather detailed vocabulary no doubt reflects the importance of bodies of water in our social and economic practices, from shipping to cruising.

As another example, consider sitting objects, which are also important to English speakers, probably because of the extensive industry developed over time to produce such objects. Table 8.1 contains a few examples of how English vocabulary is specialized in this domain.

Again, this specialized vocabulary presents us with different ways to view sitting objects. One word would actually suffice practically; but for whatever cultural reason, this type of vocabulary serves classification needs that are probably connected to the action of sitting in social situations.

8.3 Ethnosemantics

The discussion of specialized vocabularies falls technically under the category of *ethnosemantics*, or the study of semantic systems in terms of their culture-specific implications. It was Franz Boas (Chapter 1) who established the principles of ethnosemantic research, emphasizing the study of language as a tool of understanding different cultures.

Data is gathered by fieldwork and basic ethnographic methods (Chapter 1). This implies that the analyst has to enter into contact with members of a specific culture in order to glean how the language allows its speakers to understand and interpret their particular reality. Ethnosemantics has developed several techniques to classify and organize the data collected ethnographically; one of these is *componential analysis*. The technique involves decomposing the meaning of lexemes into constituent elements as we shall see in the next section.

8.3.1 Componential Analysis

Consider these word sets:

1   father, mother, son, daughter
2   bull, cow, calf (male), heifer
3   dog (male), dog (female), pup (male), pup (female).

Table 8.1 Sitting Objects in English

Object	Distinguishing features (among others)
chair	sits one person, with a back
stool	sits one person, without a back
sofa	sits more than one person, with a back, soft
bench	sits more than one person, with a back, hard
lawn chair	sits one person, with a back that can be reclined
armchair	sits one person, with a back, soft

If we contrast the items in these sets with words such as *bread, milk, sword*, and *car*, we can easily see that they all share the property of animacy (that is, they refer to animate referents). Hence, the feature [+animate] would appear to be a basic component of their meaning. Now, comparing the items in set (1) with those in (2) and (3) we can see that they are kept distinct by the feature [±human]; and comparing the items in (2) and (3) it appears that further distinctions, [±bovine] and [±canine], are needed. Within each set, what keeps the first two items separate from the second two is the feature [±adult]. Finally, [±male] and [±female] are needed to ensure that all items contrast by at least one feature. We can show which distinctive semantic features are built into, or absent from, each word as Table 8.2.

The chart now makes it possible to show what differentiates, say, *mother* from *daughter* or *heifer* from *dog (female)*, in a precise manner. Although this is a useful way of establishing the differential meanings of lexical items, it can also produce anomalous results. The difference above between *heifer* and *dog (female)* can be given as either [+bovine] versus [-bovine] or as [-canine] versus [+canine]. There really is no way to establish which one is, conceptually, the actual trigger in the opposition. Moreover, when large numbers of words are decomposed in this way, it becomes obvious that to keep them distinct one will need quite a vast array of semantic features. The whole exercise would thus become artificial and convoluted. One might need as many features as words.

But componential analysis is nonetheless useful as a rudimentary organizing grid to classify lexical-semantic data collected in context. Generational differences in kinship systems such as the ones discussed in the previous section can now be mapped against one another in terms of specific semantic features.

Table 8.2 Componential Analysis

	animate	human	bovine	canine	adult	male	female
father	+	+	−	−	+	+	−
mother	+	+	−	−	+	−	+
son	+	+	−	−	−	+	−
daughter	+	+	−	−	−	−	+
bull	+	−	+	−	+	+	−
cow	+	−	+	−	+	−	+
calf (male)	+	−	+	−	−	+	−
heifer	+	−	+	−	−	−	+
dog (male)	+	−	−	+	+	+	−
dog (female)	+	−	−	+	+	−	+
pup (male)	+	−	−	+	−	+	−
pup (female)	+	−	−	+	−	−	+

Take, for instance, English kinship terms. In it, [gender] is a commonly used classificatory semantic feature—*mother-father, sister-brother*—as are [lineal, collateral relations]—*mother-aunt, son-nephew*. In Iroquois, kinship terms show similar distinctive features in the conceptual domain of generational and gender distinctions. But there are differences. Iroquois uses separate terms for older and younger siblings: older sister (*ahsti*)-versus-younger sister (*kheke*); older brother (*hahsti*)-versus-younger brother (*heke*). And it groups together lineal categories: father and father's brother (*hanih*); mother and mother's sister (*noyeh*).

Consider as one further example, the language spoken by the traditional Papago people of Arizona, which has a sophisticated core vocabulary for referring to plants, based on categories reflecting the environment in which the Papago lived historically:

- trees = "stick things"
- cacti = "stickers"
- cultivated seasonals = "things planted from seeds"
- wild seasonals = "growing by themselves"
- unlabeled = "wild perennials that are not cacti, trees, or bushes"

These show that the features [stick figure], [planting] and [growth] are essential in how the Papago speak about and perceive plants.

8.3.2 Schemas

The notion of *cultural schema* (CS) is sometimes used within ethnosemantics (Nishida 1999), defined as a unit of cultural knowledge that people use when they interact with members of the same society in certain situations and talk about certain topics (Malcolm and Sharafian 2002). CSs are thus structures of information derived from cultural experiences that allow people to interpret the world in communal ways. The main types of CSs according to Nishida (1999) are as follows:

1   *Fact-and-concept schemas*: These encode general information about the world, such as the fact that New York is a city in America, or the fact that automobiles are vehicles with (generally) four wheels and a motor.
2   *Person schemas*: These refer to people and their personality traits, and are typically encoded by adjectives and other qualitative lexemes: *shy, outgoing, cute, intelligent*. They are portrayals of personality features that are steeped in cultural experiences and traditions.
3   *Self schemas*: These refer to how people see themselves, and thus to how they expect others to see them. Personal pronouns (*I, you*), for instance, allow people to juxtapose themselves against others through deictically based reference.

4   *Role schemas*: These refer to social roles that condition sets of behaviors in given situations. These are encoded by registers and specific styles.
5   *Context schemas*: These refer to how certain contexts can change linguistic meanings and how it is possible to adapt to these.
6   *Procedure schemas*: These refer to the relevant sequences of events that apply in common situations. At a restaurant, the order of speech mirrors the order in which dishes are served.
7   *Strategy schemas*: These involve the language used to solve problems. Pedagogical discourse is full of strategy schemas. For instance, a music teacher might say "bring this up" in order to get a student to play an instrument louder.
8   *Emotion schemas*: These are schemas that contain affective information, such as "I love you with all my heart."

CS theory and conceptual metaphor theory appear to share many notions (Chapter 2). Recall that a metaphorical statement such as "That person is a snake" connects two referents: (1) "that person" and (2) "a snake." The linkage of the two is guided by a mental schema that infers similarities between the two referents, encoded in the conceptual metaphor, *people are animals*. The schema engenders a perspective of personality that literal language cannot possibly convey—a perspective that is based on cultural experiences and representations of snakes as dangerous reptiles. The reason why we speak this way, claims Lakoff (1987), is because we unconsciously perceive qualities in one domain (the animal kingdom) as coexistent in another domain (human personality).

8.4 Language and Mind in Cyberspace

The study of the language–mind nexus today has been extended to cyberspace. A premise of the WH inheres in seeing the various subsystems of language not as autonomous phenomena, to be studied in and of themselves, but also in relation to the media environments in which they occur.

Cyberspace is one of those environments. Like never before, the new technologies allow us to collect or mine linguistic data and to make much more accurate assessments of patterns within the data. At the same time, it behooves linguists to deconstruct any dangers that new media might harbor. In George Orwell's (1903–1950) 1949 novel, *Nineteen Eighty-Four*, the government, like a "big brother," watches and monitors every move its citizens make in order to detect any signs of unrest or nonconformity. To control the minds of citizens, big brother impels them to use what Orwell calls Newspeak—a form of language meant to manipulate thought. Orwell's warning is thus a Whorfian one; it has become particularly relevant in the current world, where data mining has become common, allowing agencies to compile information on individuals, without them knowing it.

8.4.1 The WH and the Online World

If different languages encode different conceptual categories, which may affect the way people think, then the changes that are taking place in online culture should have an impact on existing worldviews. Lanchantin, Simoëos-Perlant, and Largy (2012) examined the instant messages of 32 French-speaking students aged 13. They found that the students used a form of "graphemic cognition" that translates sounds into letters and expressions. In other words, digital writing practices guided the structure of their messages. In contrast, Tagliamonte and Denis (2008) collected data from traditional and digital texts of English-speaking adolescents between the ages of 15 and 20, noting that there were no differences in how the languages were used to encode the same referents. But Baron (2010) contested this pattern of findings suggesting that the use of words is reduced as much as possible in digital writing, making it vastly different, and thus influencing the content of messages.

Huang, Yen, and Zhang (2008) looked at the effects of emoticons on users of instant messages (IMs). The results showed that emoticon use had a positive effect on personal interaction, perceived information richness, and the perceived usefulness of a communication. The findings suggested, therefore, that emoticons were not just decorative devices, but also a way of involving people cognitively and emotionally that may have little or no corresponding structures in print writing. The same can probably be extended to the use of emoji (previous chapter).

Zappavigna (2011) explored how language is used to build a community via Twitter. A corpus of 45,000 tweets was collected in the 24 hours after the announcement of Barack Obama's victory in the 2008 US presidential election. Zappavigna looked at the evaluative language used in tweets. She found that the hashtag itself had extended its meaning to operate as a linguistic marker referencing the target of evaluation in a tweet (#Obama). This rendered the language searchable and used to upscale the values expressed in the tweet. Zappavigna concluded that there is now a new perception of communication that she labeled "searchable talk." The subtext is: "Search for me and affiliate with my value!"

8.4.2 Big Data

Large datasets, known as *big data*, can be analyzed computationally to reveal patterns, trends, and conceptual associations. The use of such data has enormous implications for privacy as well as implications regarding the threat of manipulation by those who compile such data, such as government agencies, advertisers, and the like. Big data are used to predict behavior and to spot trends. For this reason, they are also used for benevolent purposes, such as preventing crime and diseases. The main sources for big data collection include:

1   *Streaming data*, analyzed as they arrive allowing analysts to make decisions on what to keep and what to discard.
2   *Social media data*, organized by algorithms designed to mine from the data some required pattern.
3   *Publicly available data*, including data obtainable from the US government's data.gov, the CIA's World Factbook or the European Union's Open Data Portal.

Studying the relation between data collected algorithmically and language is something that is gaining ground in sociolinguistics (Hiltunen, McVeigh, and Säilly 2017). A particularly relevant area is the connection between the world of global communications and evolving forms of intelligence via patterns in the big data. Derrick de Kerckhove (1997) claimed a few decades ago that the global village, based on the Internet, has provided a critical mass in the emergence of a new form of intelligence, called *collective intelligence*, which means that the sum total of the ideas of people are perceived as more important than those of any one individual. He speculated that we have undergone one of the greatest evolutionary leaps in the history of our species. The architecture of connected intelligence resembles that of a huge brain whose cells and synapses are encoded in software and hardware that facilitate the assemblage of minds. In this environment, we are all just one part of the collective mind, whose ideas are carried by software and hardware systems that overlap with them and with relevant data and information.

Today, cyberspace contains an infinitude of documents, databases, electronic publications, etc. The miasma of information it contains made it immediately obvious, shortly after its introduction, that appropriate technology was needed to locate specific types of information. This led to the development of uniform resource locator (URL) technology. Using software that connects a computer to the Internet a user can select a URL that contains information. The computer then contacts that address, making the information available to the user. With millions of separate URLs, classification and indexing have clearly become critical Internet functions. Indexing services—located on the Internet itself—enable users to search for specific information by entering the topic that interests them.

The transfer of large databases onto the Internet has created a new way of viewing and organizing the classification of information. People can post their own messages, opinions, commentaries, and ideas on any subject imaginable on websites, on personal blogs, etc. It has also become a primary reference tool with online dictionaries, encyclopedias, etc. Unlike printed texts, Internet pages can be updated constantly and, thus, are never out of date. Cyberspace is fast becoming a common space to which people will resort routinely to interact socially and intellectually. The new digital technologies have thus had a conspicuous impact on how we classify, understand, and seek information, and even how we view literature. Some digital novels allow for huge numbers of plot twists to be built into a story. They might also enable readers to observe the story unfold from the perspective of different characters. Readers may also change the story themselves to suit their interpretive fancies. In such novels, the author sets a framework for the narrative; but the actual narrative is realized by the reader. The same kind of editing power is now applicable to many (if not most) kinds of Internet documents, from web-based encyclopedias and dictionaries to online textbooks.

Despite the advent of cyberspace, there is still little doubt that our native languages influence the way we perceive the world (Deutscher 2005). The linguistic habits formed in childhood rarely leave us, although they may be shaped by new media and new modes of understanding the world. Certainly, the connections between language and mind, language and technology, and language and media are becoming ever more important in the world of big data and algorithms (a topic that will be taken up again in the next chapter).

References and Further Reading

Baron, N. S. (2010). Discourse Structures in Instant Messaging: The Case of Utterance Breaks. *Language@Internet* 7. language@internt.org/articles/2010/2651/Baron.

Boas, F. (1940). *Race, Language, and Culture.* New York: Free Press.

Carmichael, L., Hogan, H. P., and Walter, A. A. (1932). An Experimental Study of the Effect of Language on Visually Perceived Form. *Journal of Experimental Psychology* 15: 73–86.

Conklin, H. (1955). Hanonóo Color Categories. *Southwestern Journal of Anthropology* 11: 339–344.

De Kerckhove, D. (1997). *Connected Intelligence: The Arrival of the Web Society.* Toronto: Somerville.

Deutscher, G. (2005). *Why the World Looks Different in Other Languages.* New York: Henry Holt.

Hiltunen, T., McVeigh, J., and Säilly, T. (2017). How to Turn Linguistic Data into Evidence. *Studies in Variation, Contacts, and Change in English* 19. www.helsinki.fi/varieng/series/volumes/19/introduction.html.

Huang, A. H., Yen, D. C., and Zhang, X. (2008). Exploring the Potential Effects of Emoticons. *Information & Management* 45: 466–473.

Kramsch, C. (1998). *Language and Culture.* Oxford: Oxford University Press.

Lakoff, G. (1987). *Women, Fire, and Dangerous Things: What Categories Reveal About the Mind.* Chicago: University of Chicago Press.

Lanchantin, T., Simoëos-Perlant, A., and Largy, P. (2012). The Case of Digital Writing in Instant Messaging: When Cyber Written Productions Are Closer to the Oral Code Than the Written Code. *Psychology Journal* 10: 187–214.

Langacker, R. W. (1987). *Foundations of Cognitive Grammar.* Stanford, CA: Stanford University Press.

Langacker, R. W. (1990). *Concept, Image, and Symbol: The Cognitive Basis of Grammar.* Berlin: Mouton de Gruyter.

Langacker, R. W. (1999). *Grammar and Conceptualization.* Berlin: Mouton de Gruyter.

Levine, R. (1997). *A Geography of Time: The Temporal Misadventures of a Social Psychologist or How Every Culture Keeps Time Just a Little Bit Differently.* New York: Basic Books.

Lucy, J. (1996). The Scope of Linguistic Relativity: An Analysis and Review of Empirical Research. In: J. Gumperz and S. Levinson (eds.), *Rethinking Linguistic Relativity*, pp. 37–70. New York: Cambridge University Press.

Malcolm, I. G. and Sharafian, F. (2002). Aspects of Aboriginal English Oral Discourse: An Application of Cultural Schema Theory. *Discourse Studies* 4: 169–181.

Martin, L. (1986). Eskimo Words for Snow: A Case Study in the Genesis and Decay of an Anthropological Example. *American Anthropologist* 88: 418–423.

McLuhan, M. (1964). *Understanding Media: The Extensions of Man*. London: Routledge.

McWhorter, J. H. (2016). *The Language Hoax*. Oxford: Oxford University Press,

Mill, J. (1878). *Analysis of the Phenomena of the Human Mind*. London: Longman.

Nishida, H. (1999). Cultural Schema Theory. In: W. B. Gudykunst (ed.), *Theorizing About Intercultural Communication*, pp. 401–418. Thousand Oaks, CA: Sage.

Ottenheimer, H. J. (2013). *The Anthropology of Language: An Introduction to Linguistic Anthropology*. Belmont, MA: Wadsworth.

Pullum, G. (1991). *The Great Eskimo Vocabulary Hoax and Other Irreverent Essays on the Study of Language*. Chicago: University of Chicago Press.

Ray, V. (1953). Human Color Perception and Behavioral Response. *Transactions of the New York Academy of Sciences* 16.

Sapir, E. (1921). *Language*. New York: Harcourt, Brace, & World.

Tagliamonte, S. A. and Denis, D. (2008). Linguistic Ruin? Lol! Instant Messaging and Teen Language. *American Speech* 83: 3–34.

Trask, R. (1999). *Language: The Basics*. London: Routledge.

Whorf, B. L. (1956). *Language, Thought, and Reality*, J. B. Carroll (ed.). Cambridge, MA: MIT Press.

Zappavigna, M. (2011). Ambient Affiliation: A Linguistic Perspective on Twitter. *New Media & Society* 135: 788–806.

9 Language, Media, and Social Evolution

As illustrated throughout this book, the overall objective of sociolinguistics is to study the synergy that exists among language, society, culture, and verbal interaction. Everything from conversations, honorifics, slang, and text messaging to bilingualism and language maintenance in immigrant communities is of interest to sociolinguistics, which also has in its purview the effects of media of all kinds on language and social evolution. Take, for example, an electronic writing medium such as blogging, which has largely replaced the traditional print article. Blogs originated in the chat groups of the early Internet, some of which go as far back as bulletin boards. It is estimated that there are more than 100 million blogs worldwide, covering the entire gamut of human interest, from politics to pop culture.

Blogs have several advantages over traditional print articles. First, they have the ability to reach a broad (and potentially international) readership instantaneously and cheaply, whereas print articles take more time to release, have a circumscribed circulation, and entail many more costs to publish. Blogs are edited online directly and thus can be updated continuously, whereas print articles need to be revised and republished over a period of time. Blogs can be maintained permanently on websites and indexed in any way one wishes (in the order in which they were written, according to theme, and so on). Feedback is rapid, because most blogs allow for readers to respond and leave comments to which the blogger can reply in turn. Comments are the basis for the trackback feature, which transmits alerts to previous commentators. In addition, permalinks allow users to comment on specific posts rather than on entire blogs, and this, in turn, allows the blog to create an archive of past posts.

The advent of blogging has had sociopolitical consequences, as evidenced by various events in the new millennium (Rodzvilla 2009). In one highly publicized case, bloggers critiqued the comments made by US Senate majority leader Trent Lott at a party in honor of Senator Strom Thurmond. Lott suggested that Thurmond would have made the ideal president. The bloggers portrayed this as implicit approval of racial segregation, because Thurmond had seemingly promoted it in his 1948 presidential campaign, as documents recovered by the bloggers showed. The mainstream media had never reported on this story until after the bloggers broke it. Lott stepped down as majority leader, likely because of the blogs. As this one single example shows, blogs and social media have become sources of influence in political matters, shaping public opinion.

Clearly, language, society, and media (old and new) are variables in a sociolinguistic equation—when one of these changes in the equation, so too do the others. Sometimes the trigger for change might be the language itself; other times it may be the medium; and other times still it may be social change. This final chapter will look at aspects of this equation.

9.1 Medium and Language

The Internet-based global village in which we live has heightened sensitivity to the plight of others across the world. Digital media offer an effective means for bringing about social justice, as the #MeToo movement against sexual harassment and sexual assault has shown. Of course, philanthropy and social justice are not inventions of the digital age—they have always been a part of human history. But because of the global reach of digital media, today they can be promoted more broadly than in the past. By the same token, the dangers of the digital world are rather stark, including the spread of hate memes and fake content spreading just as broadly throughout cyberspace.

Digital media may also be changing many of the traditional social rules and patterns of behavior. Tossell et al. (2012), for example, studied the use of emoticons in text messages aiming to determine how the genders differed in the frequency and variety of their usage. Previous research had found small and sundry differences in emoticon use between genders, suggesting that technology was closing the gender gap in communicative behaviors. Tossell et al. confirmed this, discovering that males used as diverse a range of emoticons as the females. This neutralization of gender-based patterns may have spread to the offline world. A similar pattern of findings emerged from a study conducted by Ilona Vandergriff in 2013. Similarly, Huffaker and Calvert (2005: 19) found that "blogs operated by young males and females are more alike than different" and that females no longer use "language that is more passive, accommodating, or cooperative." These studies appear to document how social change is being mirrored in, and perhaps even influenced by, the language and modalities of interaction brought about by digital media.

In a comprehensive study, Varnhagen, Mcfall, and Pugh (2010) collected instant messaging texts over a one-week period from adolescents in order to examine the evolution of communicative competencies in online and offline interactions. The researchers gave the subjects a writing task to be carried out in the two contexts and found that shortcuts, abbreviations, acronyms, unique spellings, and emoticons were most prevalent in the instant message texts, as expected; however, they found that punctuation and spelling errors were relatively uncommon in the written assignments. They concluded that the digital medium does not have a deleterious effect on conventional literacy. This suggests, more broadly, that we are developing a new adaptive form of communicative competence, shaped by the medium used and its related contextual factors (as discussed already in previous chapters).

9.1.1 Language and Virtual Communities

Because of digital media, the sociolinguistic study of speech communities has been expanded accordingly to include virtual communities (also as mentioned previously). A virtual community (VC) is a "social aggregation that emerges from the Net when enough people carry on public discussions long enough, with sufficient human feeling, to form webs of personal relationships in cyberspace" (Rheingold 1993: 5). Unlike real-world speech communities, VCs lack the commitment, longevity, and accountability among members that would make them qualify as communities in the traditional sense. As Manuel Castells (2001: 389) has put it, VCs "do not follow the same patterns of communication and interaction as physical communities do. But they are not 'unreal,' they work in a different plane of reality." Some of the aspects of VCs that are now targets of sociolinguistic research are the following (Preece, Maloney-Krichmar, and Abras 2003; Gruzd, Wellman, and Takhteyev 2011):

1   VCs involve regular communication around a shared purpose or interest.
2   Linguistic and social practices are based on this interest, including the development of specialized vocabularies and sociolects, as for example, twitterlects.
3   The construction (or reconstruction) and negotiation of identities occurs within the VCs and these are mapped against offline identities.
4   VC linguistic norms develop spontaneously in order to allow members to organize interactions and to make conversation and dialogue fluid and efficient.
5   Social rituals are developed to maintain social distinctions of various kinds (and not necessarily based on real-world class and social backgrounds).
6   VCs are organized around "a shared, negotiated, and fairly specific enterprise" (Meyerhoff 2006), and thus occasional users of the same site may not truly be part of the enterprises, but just onlookers.
7   VCs are self-sustaining because they are open to newcomers. On Twitter, for instance, any user can start following any other user without requiring the other to follow them back.

The study of VCs has also led to an expansion of research methods and data collection techniques (Chapter 1). Some of these are listed below:

1   *Online interviews* are conducted through computers screens, allowing researchers to gather the same kind of information about VCs that applies to real-life speech communities.
2   *Social media ethnography* is the method whereby a researcher joins a specific VC group and observes reactions to communicative events from within the group.
3   *Big data* sources (Chapter 8) now can help collect data on VCs easily.
4   *Data-mining techniques* provide information on usage habits, while at the same time providing information on how conversations are unfolding in specific VCs.

9.1.2 Convergence

The arrival of new media via the Internet has brought about a phenomenon known generally as convergence. The term is used with several meanings, such as the erosion of traditional distinctions among media due to concentration of ownership, globalization, and audience fragmentation, and the process by which formerly separate technologies such as television and the telephone are brought together through digitation. For example, the Internet has permitted media convergence, because it can deliver digitized print, images, sound, voice, and data equally well.

Henry Jenkins (2006) has broken down the meanings of convergence as shown:

1   *Technological convergence*, or the digitization of content allowing for its distribution without any of the previous quality filters, so that anyone can record, videotape, and upload content.
2   *Economic convergence*, whereby mega-companies buy up media content and distribute it broadly throughout cyberspace.
3   *Social convergence*, which implies that many of the traditional distinctions people reared in different social contexts are being attenuated, influenced by technological and economic convergence.
4   *Cultural convergence*, which means that some traditional cultural distinctions are becoming less marked in the global village.
5   *Global convergence*, which means that in the global village there is an admixture of hybrid cultural products arising from global exchanges.

The term convergence is also used in sociolinguistics to describe how people use various media to make messages. For example, studies of selfies have shown that they involve a new way to enact the presentation of Selfhood, which may have psychological implications (Balakrishnan and Griffiths 2018). This type of convergence, where the visual and the textual are merged, is a powerful form of communication. It implies a new kind of competence that may be called simply multimedia competence, defined as the ability to merge various media in the construction of messages and in the enactment of social interactions.

9.2 Mediation

The foregoing discussion was meant to emphasize that communication today is shaped by changes in media, more so than at any other time in the past. In a way, we are undergoing a second paradigm shift with the first one being the advent of alphabets (McLuhan 1964).

The first alphabets appeared in Phoenicia and other Semitic-speaking areas of the ancient world around 1000 BCE (Chapter 7). McLuhan saw this event as igniting a cognitive revolution because, for the first time in human history, symbols were used to represent words. Called the "alphabet principle" it changed the sensory environment for knowledge-making, from acoustic to visual. Writing is a displacement from a direct sensory experience of the world to one mediated by symbols. The process of recording ideas, knowledge, or messages in some physical way (through pictography or alphabets) involves mediation (McLuhan 1964). In effect, communication and society evolve in tandem with any new medium introduced into the society for realizing the former.

The alphabet mediates how we perceive knowledge. In alphabetic writing we do not "see" a referent directly through some picture (as in pictography), but rather we reconstruct it through phonemic symbols. So, when we read a word such as *cat* we must extract from the letters the sounds they represent. As a result, alphabetic writing adds a level of abstraction that is not present in processing stimuli and images directly through sensory channels.

It was McLuhan who originated the idea of *mediation*, or the notion that media influence how people understand the world. This is why digital media have come to play crucial roles in society, shaping how people come to understand themselves. McLuhan also realized that changes in media lead to changes in knowledge-storing and knowledge-making systems.

9.2.1 Digital Media

As E. Gabriella Coleman (2010: 488) has aptly put it, "digital artifacts have helped engender new collectivities." She goes on to argue that these have had a significant impact on everyday life:

> Digital media feed into, reflect, and shape other kinds of social practices, like economic exchange, financial markets, and religious worship. Attention to these rituals, broad contexts, and the material infrastructures and social protocols that enable them illuminates how the use and production of digital media have become integrated into everyday cultural, linguistic, and economic life.

Digital media have led to a paradigm shift (Cheney-Lippold 2017). Already in the late 1990s, Manuel Castells (1999) argued that the digital age had induced a tension that he labels the net-versus-the self. The former constitutes the organizational structures that have emerged on the Internet, and the latter, the people's attempts to establish their identities (religious, ethnic, sexual, territorial, or national) in terms of those structures.

9.2.2 Media Literacy

As discussed (Chapter 7), a new, complex form of literacy, called *media literacy*, has emerged in the global village, defined as knowledge of how the media work and how they might influence perspective and understanding—similar to how print literacy permits people to better understand written texts in all their dimensions (psychological, social, etc.). Functional literacy, as discussed, is the ability to extract meaning from print. This is developed through formal schooling. Today, such literacy has merged with media literacy to produce a set of subliteracies that have become critical to coping with everyday life. This has led to an expanding awareness of the relation between language and the world:

1 *Multilingualism literacy*: awareness of different languages on the Internet and thus of different literacy practices and what they entail.
2 *Digital media literacy*: awareness of the role of new media on traditional literacy and other traditional social practices.
3 *Online communication literacy*: awareness of how language and writing are evolving in new online contexts.
4 *Stylistic diffusion literacy*: awareness of the spread of slangs and jargons from online culture to VCs, producing new forms of high and low sociolects.
5 *Mobile literacy*: awareness of how texts are to be written on mobile devices. There are now text-messaging poetry competitions, with the mobile system producing a channel for exploiting linguistic creativity. The cellphone has generated a new literary genre—"cellphone novels" consisting of chapters that readers download in short installments. They are novels in the traditional sense, but without editing or rewriting.
6 *Blog literacy*: awareness of new forms of blog-based multimodal writing, including photoblogs, videoblogs, audioblogs, and moblogs. These have brought about new linguistic and stylistic conventions and might continue to change literacy practices in the future.
7 *Virtual community literacies*: as discussed above, awareness of how language use varies according to VC, from Twitter to role-playing gaming communities.
8 *Email literacy*: awareness that this medium that is closest to traditional print literacy practices. It is the medium used by businesses, schools, and other institutions and thus more sensitive to formal registers than other types of computer-mediated-communication.
9 *Instant messaging literacy*, which has developed its own form of informal language, although with corrective devices such as iPhones and

Smartphones that make spelling more complete, it is evolving more and more into traditional literacy practices.

10   *Visual literacy*, which involves knowledge of how to construct or communicate messages via media such as Instagram and Snapchat, among others.

11   *Screen literacy*, which involves adapting speech patterns in screen media such as Skype and Facetime.

Overall, media literacy can be defined as the ability to extract and use relevant information in multiple formats from a wide range of sources via media convergence. It thus encompasses technological and information-gathering abilities, that go beyond traditional ways of collecting and using information.

9.3 Communicative Competence Expanded

The notion of communicative competence is a key one in sociolinguistics (as we have seen), alluding to knowledge of the linguistic resources required to effectuate verbal interaction in a socially appropriate way. The world of social media, with its emoji, hashtags, and memes, has led to an expansion of the notion of communicative competence as it was originally formulated, refashioned to take into account how communication unfolds in different VCs and in social media generally (Gillen and Merchant 2013).

An important feature of Twitter, for example, is the fact that the individual user can choose whose tweets to read and whose to filter out. An individual Twitter account allows people to search for and select others to follow, and this selection determines whose tweets show up on one's own page. This gives the individual a personal point of view and control over a social network that are not possible to realize in real space, at least to the same extent. To participate in Twitter is to enter into a different kind of discursive relationship with others and to expect more flexibility in style than in F2F contexts.

There are thus now two types of communicative competence, real-world communicative competence (RCC) and digital communicative competence (DCC), with the two blending into a general meta-communicative competence. There is some evidence that DCC is weaker in older netizens. A study by Stapa (2012), for example, investigating the language features and patterns of online communication among Malaysian Facebook users found that there is an age gap that differentiates the young users from the older generations who are not used to online communication patterns. After examining Facebook conversations among 120 young Malaysians from different ethnic groups, mother tongues, and cultural background, the study found that DCC involves a new sense of linguistic identity that is not found among older users. Needless to say, as young netizens age, it will be interesting to see how many of the characteristics that now define DCC will be carried over into subsequent life and transmitted to subsequent generations.

9.3.1 Conversation Analysis in Cyberspace

A key methodology of sociolinguistics is, as discussed, conversation analysis (Chapter 6). Conversations that take place in online contexts are now studied with the same tools of traditional CA, which has been expanded somewhat to take media literacy and its various subliteracies into account. Text messaging (TM), for example, is constructed in real time, since both users can conduct a back-and-forth exchange, but since it involves a different medium of delivery various linguistic features emerge that apply to TM in contrast to F2F conversations. The question that is relevant in this case is the following one: Are online conversations serving the same kinds of social functions as offline ones? Research in this domain suggests that conversation varies according to: (1) function of the speech act, (2) device constraints on conversations, (3) special linguistic forms (such as netlingo), and (4) profile of the participants. This means that conversational structures in cyberspace are less habitual and predictable, and evolving at a more rapid pace than ever before.

In a relevant and relatively early study, Pampek, Yermolayeva, and Calvert (2009) found that people used Facebook as part of a daily routine and that they communicated on Facebook using a one-to-many style, in which they were the creators disseminating content to their friends. Even so, they spent more time observing content on Facebook than actually posting content. As the study suggested, the motivations for communicating in social networks is the same as the motivation for communicating in general—to socialize, to present oneself to others, and to gain understanding of things. The forms of communication may have changed, but the motivations seem to be the same ones. Another early study at the University of Kansas posted a video on YouTube asking the question: "Why do you use YouTube"? The research project received 370 video responses (Wesch 2007). The top 10 answers are as follows:

1   to connect with others or to be social
2   for fun or entertainment
3   simply because they like it
4   to express their opinions
5   to be creative
6   because they are bored ("nothing better to do")
7   because it is more "real" or authentic than commercial productions
8   because they hoped they might become famous
9   to see what other people think of them
10   because they are addicted to social media.

The results were significant in attenuating some common assumptions about YouTube as a site simply for video watching. People go on YouTube to socialize. This suggests that the main motivation to enter into digital spaces is social. YouTube now has educational uses, and many schools use it to deliver classes, lectures, and the like. Online learning communities have been called "adhocracies," or learning organizations with few fixed structures or established relationships among interlocutors. In other words, an adhocracy is the polar opposite of the contemporary university (which preserves rigid territories between disciplines and departments). McKinney (2006) argues that YouTube is an example of how VCs emerge spontaneously, without connection to historical ingroup associations.

The point of the foregoing discussion is to emphasize the role of mediation in shaping communicative competence and in effectuating social change. Whereas it has always been a factor in the language–media–society equation mentioned at the start of the chapter, it has become particularly prominent and powerful today. It will have to be seen what will happen as future technologies make different kinds of media available. One thing will be for certain, they too will change the dynamics of the equation.

9.3.2 Human –Machine Interaction

An emerging area of interest involves human–machine interaction, connecting sociolinguistic research with the cognitive sciences and artificial intelligence (AI) research (for an overview, see Guzman 2018). The questions that such interaction involves are truly significant reaching into the nature of communication itself and what it means to construct messages and expect them to be understood. This is a topic that can only be broached schematically here.

One of the first experiments in human–machine interaction is known as the Eliza Project, and is worthwhile revisiting here. The project was carried out by Joseph Weizenbaum in 1966, with a program he called ELIZA. The program was designed to mimic the speech that a psychotherapist would use. ELIZA's questions such as "Why do you say your head hurts?" in response to "My head hurts" were perceived by subjects as being so realistic that many believed that the machine was actually alive. But, as Weizenbaum wrote a decade later, ELIZA was a parodic imitation of psychoanalytic speech; it had no consciousness of what it was saying.

ELIZA gave momentum to natural language programming (NLP). It was shortly after that NLP algorithms emerged, with each one coming closer and closer to producing human speech that verged on verisimilitude. The early NLP languages were constructed with versions of BASIC. Here is an example:

What's your name?
Jennifer.
Hello Jennifer. How many children do you have?
Two.
Do you want more children?
Yes.
How many children do you want?
One.

Do you want more children (after that)?

No.

Goodbye, Jennifer.

Without going into details here, this dialogue would be translated into machine language that converts natural language forms into symbolic representations. NLP uses sophisticated logical, probabilistic, and neural network systems that can effectively carry out verisimilar conversations.

The probabilistic aspect of NLP is a central one, given that many aspects of human communication involve uncertainty. Today algorithms can be designed to be much more flexible and thus more similar to human conversation. This type of analysis, named after English mathematician Thomas Bayes (1702–1761), describes how the conditional probability of each of a set of causes for a given outcome can be computed from the probability of each cause and the conditional probability of the outcome of each cause. The Bayesian approach turns strict algorithmic logic (a set of sequential rules) into a probabilistic one, enabling rules and rule systems to be adaptive and flexible. In this framework, a prior hypothesis is updated in the light of new relevant observations or evidence, and this is done via a standard set of algorithmic procedures. But the problem of understanding nevertheless comes up—how does the human mind interpret verbal information, rather than just process it?

AI has developed powerful algorithms that define deep learning and which study how computers can learn from huge amounts of data. An everyday example of a deep learning system is the one that distinguishes between spam and non-spam emails on servers, allocating the spam ones to a specific folder. It can also determine the sense of, say, an ambiguous word on the basis of word collocations in a text. A collocation is a sequence of words that typically co-occur in speech more often than would be anticipated by random chance. Collocations are not idioms, which have fixed phraseology. Phrases such as *crystal clear, cosmetic surgery*, and *clean bill of health* are all collocations. Whether the collocation is derived from some syntactic (*make choices*) or lexical (*clearcut*) criterion, the principle underlying collocations—frequency of usage of words in tandem—always applies. And it is this principle that undergirds some predictive algorithms.

The promise of human–machine interaction can be traced to the science of *cybernetics*, or the study of control and communication in humans, machines, and animals, founded by Norbert Wiener in his book *Cybernetics, or Control and Communication in the Animal and the Machine*, published in 1948, although the ideas go back to antiquity. The term cybernetics comes originally from the Greek word *kybernetikos*, meaning "good at steering," in reference to the skill of helmsmanship. The same word was used in 1834 by the physicist André-Marie Ampère to denote the study of government in his classification system of human knowledge. Ampère had probably taken it from Plato, who used it to signify the governance of people. Wiener subsequently popularized the social implications of cybernetics, drawing analogies between machines (robots and computers) and humans in his best-selling 1950 book, *The Human Use of Human Beings: Cybernetics and Society*. Wiener saw a common ground among the various forms of intelligence—human, animal, and artificial.

Examining cybernetic systems involves understanding how they communicate. Mechanical systems communicate via signals of various types; animals via signals based on their specific biology; and humans via (1) gesticulation (hands and bodily actions); (2) vocal organs (oral language) (3) writing (pictographic, alphabetic, etc.); (4) visuality (painting, sculpting, etc.); (5) mechanical means (radio, computers, etc.); (6) vocalizartion (singing); and (7) body language (gestures, facial expressions, etc.). In human communication, exchanges can be interpersonal (between human beings), group-based (between some individual or medium and groups), and mass-based involving communication systems that encompass entire societies. No other communication system, for now, can approach this level of complexity and versatility.

Two related areas of cybernetic research are robotics and automata theory, both of which dovetail with research in AI and computer engineering. Robotics can be defined as the science of machines engineered to carry out activities that mimic human activities (or even replicate them). Engineers have developed sophisticated mobile robots equipped with cameras for sight and sensors for touch. One of the first robots, named Elektro, was made in 1937 by the Westinghouse Electric Corporation. Elektro was humanoid in appearance—it could walk and move its arms and head by voice command, speak around 700 words (through a record player built into it), and smoke cigarettes. But Elektro did not have advanced AI, and thus could not learn to adapt to its environment and learn to do new tasks through deep learning algorithms.

A typical robot today is programmed with a set of algorithmic instructions that specify precisely what it must do and how to do so. The instructions are stored in the robot's computer control center, which, in turn, sends commands to the motorized joints, which move various parts of the robot, constituting so-called servomechanism and feedback systems. Most robot algorithms are based on data-mining information, which is converted into knowledge network systems to produce knowledge representation. In some instances, the algorithm attempts to generalize from certain inputs in order to generate, speculatively, an output for previously unseen inputs. In other cases, the algorithm operates on input where the desired output is unknown, with the objective being to discover structure in the information. In effect, robot algorithms are designed to predict new outputs from specific test cases. They mimic the same kinds of inductive learning patterns by the human brain, that is, the extraction of patterns on the basis of specific cases. The goal has been (and achieved in many cases) robots that acquire skills through autonomous exploration of specific cases and through interaction with human teachers.

A basic design principle of robots is called "degrees of freedom," which refers to the different ways that the robot can move—up and down, in and out, side to side, tilt, rotate, etc. Part of the relevant algorithm is designed so that the robot can use camera images of the environment to determine movement. Robots can also use satellite navigation systems to move around and to perform actions such as picking things up, moving them around, etc. House robots are now designed to communicate through a speaker, take voice commands, and to use a Wi-Fi computer for adapting information to the state of events. The robot that has the apparent capacity to interact purposefully with humans is called a *cobot*. In contrast to traditional robots, which are designed to operate autonomously or with limited guidance, cobots have the ability to respond to situations through learning algorithms that are stored in their memory system. Interestingly, cobots have been found to develop word-to-meaning mappings without grammatical rules—a very important finding to say the least. Suffice it to say here that research on cobots is allowing us to understand how the mechanisms of language operate; however, so far it has told us virtually nothing about how the human brain extracts meaning from language and then applies it to discover the world in new, not automatic, ways.

9.4 How to Speak to an Alien

In a 2016 movie called *Arrival*, a linguistics professor named Louise Banks is charged with the task of developing a language for communicating with aliens who have landed on earth, a pair of extraterrestrials whose spacecraft landed in Montana; to do otherwise could threaten humanity. Although it is a science fiction movie, it raises fundamental questions about the nature of human language and its role in the human species. It presents a fictional framework for concluding the present textbook.

The problem Banks faces is that even if a set of symbols could be devised to communicate with the aliens, they would be imbued with human meanings and thus are unlikely to be understood by the alien species. We would not know how they think and what they would make of our linguistic symbols. Words are capsules of thought derived from human experiences. They are not just devices carrying information; they are signs that encode our interpretations and evaluations of the world. So, we cannot be sure what interpretation a linguistic signal or cue will elicit in the aliens (if any). Incidentally the study of what it means to potentially communicate with aliens has a technical name—*astrolinguistics* (Ollongren 2012). It is defined as the investigation of potential common elements of a *lingua cosmica* that could be understood presumably by extraterrestrial intelligences, exploring concepts central to core linguistic theory. Banks actually makes astrolinguistic communication look easy in the movie, using a blend of linguistic cues with mathematical and scientific symbols. The assumption is that alien species would understand the same kind of information that humans do—an unlikely one.

The movie makes it obvious that for aliens to understand a human message, they would also need the instructions of how to do it. We would have to teach them grammar, vocabulary, writing, and mathematics. We would also have to teach them about markedness systems in language that signal socially indexed information. But then, we would also have to teach them how to read the instructions—leaving us in a vicious circle. There really is no "Rosetta Stone" for astrological communication. Even mathematics would likely be different in astral civilizations, if such civilizations exist. The world has become smaller because of Internet technologies. It is now routine to communicate with people across the globe almost instantaneously, regardless of their national origins. This has changed the rules of social interaction and communication radically. In a sense, the new forms of communication are "astrolinguistic," because they imply finding patterns in language that will relate to all humans everywhere, even though this may turn out to be unsuccessful.

Seargeant and Tagg (2011) introduced the idea of "hybrid languages" to describe how languages are evolving online, where English and Thai, for example, are becoming amalgamated, with one and the other being used in a collage of forms and meanings. Hybridization seems to be an emergent property of expanding communicative competencies.

No matter how scientific, fact based, or theoretically sound an account of the connection between language, mind, culture, society, and new media might appear or might be purported to be, no science can ever truly account for the remarkable phenomenon that we call language. We might be able to describe what the bits and pieces are like and how they mesh together; but we will never be able to put into an overall theory all there is to know about language. The goal of the linguist is to figure out how the pieces of the language puzzle fit together to produce meaning, but this tells us nothing about why we need meaning in the first place, or what relevance it has to human survival.

The research in sociolinguistics has shown that diversity is the norm, but that diversity reflects differentiated attempts to solve similar problems of meaning across the world. It shows how we come up with different solutions according to situation, time, and place. The fact that we can understand one another shows how much we are really all one race, seeking similar solutions and outcomes to the experience of existence.

References and Further Reading

Balakrishnan, J. and Griffiths, M. D. (2018). An Exploratory Study of "Selfitis" and the Development of the Selfitis Behavior Scale. *International Journal of Mental Health and Addiction* 16: 722–736.

Castells, M. (1989). *The Informational City: Information Technology, Economic Restructuring, and the Urban Regional Process*. Oxford: Wiley-Blackwell.

Castells, M. (1996). *The Information Age: Economy, Society, and Culture*. Oxford: Wiley-Blackwell.

Castells, M. (2001). *The Internet Galaxy*. Oxford: Oxford University Press.

Cheney-Lippold, J., (2017). *We are Data: Algorithms and the Making of our Digital Selves*. New York: New York University Press.

Coleman, E. G. (2010). Ethnographic Approaches to Digital Media. *Annual Review of Anthropology* 39: 487–505.

Gillen, J. and Merchant, G. (2013). Contact Calls: Twitter as a Dialogic Social and Linguistic Practice. *Language Sciences* 35: 47–58.

Gruzd, A., Wellman, B., and Takhteyev, Y. (2011). Imagining Twitter as an Imagined Community. *American Behavioral Scientist* 55(10): 1294–1318.

Guzman, A. L. (2018). *Human-Machine Communication: Rethinking Communication, Technology, and Ourselves*. New York: Peter Lang.

Huffaker, D. A. and Calvert, S. L. (2005). Gender, Identity, and Language Use in Teenage Blogs. *Journal of Computer-Mediated Communication* 10. http://jcmc. indiana.edu/vol10/issue2/huffaker.html.

Jenkins, H. (2006). *Convergence Culture: Where Old and New Media Collide*. Cambridge, MA: MIT Press.

McKinney, J. (2006). Why YouTube Works. *Unsought Input*. www.unsoughtinput. com/index.php/2006/08/21/.

McLuhan, M. (1964). *Understanding Media: The Extensions of Man*. London: Routledge.

Meyerhoff, M. (2006). *Introducing Sociolinguistics*. London: Routledge.

Ollongren, A. (2012). *Astrolinguistics: Design of a Linguistic System for Interstellar Communication Based on Logic*. New York: Springer.

Pampek, T. A., Yermolayeva, Y. A., and Calvert, S. A. (2009). College Students' Social Networking Experiences on Facebook. *Journal of Applied Developmental Psychology* 30: 227–238.

Preece, J., Maloney-Krichmar, D., and Abras, C. (2003). History of Online Communities. In: K. Christiansen and D. Levinson (eds.), *Encyclopedia of Community*, pp. 1023–1027. Thousand Oaks, CA: Sage.

Rheingold, H. (1993). *The Virtual Community*. Cambridge, MA: MIT Press.

Rodzvilla, J. (ed.) (2009). *We've Got Blog: How Weblogs Are Changing Our Culture*. New York: Basic Books.

Savas, P. (2011). A Case Study of Contextual and Individual Factors That Shape Linguistic Variation in Synchronous Text-Based Computer-Mediated Communication. *Journal of Pragmatics* 43: 298–313.

Seargeant, P. and Tagg, C. (2011). English on the Internet and a "Post-Varieties" Approach to Language. *World Englishes* 30: 496–514.

Stapa, S. H. (2012). Understanding Online Communicative Language Features in Social Networking Environment. *GEMA Online Journal of Linguistic Studies* 12: 817–830.

Tossell, C. C., Kortum, P., Shepard, C., Barg-Walkow, L. H., Rahmati, A., and Zhong, L. (2012). A Longitudinal Study of Emoticon Use in Text Messaging from Smartphones. *Computers in Human Behavior* 28: 659–663.

Vandergriff, I. (2013). Emotive Communication Online: A Contextual Analysis of Computer-Mediated Communication (CMC) Cues. *Journal of Pragmatics* 51: 1–12.

Varnhagen, C., Mcfall, P., and Pugh, N. (2010). Lol: New Language and Spelling in Instant Messaging. *Reading and Writing* 23(6): 719–733.

Weizenbaum, J. (1966). ELIZA—A Computer Program for the Study of Natural Language Communication between Man and Machine. *Communications of the ACM* 9: 36–45.

Wesch, P. (2007). Why Do YouTube?—Video Response Analysis Digital. *Ethnography*. http://mediatedcultures.net/ksudigg/?p=82.

Wiener, N. (1948). *Cybernetics, or Control and Communication in the Animal and the Machine*. Cambridge, MA: MIT Press.

Wiener, N. (1950). *The Human Use of Human Beings: Cybernetics and Society*. Boston, MA: Houghton-Mifflin.

Exercises and Discussions

Chapter 1

1 This chapter mentions some features that all languages have in common. Can you think of others?

2 Why is the difference between language and speech a relevant one for sociolinguistics?

3 Each language has a system of distinctive sounds, called phonemes. Sometimes, differences in phonemes may signal some social or dialect difference.

Example: the *a* in *tomato*

It can be produced by opening the mouth to the maximum, as in *bah*, or else by opening it in a more lateral way, as in *pay*. Both sounds are used in pronouncing *tomato* but may reflect regional differences or perhaps even differences in individual pronunciation.

Can you think of others in English? If so, explain them in your own words.

4 Each language has meaning-bearing units known as morphemes. Part of linguistic analysis is the segmentation of words into morphemes. Segmentation is also a method for diagnosing anomalies in word formation.

Example: unlegitimate

The morpheme /un-/ (known as a prefix) is not used with *legitimate*. The acceptable prefix in this case is /il-/: *illegitimate*. However, /un-/ is used with other words: *unmistakable, unforgettable*.

Using this kind of morphemic diagnosis, what is anomalous about:

(a) uncorrect?
(b) churchs?
(c) mouses?

5 Each language has strategies for conducting meaningful social interaction. The following are English utterances that have been constructed

anomalously from the standpoint of usage. Using simple explanations, indicate what is improper about them.

Example: My name is Mr. Bill

In polite speech, titles (known as *honorifics*) are used with a complete name or with a surname, not a first (or given) name (unless there is a specific reason to do so): "My name is Mr. Bill Smith" or "My name is Mr. Smith." The given utterance is an acceptable one if used, for example, by a speaker attempting to be humorous or facetious with friends.

(a) Glad to make your acquaintance, Mr. Jones. How the heck are you?
(b) Mother, tell your husband that I am going out!
(c) (Phone communication) Hello, who is it? I'm Mary.
(d) (Text message to a close friend) Dear Mary, how are you feeling today?

6   What do the following forms indicate socially or culturally?

Example: Titles (Mr., Mrs., Prof., Dr.)

Some titles have the general social function of showing respect or deference when addressing certain socially esteemed people such as professors and doctors. Some titles reveal gender-coded differences. *Mrs.* indicates that a woman is married. The corresponding *Mr.* title has no similar information built into it. This reveals an unconscious differential perception of gender.

(a) Greeting protocols (Hello, Goodbye, How's it going? What's up?)
(b) Surnames or family names (Smith, Johnson)
(c) CMC forms such as *u* for *you* or *lol* for *laugh out loud*.

7   Comment on what each excerpt means in terms of the ideas discussed in this chapter.

From Ferdinand de Saussure, *Cours de linguistique générale* (1916):

A scientific study will take as its subject matter every kind of variety of human language: it will not select one period or another for its literary brilliance or for the renown of the people in question. It will pay attention to any tongue, whether obscure or famous, and likewise to any period, giving no preference, for example, to what is called a classical period, but according equal interest to so-called decadent or archaic periods. Similarly, for any given period, it will refrain from selecting the most educated language, but will concern itself at the same time with popular forms more or less in contrast with the so-called educated or literary language, as well as the forms of the so-called educated or literary language. Thus linguistics deals with language of every period and in all the guises it assumes.

From Franz Boas, *The Methods of Ethnology* (1920):

At the present time, at least among certain groups of investigators in England and also in Germany, ethnological research is based on the concept of migration and dissemination rather than upon that of evolution. A critical study of these two directions of inquiry shows that each is founded on the application of one fundamental hypothesis. The evolutionary point of view presupposes that the course of historical changes in the cultural life of mankind follows definite laws which are applicable everywhere, and which bring it about that cultural development is, in its main lines, the same among all races and all peoples. Opposed to these assumptions is the modern tendency to deny the existence of a general evolutionary scheme which would represent the history of the cultural development the world over.

From Benjamin Lee Whorf, *Language, Thought, and Reality* (1956):

Every normal person in the world, past infancy in years, can and does talk. By virtue of that fact, every person—civilized or uncivilized—carries through life certain naive but deeply rooted ideas about talking and its relation to thinking. Because of their firm connection with speech habits that have become unconscious and automatic, these notions tend to be rather intolerant of opposition. They are by no means entirely personal and haphazard; their basis is definitely systematic, so that we are justified in calling them a system of natural logic—a term that seems to me preferable to the term common sense, often used for the same thing... . The world is presented in a kaleidoscopic flux of impressions which has to be organized by our minds—and this means largely by the linguistic systems in our minds. We cut nature up, organize it into concepts, and ascribe significances as we do, largely because we are parties to an agreement to organize it in this way—an agreement that holds throughout our speech community and is codified in the patterns of our language. The agreement is, of course, an implicit and unstated one, but its terms are absolutely obligatory; we cannot talk at all except by subscribing to the organization and classification of data which the agreement decrees.

Chapter 2

1   Explain the social implications associated with each title.

   (a) Miss
   (b) Ms.
   (c) Prof. (Professor)
   (d) Dr. (Doctor)
   (e) Rev. (Reverend)
   (f) Madam
   (g) Sir

2   In many societies, men and women are expected to use different forms of speech. In English, too, certain mannerisms of speech appear to be gender coded. If so, how might women and men intentionally differentiate them-selves (if they so desire) to communicate the following things in English?

(a) Politeness with a stranger
(b) Excusing oneself among friends
(c) Inviting a new romantic partner out for a date

3   The following terms and expressions use *man* indicating that the mas-culine gender is the unmarked one. What terms are currently used (or should be used if there are none) in their place to eliminate the mark-edness bias implicit in them?

(a) fireman
(b) postman
(c) mankind
(d) manpower
(e) man and wife
(f) men of letters
(g) manmade

4   Give examples of different pronunciation or vocabulary between any variant of English and Standard English that signal differences in social class.

5   Create a short message in netlingo and then discuss its particular char-acteristics (abbreviations, acronyms, and so on).

6   Provide the denotative meaning of each of the following words and then use each one in a sentence that exemplifies a connotative meaning. For example, the denotative meaning of the word *cat* is "small feline with retractile claws and whiskers, and that emits sounds called purring, hissing, and meowing." A connotative use of the word can be seen in "They always play cat and mouse," a sentence that implies a series of cunning strategies designed to thwart an opponent:

(a) dog
(b) blue
(c) way
(d) right
(e) ground

7   Give examples of current memes and what they mean socially and culturally.

8   The following excerpt is from P. Eckert and S. McConnell-Ginet, *Language and Gender* (2003):

We are surrounded by gender lore from the time we are very small. It is ever-present in conversation, humor, and conflict, and it is called upon to explain everything from driving styles to food preferences. Gender is embedded so thoroughly in our institutions, our actions, our beliefs, and our desires, that it appears to us to be completely natural. The world swarms with ideas about gender—and these ideas are so commonplace that we take it for granted that they are true, accepting common adage as scientific fact. As scholars and researchers, though, it is our job to look beyond what appears to be common sense to find not simply what truth might be behind it, but how it came to be common sense. It is precisely because gender seems natural, and beliefs about gender seem to be obvious truths, that we need to step back and examine gender from a new perspective. Doing this requires that we suspend what we are used to and what feels comfortable, and question some of our most fundamental beliefs. This is not easy, for gender is so central to our understanding of ourselves and of the world that it is difficult to pull back and examine it from new perspectives. But it is precisely the fact that gender seems self-evident that makes the study of gender interesting.

Do you think gender differences are based primarily in biology or in culture? Explain your position.

9   The following excerpt is from G. Lakoff, *The Contemporary Theory of Metaphor* (1979):

Imagine a love relationship described as follows: Our relationship has hit a dead-end street. Here love is being conceptualized as a journey, with the implication that the relationship is stalled, that the lovers cannot keep going the way they've been going, that they must turn back, or abandon the relationship altogether. This is not an isolated case. English has many everyday expressions that are based on a conceptualization of love as a journey, and they are used not just for talking about love, but for reasoning about it as well. Some are necessarily about love; others can be understood that way: Look how far we've come. It's been a long, bumpy road. We can't turn back now. We're at a crossroads. We may have to go our separate ways. The relationship isn't going anywhere. We're spinning our wheels. Our relationship is off the track. The marriage is on the rocks. We may have to bail out of this relationship. These are ordinary, everyday English expressions. They are not poetic, nor are they necessarily used for special rhetorical effect. Those like Look how far we've come, which aren't necessarily about love, can readily be understood as being about love.

Can you give other examples of conceptual metaphors connected with *love*?

10 The following excerpt is from R. Hudson, *Sociolinguistics and the Theory of Grammar* (1986):

The choice of forms depends inter alia [among other things] on the speaker's "social knowledge," which includes their classification of the speaker according to social categories. This classification need not be categorical—indeed, there is now ample evidence that people often classify themselves and others as members of some group to varying degrees... . It also depends on the speaker's intentions, which include such questions as how badly they want to be classified as a member of some social group, or how much they want the hearer to like them. This too is clearly a matter of degree and can influence the quantitative distribution of sociolinguistic variants in speech.

Is there a difference between social knowledge and communicative competence? If so, how so? If not, why not?

11   The following excerpt is from E. R. Thomas, *Phonological and Phonetic Characteristics of African American Vernacular English* (2007):

Some special considerations relate to AAVE. First, AAVE is often distinguished from African American English (AAE). AAVE relates specifically to a vernacular form, spoken principally by working-class African Americans. AAE refers to the speech of all African Americans, including middle-class African Americans. Middle-class AAE most often lacks the more stigmatized morphosyntactic variants, although some middle-class speakers may employ them for stylistic effect or to express solidarity. Most pronunciation variables are not as stigmatized, however, and, for many of them, there may be no meaningful distinction between AAVE forms and AAE forms... . Third, AAVE (and AAE) have a unique migration history. They originated in the South, and specifically in the Coastal Plain and Piedmont sections of the South, and were at first tied to a rural lifestyle. However, beginning before World War I and continuing through World War II, the Great Migration occurred in which large numbers of African Americans migrated to cities outside the South in order to find work and to escape Jim Crow laws. A result was that the focus of African American culture shifted to urban life.

What social functions do you think AAVE encompasses?

12   The following excerpt is from S. M. Wilson and L. C. Peterson, *The Anthropology of Online Communities* (2002):

Analyzed through the lens of contemporary approaches in ethnographies of communication, research in multilingual, multisited internet experiences would contribute to debates in the literature which seeks to position studies of mediated communication and technology in local social and communicative practices. Such research might help our understanding of the ways in which speakers incorporate new technologies of communication from existing communicative repertoires, and these technologies influence new and emerging cultural practices. In this sort of investigation, researchers must ask: Where do community members situate computers and other communication and information technologies in their daily lives? How are the tools of new media changing the contexts and frames of communicative practices? Are new forms of communicative competence developing as a consequence of new media tools in offline speech communities? How does technology enhance or displace discourses and practices of tradition? How might new technologies alter novice-expert relations? How do linguistic structures of online interactions affect offline practice?

Design an online study accessing social media sites to determine if there are differences in the language used by males and females, paying special attention to vocabulary and grammar.

Chapter 3

1   Below are some spelling and vocabulary differences between American and British English.

American spelling	British spelling
color	colour
odor	odour
center	centre
program	programme
analyze	analyse
recognize	recognise

American vocabulary	British vocabulary
mail	post
gasoline	petrol
TV	telly
friend	mate
elevator	lift
subway	underground

Can you provide other examples, not only in spelling and vocabulary, but also in other areas of language, such as pronunciation or grammar?

2   Now, provide differences between Standard American English and any regional dialect of which you may be aware.

3   Pidginization is the process of simplifying utterances for communicative purposes, such as when speaking to people who are not native speakers or

when speaking to children. In English, this involves mainly the elimination of morphological detail. For example, the sentence "She is going to the store tomorrow" is pidginized to "She go store tomorrow" without any loss of meaning. How would you pidginize the following sentences?

(a) They will be going to the mall this afternoon.
(b) I had already arrived yesterday when you called.
(c) I don't know where I put the book that you had given me yesterday.
(d) Your friends had already been taking that subject at school.

4   Each of the following English words was borrowed from another language. Using an etymological dictionary, indicate the source language and explain the nativization process involved:

(a) cipher
(b) algorithm
(c) education
(d) naïve
(e) cinema

5   Read the following excerpt from "How a Dialect Differs from a Language," *The Economist* (2013):

Two kinds of criteria distinguish languages from dialects. The first are social and political: in this view, "languages" are typically prestigious, official and written, whereas "dialects" are mostly spoken, unofficial and looked down upon. In a famous formulation of this view, "a language is a dialect with an army and a navy." Speakers of mere "dialects" often refer to their speech as "slang," "patois" or the like. (The Mandarin Chinese term for Cantonese, Shanghaiese and others is fangyan, or "place-speech.") Linguists have a different criterion: if two related kinds of speech are so close that speakers can have a conversation and understand each other, they are dialects of a single language. If comprehension is difficult to impossible, they are distinct languages. Of course, comprehensibility is not either-or, but a continuum—and it may even be asymmetrical. Nonetheless, mutual comprehensibility is the most objective basis for saying whether two kinds of speech are languages or dialects. By the comprehensibility criterion, Cantonese is not a dialect of Chinese. Rather it is a language, as are Shanghaiese, Mandarin and other kinds of Chinese. Although the languages are obviously related, a Mandarin-speaker cannot understand Cantonese or Shanghaiese without having learned it as a foreign language (and vice-versa, though most Chinese do learn Mandarin today). Most Western linguists classify them as "Sinitic languages," not "dialects of Chinese."

Can you give examples of languages that are mutually intelligible yet belong to different nations and thus are not considered to be dialects of each other?

6   Read the following excerpt from A. Hudson, *Outline of a Theory of Diglossia* (2002):

Diglossia, in its ideal form, may be conceived of as the quintessential example of linguistic variation where linguistic realization as opposed to language acquisition—here, grossly oversimplified, the use of H or L— is a function solely of social context, and not of social identity of the speaker. In diglossia, it is context, not class, or other group member- ship, that controls use. Sociolinguistic situations therefore may be com- pared to each other in terms of the degree to which the variation between two or more alternants in their respective code matrices is determined by social context, as opposed to the social identity of the speaker, and in situations such as those described for Switzerland, Greece, most Arabic-speaking countries, and numerous other cases, the bulk, if not all, of the variance in the use of H and L appears to be explained by situational context.

Does diglossia exist in the US? Would you consider Spanglish-versus- Standard Spanish to be a diglossic dichotomy? What about Standard American English-versus-African American Vernacular English?

7   Read the following excerpt from J. Cummins *Bilingualism and Minority- Language Children* (1981):

Minority language children pick up L2 in much the same way in the street and/or in school. First, there is a period which can range from several days to several months when the child says very little in L2 but tries to decipher the L2 utterances of others through linking up the utterance with the meaning of the situation. Then words and phrases will be tried out and the effects of these utterances will be observed. Utterances which are not appropriate or don't have the expected effects will be modified until gradually the words and the rules for combining them (grammar) begin to fit together into an organized system that gradually approximates that of a native-speaker of L2. The amount of time necessary to acquire mastery of a second (or first) language will depend on the extent to which individuals have the opportunity and inclination to interact with competent users of the language. It is thus not surprising that immigrant children usually learn the second lan- guage more rapidly than their parents since, typically, they have much more exposure to the language than their parents.

How would you define a minority language? What minority languages are there in the US?

8   Read the following excerpt from A. Hudson, *Outline of a Theory of Diglossia* (2002):

The association between diglossia and literacy, in the sense of both the incidence of individual literacy skills and the existence of a literary tradition, is not an accidental one, since social stratification of literacy may give rise to the independent development of two or more increasingly divergent language varieties. As the linguistic varieties become more divergent, more extensive training is required for the mastery of the literary variety, a development that in turn confers additional prestige upon it: "With the development of writing and a complex and introspective literature, the language variety so employed will often be accorded such high value because of the recorded nature of the medium and the need to be trained to read and write it" (Abrahams 1972:15).

How would you define literacy today? What about online literacy?

9   Read the following excerpt from R. Page, *The Linguistics of Self-Branding and Micro-Celebrity in Twitter: The Role of Hashtags* (2012):

Within the linguistic marketplace of Twitter, hashtags are a crucial currency which enables visibility and projects potential interaction with other members of the site. Hashtags can be used to make a term searchable and therefore visible to others who are interested in tweets written about the same topic. When a hashtag is used with sufficient frequency, it may be listed in the "trending topics" sidebar of the Twitter site, hence promoting a topic or term (and hence the tweets and their authors) to an audience which extends far beyond the follower list of the person who used the hashtag. For a hashtag to achieve a rank in the trending topics list is taken as a signal of status and influence. For example, fans of the pop star Justin Bieber notoriously manipulated Twitter's trending topics in order to demonstrate the popularity of the singer and the influence of his fan base.

Do you have a hashtag? Explain its characteristics using some of the insights found in this reading. Why do you think hashtags have become so popular?

10 In your own words explain the difference between a dialect and a standard language.

Chapter 4

1   Each word, expression, or protocol below is part of formal language. Change each one to a corresponding informal form:

(a) residence
(b) advertisement

(c) soft drink
(d) adhesive
(e) greetings
(f) hello
(g) goodbye

2　Give examples of current adolescent or urban slang, explaining what linguistic process is involved (hedging, tagging, and so on).

3　How much jargon do you know from the various professions?

(a) Lawyer talk
(b) Professor talk
(c) Doctor talk

4　Correct the following utterances in a stylistically appropriate fashion.

(a) The journey was taken by Bob. It was not taken by me, neither was it my intention to do so. The journey preparations were accomplished quickly. The journey was taken by Bob for several reasons. These reasons were necessitated by stressful situations.

(b) The experiment was, like, good. I knew I was going to get a chemical reaction. I thought I would get salt. But I got something else instead. I will try the experiment again.

5　From Twitter sites, collect markers (abbreviations, emoji, and so on) that you can associate with some social variable (gender, age, class).

6　Read the following excerpt from D. Hymes, *On Communicative Competence* (1971):

The internalization of attitudes towards a language and its uses is particularly important (Labov, 1965, pp. 84–85, on priority of subjective evaluation in social dialect and processes of change), as is internalization of attitudes toward use of language itself (e.g. attentiveness to it) and the relative place that language comes to play in a pattern of mental abilities (Cazden 1966), and in strategies—what language is considered available, reliable, suitable for, vis-à-vis other kinds of code. The acquisition of such competency is of course fed by social experience, needs, and motives, and issues in action that is itself a renewed source of motives, needs, experience. We break irrevocably with the model that restricts the design of language to one face toward referential meaning, one toward sound, and that defines the organization of language as solely consisting of rules for linking the two. Such a model implies naming to be the sole use of speech, as if languages were never organized to lament, rejoice, beseech, admonish, aphorize, inveigh (Burke 1966:13), for the many varied forms of persuasion, direction, expression and symbolic play. A model of language must design it with a face toward communicative conduct and social life.

Explain in your own words why social cues are embedded in language
and how these can be used to detect social variables in online messages.

7   Read the following excerpt from D. W. Lee, *Genres, Registers, Text
Types, Domains, and Styles: Clarifying the Concepts and Navigating a
Path Through the BNC Jungle* (2001):

One way of making a distinction between genre and text type is to say
that the former is based on external, non-linguistic, "traditional" criteria while the latter is based on the internal, linguistic characteristics of
texts themselves (Biber 1988: 70 & 170; EAGLES 1996). A genre, in this
view, is defined as a category assigned on the basis of external criteria
such as intended audience, purpose, and activity type, that is, it refers to
a conventional, culturally recognised grouping of texts based on properties other than lexical or grammatical (co-)occurrence features, which
are, instead, the internal (linguistic) criteria forming the basis of text
type categories. Biber (1988) has this to say about external criteria.
Genre categories are determined on the basis of external criteria relating
to the speaker's purpose and topic; they are assigned on the basis of use
rather than on the basis of form (p. 170). However, the EAGLES (1996)
authors would quibble somewhat with the inclusion of the word topic
above and argue that one should not think of topic as being something
to be established a priori, but rather as something determined on the
basis of internal criteria (i.e., linguistic characteristics of the text).

Classifying texts is a difficult task. How would you classify the following texts, using simple distinctions such as formal-versus-informal,
slang-versus-standard, and so on?

(a) An email to a teacher
(b) A tweet to a follower
(c) A text message to a friend
(d) An essay in sociolinguistics

8   Read the following excerpt from J. B. Walther, *Interaction through
Technological Lenses: Computer-Mediated Communication and Language* (2012):

In remarking on communication technology, social psychology, and
language since the appearance of our special issue, I wish to frame certain observations in light of an issue that has remained central
throughout the evolution and diffusion of this field: the influence of
different communication systems on the restriction or provision of nonverbal cue systems that may accompany language in online interaction.
Certainly there are other meta-constructs in the field of communication
technology research. Yet some, if not most, of the field's most enduring

issues have concerned the psychological and communication effects that occur on and through language when people do or do not see or hear one another, without the nonverbal elements of communication on which so much otherwise often relies. Research alternatively describes the restriction of technology-mediated communication to language as a constraint or a liberation.

Summarize the argument made in your own words. Then, indicate what features of CMC differ from F2F communication.

9   Read the following excerpt from C. Danescu-Niculescu-Mizil, M. Gamon, M., and S. Dumais, *Mark My Words! Linguistic Style Accommodation in Social Media* (2011):

Twitter conversations are unlike those used in previous studies of accommodation. One of the main differences is that these conversations are not face-to-face and do not happen in real-time. Like with email, a user does not need to immediately reply to another user's message; this might affect the incentive to use accommodation as a way to increase communication efficiency. Another difference is the (famous) restriction of 140 characters per message, which might constrain the freedom one user has to accommodate the other. It is not a priori clear whether accommodation is robust enough to occur under these new constraints.

Indicate what style differences there might be among the four kinds of communication environments:

(a) text messaging
(b) Twitter
(c) Facebook
(d) Instagram

10   Read the following excerpt from J. Gillen and G. Merchant, *Contact Calls: Twitter as a Dialogic Social and Linguistic Practice* (2013):

Twitter is currently achieving a new level of institutionalisation as it features in legal cases, debates about privacy, and political intrigue. It is, like the social networking site Facebook, a commercial success, a triumph of marketing that was fortunate in striking a complementary note with other applications, software and hardware innovations, so that it quickly captured the public imagination. In the first few years after its launch in 2006 it spawned more than 50,000 third-party applications (Potts and Jones 2011). The microblogging tool Twitter is in some ways a "conversation"—at once democratic, in that everybody can join, ostensibly on equal footing, and a powerful, way of communicating one's message in an age of "networked individualism" (Wellman

2001). It will not, we think, be difficult to argue that "tweeting" is a significant social practice worthy of attention: even if some people wholly shun participation themselves, they will, in a variety of contexts, have become aware that Twitter is impinging on many areas of life that touch upon the mass media. The use of Twitter is clearly more than peripheral in diverse social spheres, including revolutionary movements, the dalliances of celebrities, government, industrial disputes and international sporting events (Attia et al. 2011; Cottle 2011; Jones and Salter 2011; Zappavigna 2012).

What do you think the term "dialogic" means in this case? How would you characterize socially based dialogue online?

Chapter 5

1   Read the following excerpt from K. Gibson, *English Only Court Cases Involving the U.S. Workplace: The Myths of Language Use and the Homogenization of Bilingual Workers' Identities* (2004):

Language—both code and content—is a complicated dance between internal and external interpretations of our identity. Within each community of practice, defined by Eckert and McConnell-Ginet (1999: 185) as groups "whose joint engagement in some activity of enterprise is sufficiently intensive to give rise over time to a repertoire of shared practices," certain linguistic (among other) practices are understood by the members to be more appropriate than others. While monolingual speakers are restricted to altering the content and register of their speech, bilingual speakers are able to alter the code, as well as content and register, of their language dependent upon the situation. Speakers who embrace the identity of a particular community will engage in positive identity practices, while those who reject the identity will use negative identity practices to distance themselves from it (Bucholtz 1999). However, this framework only takes into account the intentions of the speaker, and neglects the role of the hearer. Conflict arises when the hearer has a different understanding of the speaker's identity than the one the speaker desires. The tension is further compounded when the hearer is in a position of power and can not only misinterpret the desires of the speaker, but can actively thwart this expression, forcing the speaker into an entirely different, perhaps unwanted, identity. This plays out daily in the workplaces of America, where English Only policies are enforced to maintain the powerful hearers' view that good workers speak English among themselves and refrain from other, inappropriate, languages.

If you speak another language and consider yourself bilingual, do you sense a shift in personality when you switch languages?

2   Read the following excerpt from A. Patel, *Slang Words: What Are Young People Saying These Days?* (2012):

"Moss," "merked," "reach" and "dip." If you have no idea what those words mean, don't beat yourself up too much—this is just everyday teenage lingo. Teens tend to have a language of their own, but if you feel like infiltrating the crowd (or even just trying to understand some tweets), we have a guide to help you sort through the jargon. And with the holidays just around the corner, it could be useful to pick up a few key phrases to blend in with the younger folks at your holiday dinner—without looking completely out of place. Last year, our teenage slang list included words and phrases like "epic fail," "photobomb" and "lipdub," which just goes to show that some things never change—they just get reused over and over again. But 2012 also brought about mainstream recognition for a few words, like "f-bomb," "seting," "bucket list" and the Oprah-inspired "aha moment," which were all added to the Merriam-Webster Dictionary's 2012 list.

Do you know any of the slang items mentioned? If so, explain them in your own words.

3   Identify the source language and original meaning from which the following names are derived.

(a) Christopher
(b) Danielle
(c) Alexander
(d) Sarah
(e) Jamal
(f) Lucy
(g) Laura
(h) Hugh

4   Identify the source and meanings of the following surnames.

(a) Rivers
(b) Singer
(c) Cardinal
(d) Dickenson
(e) Woods
(f) Fox
(g) Hill
(h) Bergman

5   What aspects of contemporary English speech (words, phrases, mannerisms, protocols) would you consider to be part of hip talk?

6   Read the following excerpt from F. Grosjean, *Life as a Bilingual: Living with Two Languages* (2011):

> Bilingual 1 "When I'm around Anglo-Americans, I find myself awkward and unable to choose my words quickly enough... . When I'm amongst Latinos/Spanish-speakers, I don't feel shy at all. I'm witty, friendly, and ... I become very out-going."
>
> Bilingual 2 "In English, my speech is very polite, with a relaxed tone, always saying "please" and "excuse me." When I speak Greek, I start talking more rapidly, with a tone of anxiety and in a kind of rude way... ."
>
> Bilingual 3 "I find when I'm speaking Russian I feel like a much more gentle, 'softer' person. In English, I feel more 'harsh,' 'businesslike'."

> Could it be that bilinguals who speak two (or more) languages change their personality when they change language? After all, the Czech proverb does say, "Learn a new language and get a new soul."
>
> Do you think that speaking one of their languages makes a bilingual feel differently?

7   Read the following excerpt from M. Warschauer, *Language, Identity and the Internet* (2000):

> As it turns out, though, the fears of an English-dominated Internet were premature. Recent analysis indicates that the number of non-English websites is growing rapidly and that many of the more newly active Internet newsgroups (e.g., soc.culture.vietnamese) extensively use the national language (Graddol 1997: 61). Indeed, by one account the proportion of English in computer-based communication is expected to fall from its high of 80 percent to approximately 40 percent within the next decade (Graddol 1997). Underlying this change of direction is a more general shift from globalization to relocalization. The first wave of globalization—whether in economics or in media—witnessed vertical control from international centers, as witnessed for example by the rise of media giants such as CNN and MTV. But in more recent waves, a process of relocalization is occurring, as corporations seek to maximize their market share by shaping their products for local conditions. Thus, while CNN and MTV originally broadcast around the world in English, they are now producing editions in Hindi, Spanish, and other languages in order to compete with other international and regional media outlets.

> Do you think that the use of English on the Internet has diminished, as the author maintains? If so, what language do you think would be used in the two following situations?

(a) CMC between an English speaker and a speaker of another language who knows English.

(b) CMC between speakers of different languages, but who know English to some degree.

8 Read the following excerpt from T. Grant, *The Linguistic Cues That Reveal Your True Twitter Identity* (2013):

Twitter is awash with trolls, spammers and misanthropes, all keen to ruin your day with a mean-spirited message or even a threat that can cause you genuine fear. It seems all too easy to set up an account and cause trouble anonymously, but an emerging field of research is making it easier to track perpetrators by looking at the way they use language when they chat. The first Twitter criminal? The #TwitterJokeTrial was an early, if unfortunate, example of an apparent Twitter crime. Paul Chambers, frustrated at being prevented from visiting his girlfriend when snow disrupted transport, tweeted: "Crap! Robin Hood airport is closed. You've got a week and a bit to get your shit together otherwise I'm blowing the airport sky high!" Chambers was at first prosecuted for sending a message of "menacing character," but he later raised a successful appeal against his conviction. The message was nevertheless clear: be careful what you write, either be nice or be anonymous. Anonymous virtue? We've learned from these incidents that if you want to say something controversial or aggressive on Twitter, you'd probably better do it from an account not tied to your real name. The perceived anonymity of Twitter trolls seemed to facilitate the trolling attacks experienced by Caroline Criado-Perez and Stella Creasy MP this summer. Criado-Perez and Creasy had been running a campaign to have a woman represented on UK bank notes, and so became subject to a vitriolic misogynist attack, all via the medium of Twitter. In this case, policing has led to arrests, despite the fact that trolls opened multiple accounts to hide their identities when conducting their attacks.

If you are on Twitter, what linguistic cues do you use to identify yourself?

9 Do you think that linguistic identity is being recast in virtual spaces or is it the same identity that is being managed differently?

10 How would you characterize your own linguistic identity? If you have acquired a language other than English in childhood, point out some of its characteristics that make it unique and thus "personal" for you.

Chapter 6

1 Identify what is conversationally anomalous in each statement.

Example: Greetings Mother, see you later

Greetings normally indicate making contact, not leavetaking. It is anomalous in the above utterance, unless of course it is intended to be facetious or ironic.

(a) Madam, I gotta split!
(b) Gina, I wish to inform you that I am in love with you.
(c) Little guy, could you indicate to me what your name is?
(d) Hey little doggie, would you mind coming over here?

2   Identify each utterance as locutionary, illocutionary, or perlocutionary.

(a) Really?
(b) It's not true.
(c) My friend lives in Italy.
(d) Tell me all that you know.
(e) Quiet!
(f) What time is it?
(g) My name is Alexander.

3   How would a 17-year-old say hello to the following people?

(a) A peer
(b) A teacher
(c) Their mother or father

4   Identify the anaphoric and cataphoric devices in each of the following.

(a) Claudia likes the album I bought her yesterday.
(b) I gave it to Sarah, that is, the cup.
(c) Who ate the slice? I ate it.
(d) When did you go to Venice? I went there five years ago.

5   Make the following utterances more appropriate conversationally, using appropriate anaphoric and cataphoric devices.

(a) My sister went downtown yesterday. My sister ran into a teacher of my sister at one of the stores that my sister went to. My sister greeted the teacher and the teacher greeted my sister. My sister had not expected to see the teacher downtown, because my sister thought that the teacher never went downtown.
(b) Even though my brother will deny it, my brother is in love with Victoria. Victoria is likewise in love with my brother. But Victoria does not know yet that she is in love with my brother. My brother and Victoria go to the same school. Victoria wants to become a doctor; and my brother, even though my brother is good at math, wants to become a lawyer.

(c) Mack loves Julie. Yesterday Mack saw Julie, as Julie was walking on the street. Mack has known Julie for four years, and now Mack is in love with Julie. Mack called out to Julie, and then Mack gave Julie a kiss. Mack gave Julie a kiss because Mack loves Julie. But Julie doesn't love Mack, so Julie did not appreciate the kiss.

6   Read the following excerpts.

From P. ten Have, *Conversational Analysis Versus Other Approaches to Discourse* (2006):

The term "conversation analysis" (CA) is by now quite firmly established as the name for a particular paradigm in the study of verbal interaction that was initiated in the 1960s by Harvey Sacks, in collaboration with Emanuel Schegloff and Gail Jefferson. In CA the focus is on the procedural analysis of talk-in-interaction, how participants systematically organize their interactions to solve a range of organizational problems, such as the distribution of turns at talking, the collaborative production of particular actions, or problems of understanding. The analysis is always based on audio or visual recordings of interaction, which are carefully transcribed in detail.

From R. Wooffitt, *Conversation Analysis and Discourse Analysis* (2005):

Discourse analysis emerged in the sociology of scientific knowledge. It established a departure from realist accounts of scientists' actions to a study of scientists' accounting practices. It proposes that language is used variably. Accounts are constructed from a range of descriptive possibilities, and are intimately tied to the context in which they are produced and the functions they perform.

From P. ten Have, *Conversational Analysis Versus Other Approaches to Discourse* (2006):

The DA story, however, is completely different. In the larger sense of the term, there is an enormous variety of approaches, but not a relatively stable core set of ideas and methods. For DA, in the restricted sense as used by Wooffitt, the core idea is the intention to shift focus from the referents of discourse (for instance, a mental state such as cognition), to the discursive practices through which such referents are invoked.

From A. Gentle, *Twitter and Conversation Analysis—ho's Here?* (2009):

I believe that phone conversations for customer support have been studied quite a bit—looking for phrases that sound like triggers for anger, avoiding long pauses, and when one party overtakes a phone conversation, it's relatively easy to detect when that's happening. But with Twitter, you could have long pauses intentionally as asynchronous, IM-like conversations happen when someone gets up from their desk and returns after a business meeting, for example. Neither party is angry about that long pause, it's just an understood agreement in the Twitter medium that you may or may not be immediately responsive. How does that time factor change the "agreement" for a support exchange? Is Twitter reserved for the narcissistic whiners? Or are true relationships happening and caring, meaningful attention being paid to customers on Twitter?

Discuss the following:

(a) How is CA different from DA (discourse analysis)?
(b) What aspects of communicative competence are involved in conversations?
(c) What features of tweets are particularly interesting from a CA/DA perspective?

7   How would you rephrase the following utterances in a formal (polite) way?

Example: Come here and hurry up! → Would you mind coming here quickly?

(a) Get over here!
(b) Get lost!
(c) Give me a cup of coffee right away!
(d) You stink at telling jokes.
(e) You are rude. Cut it out!
(f) Leave me alone!

8   Identify the type of gambit used in the following utterances, along with its function:

(a) Yeah ... yeah ...
(b) I get it, you know?
(c) You agree, don't you?
(d) Allow me ...

9   Identify the communicative function(s) of each utterance. Use Jakobson's typology.

(a) Hi, Claudia. How are you?
(b) I've got a headache!
(c) See you tomorrow!
(d) Good morning.
(e) Good night.

(f) I don't like opera.
(g) Do you like Ike, as they used to say?
(h) The meaning of that word is "loving."
(i) Main Street is two blocks north of here.

10 Give examples of utterances that might be used for the following functions:

(a) instrumental
(b) regulatory
(c) interactional
(d) personal
(e) heuristic
(f) imaginative
(g) representational
(h) performative
(i) socialization

11 What aspects of gesture and facial expression do you think are crucial in F2F communication? How are these transported to online communication?

Chapter 7

1 Can you identify any modern-day pictographs or ideographs used in public signs?
2 Create your own pictographs or ideographs (as appropriate) for each of the following things:

(a) sky
(b) child
(c) love
(d) justice

3 Trace the pictographic origins of the following alphabet characters, providing a possible explanation for how each pictograph became an alphabet character:

(a) B
(b) C
(c) D
(d) I
(e) S

4 Below are some abbreviations. Do you know what they stand for? If so, explain the technique used in each case (acronymy, syllable reduction, and so on).

(a) AM
(b) ad
(c) aka
(d) BA
(e) PhD
(f) BBQ
(g) e.g.
(h) i.e.
(i) CEO
(j) email
(k) FAQ
(l) n/a
(m) UN

5 Many contemporary brands use names imitating online style to increase their appeal. How many brand names do you know that use such a style? For each one, indicate what aspect of online style was utilized.

6 The following words referring to months and days of the week have a mythic origin. Using an etymological dictionary, identify the mythical source for each one:

(a) January
(b) February
(c) Monday
(d) Tuesday
(e) Wednesday
(f) Thursday
(g) Friday
(h) Saturday

7 Read the following excerpt from F. de Saussure, *Course in General Linguistics* (1916):

Nearly all institutions, it might be said, are based on signs, but these signs do not directly evoke things. In all societies we find this phenomenon: that for various purposes systems of signs are established that directly evoke the ideas one wishes; it is obvious that a language is one such system, and that it is the most important of them all; but it is not the only one, and consequently we cannot leave the others out of account. A language must thus be classed among semiological institutions; for example, ships' signals (visual signs), army bugle calls, the sign language of the hearing-impaired, etc. Writing is likewise a vast system of signs. Any psychology of sign systems will be part of social psychology, that is to say, will be exclusively social; it will involve the same psychology as is applicable in the case of languages. The laws governing changes in these systems of signs will often be significantly similar to laws of linguistic change. This can easily be seen in the case of writing although the signs are visual signs which undergo alterations comparable to phonetic phenomena.

Saussure discusses signs as part of *semiology* (also called *semiotics*). Do you know what this discipline is? How is it related to linguistics? Would you say that the sociolinguistic study of writing and literacy is really a semiotic enterprise, or not?

8   Read the following excerpt from A. Hudson, *Outline of a Theory of Diglossia* (2002):

Gumperz's intermediate societies resemble quite closely Sjoberg's "pre-industrialized civilized societies," in which the bulk of the written tradition consists mainly of the society's sacred writings, and where writing is restricted to, and is perpetuated by, a small, educated, priestly group (Sjoberg 1964: 892). As a result, "the upper status, educated group typically employs at least two speech styles, in some cases more," all of which "differ from the speech of the common man—in the lexicon and often the phonology and grammar" (Sjoberg 1964: 893). Furthermore, the formal speech style "tends to be perpetuated over centuries with relatively little change, a phenomenon that results from the high prestige accorded it and its close tie with the written language" (Sjoberg 1964: 893).

Hudson suggests that literacy was once connected with sacredness and authority figures. Would you say that it has retained this function somewhat today, living in a secular world? Who are the authority figures today that espouse a form of literacy that we might want to emulate?

9   How is literacy valued today, in comparison to literacy in the age of print?
10 Read the following excerpt from S. Ali Dansieh, *SMS Texting and Its Potential Impacts on Students' Written Communication Skills* (2011):

As more and more students worldwide acquire and use mobile phones, so are they immersing themselves in text messaging. Such is the situation that some teachers, parents and students themselves are expressing concerns that student writing skills stand the risk of being sacrificed on the altar of text messaging. In view of the attested addictive effects of text messaging (Nokia 2002), caution must be exercised in encouraging students in its use. If not checked, students are likely to get so used to it that they may no longer realise the need for Standard English constructions even in writings that are supposed to be formal, a phenomenon O'Connor (2005) describes as "saturation." Be that as it may, it is important to eschew complacency and rather adopt conscious and pragmatic measures now so as to prevent the phenomenon from further worsening students' writing skills. All efforts must therefore be made to help students write good English whether on phone on paper.

The author takes a negative view of netlingo, backing it up with his own empirical findings. What is your take on the debate? Is texting changing literacy for the worse, or is it just another form of literacy?

11 Emoji are now part of everyday informal communications. List some of their functions, in addition to the ones indicated in the chapter.

12 Why do you think that emoji are now interpreted differentially, i.e., in a way unlike what Unicode intended?

Chapter 8

1 How many names do you know for dogs? Give the social meaning that each one elicits.

2 Make a list of the emotion(s) designated by the given color terms in English, giving a probable reason why the terms and the emotions were linked in the first place.

Example: green = envy (*You're green with envy*)

Possible reason: Green is the color of grass and an associated English proverb, "The grass is greener on the other side," may indicate that one envies what someone else has:

(a) red
(b) green
(c) yellow
(d) blue
(e) pink

3 Compare the specialized vocabularies for the categories below in any language you know other than English with the latter (English):

(a) kinship
(b) occupations
(c) plants
(d) animal
(e) spatial terms

4 Using componential analysis, establish the least number of features that will be needed to keep the following set of kinship words distinct in English:

(a) mother
(b) father
(c) son

(d) daughter
(e) brother
(f) sister
(g) grandfather
(h) grandmother
(i) uncle
(j) aunt
(k) cousin

5 Read the following excerpt from B. L. Whorf, *Language, Thought, and Reality* (1956):

When linguists became able to examine critically and scientifically a large number of languages of widely different patterns, their base of reference was expanded; they experienced an interruption of phenomena hitherto held universal, and a whole new order of significances came into their ken. It was found that the background linguistic system (in other words, the grammar) of each language is not merely a reproducing instrument for voicing ideas but rather is itself the shaper of ideas, the program and guide for people's mental activity, for their analysis of impressions, for their synthesis of their mental stock in trade. Formulation of ideas is not an independent process, strictly rational in the old sense, but is part of a particular grammar and differs, from slightly to greatly, among different grammars. We dissect nature along lines laid down by our native languages. The categories and types that we isolate from the world of phenomena we do not find there because they stare every observer in the face; on the contrary, the world is presented in a kaleidoscopic flux of impressions which has to be organized by our minds—and this means largely by the linguistic systems in our minds. We cut nature up, organize it into concepts, and ascribe significances as we do, largely because we are parties to an agreement to organize it in this way—an agreement that holds throughout our speech community and is codified in the patterns of our language. The agreement is, of course, an implicit and unstated one, but its terms are absolutely obligatory; we cannot talk at all except by subscribing to the organization and classification of data which the agreement decrees.

Summarize Whorf's ideas in your own words.
6 Can you give examples of words in other languages that cannot be translated into English and are thus borrowed? One example would be the French word *naïve*.
7 Give examples of specialized words in English that reflect modern-day living, as, for example, vocabulary associated with computers, fashion, and cars.

8   Read the following excerpt from G. Wrisley, *Rules, Language, and Reality* (2014):

> Language plays an enormously important role in our interaction with other people and with the world. We employ various words and concepts to talk about objects (tables and flowers), properties (colors and shapes), and relations (the flower is on the table, the pain is in my arm). We express feelings, ask questions, give commands, tell jokes, tell stories, sing songs, and so on. So let's return to our initial questions: How is that we're able to do all of these things with language? How is it that certain signs, symbols, and sounds are meaningful, and what exactly is their meaning? Is the word "cat" meaningful because of what it refers to—namely, those furry, meowing fleabags many of us have as pets? Is the meaning of "cat" just those animals themselves? Further, does the world determine what our concepts are to be? That is, with language do we simply try to mirror the various kinds of objects, properties, and relations that exist, or is the world "open" to different ways of conceptualizing it?

> Do you think reality is filtered by the categories of language?

9   The counterargument to the Whorfian Hypothesis is that each language encodes the same reality with different forms. Do you agree?

10 Read the following excerpt from F. Wei, W. K. Wang, and M. Klausner, *Rethinking College Students' Self-Regulation and Sustained Attention: Does Text Messaging During Class Influence Cognitive Learning?* (2012):

> Students' texting during class emerged as a partial mediator of the effect of self-regulation on sustained attention. The results showed that college students' self-regulation was negatively related to their text messaging use during class, which in turn was negatively related to their sustained attention to classroom learning, meaning that college students who possess a high level of self-regulation are less likely to text during class and are more likely to sustain their attention to classroom learning.

> Do you think that text messaging in class affects your thought processes?

Chapter 9

1   Design a study of your own, using any technique you think is appropriate, to gather data on netlingo or on emoji uses.
2   Design a study on any twitterlect to determine how it is used in a particular Twitter community.
3   What social practices do you think Twitter allows people to carry out?
4   Make a list of expressions that you use in online conversations and explain what each one means and why you use it.

5   Do you think that digital forms of language are affecting literacy negatively? If so, how so? If not, why not?

6   Do you believe that there is a synergy between online and offline communication? How do they affect one another?

7   How would you design a language for communication with extraterrestrials? Explain its features.

8   Now that you have gone through the course, give ways that you envision for using your new knowledge constructively.

Appendices

A The International Phonetic Alphabet

Alphabet characters do not always provide a consistent guide to the actual pronunciation of the sounds in words. For example, the /f/ sound in English is written in one of three ways—as *f* in *fish*, as *ph* in *phone*, and as *gh* in *tough*. Such inconsistencies in spelling are what led nineteenth-century linguists to devise a special and standardized system of notation, known as the International Phonetic Alphabet (IPA), in which one distinct symbol always stands for one and only one sound.

The IPA classifies a sound according to its particular articulatory characteristics, that is, according to how it is produced with the vocal organs (the mouth, the tongue, the teeth, and so on). For example, the symbol [f], put between square brackets (to distinguish it from the corresponding alphabet character *f*, even if they are the same) is the one used by the IPA to indicate the sound represented vicariously by the letters *f, ph,* and *gh* in the above words. Because the lower lip touches the upper teeth in the pronunciation of this sound, it is called a labiodental consonant; because it is produced by forcing the air from the lungs through the slit made by the lower lip touching the upper teeth, it is also called a *fricative*; and finally because the vocal cords in the throat are not vibrating as we produce it (compare /f/ in *fine* to /v/ in *vine* by putting your fingers over the throat), it is called *voiceless*. So, to summarize, the phonetic symbol [f] stands for a *voiceless labiodental fricative: fish* = [fiš], *phone* = [fon], *tough* = [taf]. If the [f] sound allows us to distinguish the meaning of words, as for example, *fine* from *vine*, it is then assigned "phonemic" status, indicated with slant lines: /f/. A phoneme is a sound that cues meaning differences in words.

The symbols in the IPA chart stand for the articulatory features of each sound. You will likely never have to use all the symbols, or even to understand what sounds they stand for precisely. However, a basic familiarity with phonetics may come in handy if you are going to conduct research on the relation between speech sounds and social behaviors or relations. The IPA chart is reproduced here for convenience.

THE INTERNATIONAL PHONETIC ALPHABET (revised to 2005)

CONSONANTS (PULMONIC) © 2005 IPA

	Bilabial	Labiodental	Dental	Alveolar	Postalveolar	Retroflex	Palatal	Velar	Uvular	Pharyngeal	Glottal
Plosive	p b			t d		ʈ ɖ	c ɟ	k ɡ	q ɢ		ʔ
Nasal	m	ɱ		n		ɳ	ɲ	ŋ	ɴ		
Trill	ʙ			r					ʀ		
Tap or Flap		ⱱ		ɾ		ɽ					
Fricative	ɸ β	f v	θ ð	s z	ʃ ʒ	ʂ ʐ	ç ʝ	x ɣ	χ ʁ	ħ ʕ	h ɦ
Lateral fricative				ɬ ɮ							
Approximant		ʋ		ɹ		ɻ	j	ɰ			
Lateral approximant				l		ɭ	ʎ	ʟ			

Where symbols appear in pairs, the one to the right represents a voiced consonant. Shaded areas denote articulations judged impossible.

CONSONANTS (NON-PULMONIC)

Clicks		Voiced implosives		Ejectives	
ʘ	Bilabial	ɓ	Bilabial	ʼ	Examples:
ǀ	Dental	ɗ	Dental/alveolar	pʼ	Bilabial
ǃ	(Post)alveolar	ʄ	Palatal	tʼ	Dental/alveolar
ǂ	Palatoalveolar	ɠ	Velar	kʼ	Velar
ǁ	Alveolar lateral	ʛ	Uvular	sʼ	Alveolar fricative

OTHER SYMBOLS

ʍ Voiceless labial-velar fricative
w Voiced labial-velar approximant
ɥ Voiced labial-palatal approximant
ʜ Voiceless epiglottal fricative
ʢ Voiced epiglottal fricative
ʡ Epiglottal plosive

ɕ ʑ Alveolo-palatal fricatives
ɺ Voiced alveolar lateral flap
ɧ Simultaneous ʃ and x

Affricates and double articulations can be represented by two symbols joined by a tie bar if necessary.

k͡p t͡s

VOWELS

Front Central Back

Close i • y — ɨ • ʉ — ɯ • u
ɪ ʏ ʊ
Close-mid e • ø — ɘ • ɵ — ɤ • o
ə
Open-mid ɛ • œ — ɜ • ɞ — ʌ • ɔ
æ ɐ
Open a • ɶ — ɑ • ɒ

Where symbols appear in pairs, the one to the right represents a rounded vowel.

SUPRASEGMENTALS

ˈ	Primary stress	
ˌ	Secondary stress	ˌfoʊnəˈtɪʃən
ː	Long	eː
ˑ	Half-long	eˑ
˘	Extra-short	ĕ
	Minor (foot) group	
‖	Major (intonation) group	
.	Syllable break	ɹi.ækt
‿	Linking (absence of a break)	

DIACRITICS Diacritics may be placed above a symbol with a descender, e.g. ŋ̊

̥	Voiceless	n̥ d̥		̤	Breathy voiced	b̤ a̤		̪	Dental	t̪ d̪
̬	Voiced	s̬ t̬		̰	Creaky voiced	b̰ a̰		̺	Apical	t̺ d̺
ʰ	Aspirated	tʰ dʰ		̼	Linguolabial	t̼ d̼		̻	Laminal	t̻ d̻
̹	More rounded	ɔ̹		ʷ	Labialized	tʷ dʷ		̃	Nasalized	ẽ
̜	Less rounded	ɔ̜		ʲ	Palatalized	tʲ dʲ		ⁿ	Nasal release	dⁿ
̟	Advanced	u̟		ˠ	Velarized	tˠ dˠ		ˡ	Lateral release	dˡ
̠	Retracted	e̠		ˤ	Pharyngealized	tˤ dˤ		̚	No audible release	d̚
̈	Centralized	ë		̴	Velarized or pharyngealized	ɫ				
̽	Mid-centralized	ɛ̽		̝	Raised	e̝	(ɹ̝ = voiced alveolar fricative)			
̩	Syllabic	n̩		̞	Lowered	e̞	(β̞ = voiced bilabial approximant)			
̯	Non-syllabic	e̯		̘	Advanced Tongue Root	e̘				
˞	Rhoticity	ɚ a˞		̙	Retracted Tongue Root	e̙				

TONES AND WORD ACCENTS
LEVEL CONTOUR

é̋ or ˥	Extra high	ě or ˩˥	Rising
é or ˦	High	ê or ˥˩	Falling
ē or ˧	Mid	e᷄ or ˦˥	High rising
è or ˨	Low	e᷅ or ˩˨	Low rising
è̖ or ˩	Extra low	e᷈ or ˧˦˧	Rising-falling
↓	Downstep	↗	Global rise
↑	Upstep	↘	Global fall

Figure A.1 The International Phonetic Alphabet

B A Brief Lesson in Basic Statistics

Let us assume that a sociolinguist has interviewed 25 subjects, asking them to rate, on a scale of 0 to 5, what influence they think text messaging has on the language they use offline, with 5 indicating that it has a definite effect and 0 no effect. At the end of the interview period, let's assume that the researcher has collected the following ratings, in no particular order:

1, 2, 0, 4, 1, 3, 3, 1, 2, 0, 4, 5, 2, 3, 2, 3, 2, 4, 1, 2, 3, 0, 2, 3, 1

Clearly, from looking at the ratings little seems to jut out from them. A better sense of what they indicate can be gained by grouping them into a table that lists each different rating (x) and its frequency (f) of occurrence. Such a table is called a *frequency distribution* (see Table A.1 below).

We can now easily see that there are three 0 ratings, five 1 ratings, and so on. We note that most of the subjects (7 + 6 = 13) rated the influence at 2 or 3. If we take the average of the two, we get 2.5. This is called the *central tendency* or *central location* of the distribution. The most frequently used measure of central tendency is the arithmetic average, or *mean*. The *mode* and the *median* are two other useful measures. The mode is the value that occurs most frequently. In our data it is 2 because the number 2 occurs seven times. The median is the middle value in the data. In our example, there are 25 values. If they are laid out in sequence (in order of increasing value from left to right), the median is the thirteenth number, which is 2 (see Figure A.2).

Determining the median in this case is easy to do because the total number, 25, is odd, making it possible to divide the set evenly into 12 before the middle number and 12 after. If there is an even number of values, then the median is the average of the two middle values.

The *mean* is calculated by summing all the values in the data and then dividing the sum by the number of values (25). If we do this with the set above the result is 2.16. The formula used to determine the mean reads as follows: x̄ = mean, N = number of scores in a set, x = an individual score, Σ x = sum of all the scores:

$$\bar{x} = \frac{\sum x}{N}$$

Table A.1 Frequency Distribution

x	f
0	3
1	5
2	7
3	6
4	3
5	1
	25

0, 0, 0, 1, 1, 1, 1, 1, 2, 2, 2, 2,   2,   2, 2, 3, 3, 3, 3, 3, 3, 4, 4, 4, 5

twelve   ↑   twelve

median

Figure A.2 Identifying the Median

As this simple example shows, the median, mode, and mean are typically close to each other in value. This is particularly so if the dataset is large enough or if it is truly representative. However, for most purposes the mean is probably the best method for determining the central tendency of a set of data.

Central tendency tells us very little in itself, unless we know how it relates to the individual values in the dataset. Are most values clustered tightly around the mean? Are they spread out? The spread of the values in a frequency distribution is called *dispersion*. The simplest measure of dispersion is the *range*. This is, simply, the largest score minus the smallest one. In our sample, the range is $5 - 0 = 5$. A related question is: How much dispersion is there in the data? The rating of 3 is close in value to the mean of 2.16; more specifically, it is $3 - 2.16 = 0.4$ units from the mean; contrariwise, the value of 0 is $5 - 0 = 5$ units from the mean. It we add up all these "deviations from the mean," and divide them by the total number (25), we get an average value of the deviations in the data. This is called the *standard deviation*.

The greater the standard deviation, the less reliable the data; the more the standard deviation clusters around the mean the more significant are the findings. Statistical tests have been developed to determine the significance level of the standard deviation. Let us go through schematically how the standard deviation is calculated.

First, we compute how much each rating deviates from the mean of 2.16. For example, a rating of 3 deviates from 2.16 by $3 - 2.16 = 0.84$ and the rating of 1 deviates from 2.16 by $1 - 2.16 = -1.16$. To eliminate the negative results, we can perform a clever maneuver. We simply square all the scores, which we need not do here. Then we take the average of these deviations, thus producing a "mean of deviations." Now, the reverse of squaring is taking the square root (remember that we squared the individual deviations simply to eliminate the minus signs). The result is 2.12. To summarize, the formula for computing the standard deviation is found using: SD = standard deviation, $(x - \bar{x})^2$ = the difference between each score (x) and the mean ($\bar{x}$) squared in order to eliminate the negative signs, $\Sigma (x - \bar{x})^2$ = the sum of all the differences, $\sqrt{}$ = square root of the sum, N = the total number of scores:

$$SD = \sqrt{\frac{\sum(x - \bar{x})^2}{N}}$$

The standard deviation tells us that, on average, a rating in the data will deviate from the mean by 2.12. Now: Is there some statistical test that will indicate that the same or similar result will ensue from some future experiment? There are several *significance tests* at our disposal to determine this. Their mathematical intricacies need not be described here, since these are available in basic handbooks of statistical methods. The main significance tests for the purposes of socio-linguistic analysis are the *t-test*, the *Chi square test, correlation analysis,* and *ANOVA*.

Box A.1 Basic Significance Tests

T-test: Test for comparing the means of two samples, even if they have different numbers of subjects. It compares the actual difference between two means in relation to the variation in the data (the standard deviation of the difference between the means).

Chi square: Test used to compare observed or collected data with data we would expect to obtain according to a specific hypothesis.

Correlation: Measure of the extent to which two or more variables collected from a research study fluctuate or vary together. A positive correlation indicates the degree to which the variables increase or decrease in parallel; a negative correlation indicates the opposite, namely the extent to which one variable increases as the other decreases.

ANOVA: Technique that allows the analyst to determine significance between sample groups with respect to a specific variable. ANOVA permits us to break up the sample according to the variable and then see if the result is different across samples.

C Koasati Phonemes and Alphabet (www.omniglot.com/writing/ koasati.htm)

Vowels										
a	a:/aa	i	i:/ii	o	o:/oo	u/oo	u:/uu	ą/a	į/i	ǫ/o
[a]	[a:]	[i]	[i:]	[o]	[o:]	[u]	[u:]	[ã]	[ĩ]	[õ]

Consonants								
b	c/ch	d	f/fh	h	k	l	ł/lh	
[b]	[t͡ʃʰ]	[d]	[Φ]	[h; ɦ]	[kʰ]	[l]	[ɬ]	
m	n	p	[s/š]	t	w	y	'	
[m]	[n]	[pʰ]	[s~ʃ]	[tʰ]	[w]	[j]	[ʔ]	

Figure C.1 Koasati Phonemes and Alphabet

D English Vowels

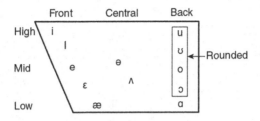

Figure D.1 English Vowels

Vowels are described in terms of the position of the tongue on its vertical (high, mid, low) or horizontal axis (front, central, back). For example, the front of the tongue is moved from low to high in pronouncing the vowel in the word *beet*, and the back of the tongue is raised in pronouncing the vowel in *boot*.

The quality of a vowel depends on whether the lips are rounded or unrounded, close together or open, or the tip of the tongue is flat or curled up (*retroflex*). In some languages, vowels can take on the quality of any nasal consonant that surrounds them in words. For instance, in French, the vowel [a] becomes nasalized, shown with the symbol [ã], before a nasal consonant—for example, the word *gant* ("glove") is pronounced [gã].

Glossary

accommodation theory   view that people adapt their speech characteristics to the situation in which they are communicating

acronym word   created from the first letters of other words; NATO is an acronym for North Atlantic Treaty Organization

adaptor   a gesture, such as head scratching, that indicates some need or state of mind

addressee   intended receiver of a verbal message

addresser   initiator of a verbal message

adjacency pair   two expressions that are found often together in conversations as part of turn taking, e.g. *What's your name?* is normally followed by *My name is ...*

affix   morpheme that is added to another morpheme, usually a root morpheme, such as /ir-/ in *irregular* and /-al/ in *national*

affricate   composite speech sound produced by a stop immediately followed by a fricative; the *ch* in *church* and the *j* in *junk*, represented phonemically by /č/ and /ǧ/ respectively

agglutinative language   language such as Turkish in which the words are constructed with more than one morpheme; the Turkish word *evlerinizden* ("from your houses") consists of the morphemes /ev-ler-iniz-den/ meaning, respectively, "house-plural-your-from"

allomorph   variant of a morpheme, and thus the actual form that a morpheme takes in a phrase /a/ and /an/ are allomorphs of the indefinite article, with /a/ used before a noun or adjective beginning with a consonant (*a boy, a new girl*) and /an/ before a noun or adjective beginning with a vowel (*an egg, an interesting hat*)

allophone   variant of a phoneme, the actual form that a phoneme takes in a word; the [l] and [ł] sounds are allophones of /l/: the latter occurs at the end of syllables and words (*will, bill*), and the former occurs in any other position within a word (*love, life*)

alphabet   system of symbols, known as letters or characters, whereby each symbol stands for a sound (or sounds) in spoken words

alveolar   sound produced when the tongue touches the area just above the upper teeth; the *t* in *trip* represented phonetically by /ţ/

alveopalatal sound produced when the tongue touches the area above the upper teeth where the hard palate begins; the *sh* in *shape*, represented by /š/

anaphoric word or particle that refers back to a word uttered or written previously in a sentence or text; *he* in *Alex says that he likes baseball*

ANOVA statistical method for analyzing variance in data

Antonym word with the opposite meaning of another word; *night* is the antonym of *day*, and vice versa

argot slang of specialized groups, especially criminal ones

asynchronous communication communication that takes place over time (not simultaneously)

bilabial sound produced by bringing both lips into contact with each other; the *p* in *pin* and the *b* in *bin*, represented phonemically by /p/ and /b/ respectively

bilingualism the use of two languages by an individual, group, or nation

borrowing process of adopting a word from another language, for general use; Italian has borrowed the word *sport* from English and English has borrowed the word *naïve* from French

bound morpheme morpheme that must be attached to another morpheme; /un-/ and /-ly/ in *unlikely*

calque word-by-word translation of a foreign phrase or expression; the title *The Brothers Karamazov* is a calque of the corresponding Russian phrase (the word order in English should be *The Karamazov Brothers*)

cant type of secretive slang used especially by criminal organizations

case form of a noun, pronoun, or adjective that indicates its syntactic relation to other words in a sentence; *he* is in the nominative (subject) case, while *him* is in the accusative (object) case

case study study that examines a particular manifestation of a phenomenon

cataphoric device word or particle that anticipates a word in a sentence or paragraph; *he* in *Although he likes Italy, Alex is not going there this year*

central tendency the main characteristic of a set of data

Chi-square test measure of how closely the frequency distribution of actual data matches that expected in theory

code switching alternating between two or more languages or varieties of language in conversation; typical speech characteristic of bilinguals

cognates words in different languages that are derived from the same source; Latin *pater* and English *father* come from the same original word in Indo-European

colloquialism word or expression that is not formal but used in ordinary conversation

communicative competence ability to use a language appropriately in social contexts

community of practice group of people who share a common goal or outlook and convey this through a common form of language

commutation test test comparing two forms that are alike in all respects except one, in order to see if a difference in meaning results; *pill-vs.-bill*

comparative grammar   early language science based on comparing forms in languages to see if they are related historically

complementary distribution   process whereby allophones of the same phoneme occur in different environments; in English [pʰ] occurs in word-initial position followed by a vowel (*pin, pill*), whereas [p] occurs in all other positions (*spin, spill, prize, cap*)

componential analysis   breaking down the meaning of words into smaller components; for example, *man is* [+male, +human], *lion is* [+male, -human]

conative function   effect a message has or is intended to have on its receiver

conceptual metaphor   generalized metaphorical formula; people are animals underlies *He's a dog* and *She's a tiger*

connotation   extensional meaning of a word; the meaning of *cool* as "attractive" rather than "fairly cold"

consonant   sound produced by means of some obstruction to the airstream emanating from the lungs; the *t* in *tough*, represented phonemically as /t/

contact   physical situation in which communication occurs

context   psychological, social, and emotional relations or situations that constrain the type of language used during communication

contrast   minimal difference between two elements; the /p/ in *pin* contrasts minimally with the /b/ in *bin*; the latter is voiced, the former is voiceless

conversation analysis   study of how conversations unfold

core vocabulary   basic vocabulary of a language, containing items such as *mother, father, son, daughter*

Creole   language that has developed from the mixture of two or more languages (a *pidgin*), becoming the first language of a group

critical period   period of childhood during which language is acquired spontaneously

cryptolect   language code used for secretive purposes

cuneiform   wedge-shaped writing used by various ancient Semitic societies that makes it possible to inscribe symbols on hard materials (such as stone)

data mining   extracting data from the Internet with appropriate algorithms

deixis   pointing out or indicating something; *up, down, here, there*

demotic   type of ancient writing that reflected everyday speech in Egypt and other areas

denotation   basic meaning of a word; the meaning of "small feline mammal" for *cat*

dental   sound produced when the tongue touches the teeth; the *d* (/d/) in *dove*

derivational morpheme   morpheme that is derived from some other morpheme; *cautiously* is derived from *cautious*

diachronic analysis   analysis of change in language

dialect   regional or social variant of a language

dialect atlas   atlas of maps showing language forms in specific regions

dialect continuum   range of dialects spoken over a given region

dialectology   study of dialects

dialogue conversation between people with a specific intent

difference minimal feature that distinguishes the meaning of forms, such as *pin* versus *bin*, whereby a single sound changes the meaning

diglossia the study of prestige in language variants within a given society

diphthong syllable containing two vowels pronounced as one segment; *quick, tweak*

discourse specific use of language in social or ideological ways

displacement evoking something not present through language

distinctive feature minimal trait in a form that serves to keep it distinct from other forms

double articulation notion that with a relatively small number of units (phonemes) one can make forms and meanings ad infinitum by combination

doublet pair of morphemes or lexemes that are associated with differential gender or class use

elaborated code notion that formal or standardized language is an elaborate social code

emotive function speaker's intent during discourse

empiricism view that we learn language from scratch through observation and imitation

ethnography method of collecting data by living among the subject group and interacting with the group in some direct way

ethnology another name for *ethnography*

ethnosemantics study of the relation between specific categories of language and cultural worldviews

face-to-face (F2F) vocal communication between interlocutors in real space

field the environment in which a speech act takes place

fieldwork research whereby the analyst collects data from the subjects

filler linguistic unit that serves a communicative function by filling otherwise silent points; *er, um*

flap sound produced by briefly striking the roof of the mouth; the *r* (r/) in *carrot*

FOXP2 gene that might be linked to a specific language impairment

frame analysis study of how communication involves presenting oneself in a specific way

free morpheme morpheme that can exist on its own; *cautious* in *cautiously*

free variation existence of two variant forms; the pronunciation of the /o/ in *tomato* as either open or close

frequency distribution the number of instances that variables take in a set of data

fricative sound produced by forcing the airstream through a narrow opening in the mouth; the *f* in *fish*, the *v* in *vine*, represented respectively as /f/ and /v/

function word word such as the *or* and that has grammatical function

gambit verbal strategy for initiating or maintaining discourse flow

genre   type of speech act, as for example, a joke or a story

gesticulant   gesture that accompanies vocal speech

gesture   communication involving hand movement

glide   sound produced by moving from one point of articulation to the next; the /w/ sound in *going*

glottal   sound produced by completely or partially closing the glottis; the /h/ in *house*

grammar   system of rules for the formation of words and sentences

ground   meaning of a metaphor

hedge   type of speech gambit that has various communicative functions (*like, ya' know*)

hieroglyphic   Egyptian pictographic and ideographic writing

homograph   word that is spelled the same as another but with a different meaning; *port* as in *The ship arrived at the port* vs. *Portuguese port is excellent wine*

homonym   word that is pronounced or spelled the same as another but with a different meaning; *learned* as in *I learned Spanish* and *learned* is in *She is a learned person*

homophone   word that is pronounced the same as another but with a different meaning; *aunt* vs. *ant*

honorific   word or expression indicating respect or class status (such as a title); *Prof., Madam, Dr.*

hypermedia   media involving multimodality and multimediality

hypertext   software system that links sites

hyponym   word that is inclusive of another; *rose* is an example of *flower*

iconic gesture   gesture accompanying vocal communication that shows the shape of something mentioned in the utterance

idealized cognitive model (ICM)   amalgam of source domains used to deliver a cultural concept

ideograph   pictograph that expresses an idea

idiolect   personal speech habits

illocutionary act   type of speech act that specifies a call to action; *Come here!* form that relates someone or something to something else in time and space; our surnames typically are indexes of our ethnic origins

infix   affix added internally in a morpheme; /-li-/ in *friendliness*

inflection   change in the form of a word; *spoken* is an inflection of *speak*

inflectional morpheme   morpheme that results from inflection

innatism   view that we are born with all we need to acquire a language

interdental   sound produced by putting the tongue between the teeth; *th* in *thing*, represented by /θ/

International Phonetic Alphabet (IPA)   the standard system of symbols used by linguists to transcribe sounds

intertexuality   texts that refer to other texts during conversation

interview   questioning subjects for experimental purposes

intonation   pitch and tone in language

irony word or statement used in such a way that it means the opposite of what it denotes; *What a beautiful day!* uttered on a stormy day

jargon slang of specialized groups (lawyers, doctors, mechanics)

labiodental sound produced by placing the upper teeth on the inside lower lip; *f* (/f/) in *funny*

language maintenance process of preserving a language or dialect

language planning legislation and official policies aiming to preserve standard languages

language shift movement away from one language to another

language spread the diffusion of one particular variant of a language over regions

langue theoretical knowledge of a language (its rules, its structure)

lateral sound produced by letting the tip off the tongue touch the alveolar ridge so that air can escape on the sides; *l* (/l/) in *love*

lexeme morpheme with lexical meaning; *logic* in *logical*

lexical field collection of lexemes that are interrelated thematically, such as sports vocabulary

lexicography science of dictionary making

lexicon set of morphemes in a language

lexicostatistics mathematical study of time depth, the length of time since two related languages became separated

lingua franca language adopted as a common language among speakers of different languages

linguistic competence abstract knowledge of a language

linguistic performance knowledge of how to use a language

linguistic profiling use of linguistic features to identify the race or ethnicity of speakers

linguistic relativity view that languages influence how people come to perceive the world

liquid consonant pronounced without friction; *l* in *love*, *r* in *right*, represented respectively as /l/ and /r/

literacy ability to read and write a language and to use it for formal expressive purposes

loanword word borrowed from another language; *cipher* was borrowed from Arabic

locutionary act speech act that entails a referential statement; *Her blouse is green*

manner of articulation how a sound is articulated

marked category form that is specific and not representative of an entire category

markedness theory that certain forms in language are basic and others derived from them

mean average in a set of data

median midpoint in a set of data

meme any bit of information that goes viral on the Internet

message   information or intent of a communication

metalingual function   language referring to language itself; *The word noun is a noun*

metaphor   process by which something abstract is rendered understandable by reference to something concrete; *Love is sweet*

metonymy   process whereby the part stands for the whole; the *White House* for "the American government"

minimal pair   pair of words such as *pill*-vs.-*bill* that differ by only one sound in the same position

mode   way in which language is used; sensory, vocal, or mechanical means of creating a message

morpheme   minimal unit of meaning; in *cautiously* there are two morphemes *cautious* and *ly*

morphology   level of language where words are formed

multilingualism   more than two languages used functionally by a particular society

multimedia   use of more than one medium to create a message (text, video, audio)

multimodality   use of various modes to create messages

mutual intelligibility   ability of speakers of the same dialect family to understand each other

myth   narrative recounting origins and various other features of early cultures in some imaginary way

name   word that identifies a person (and by extension animals, products)

nasal   sound produced by expelling the airstream partially through the nasal passage; *n* (/n//) in *near*

nativization   process whereby a loanword is reshaped phonetically to become indistinguishable from a native word

netlingo   online language with its particular compressed forms and other peculiarities

obstruent   sound produced with a degree of obstruction, such as consonants

occlusive (also *stop* or *plosive*)   sound produced by closure of the vocal tract; *p* (/p/) in *pop* and *t* in *tight*

onomastics   study of names

opposition   difference that keeps units distinct, such as the opposition between *night* and *day*

palatal   sound produced when the tongue touches the hard palate; *ch* in *chin*, represented phonemically by /č/

palatalization   process by which a sound becomes a palatal, or more like a palatal

parameter   feature of a specific language that is a manifestation of a more general innate principle

perlocutionary act   speech act that entails the request for some action; *Can you call me?*

phatic function use of language to make or maintain social contact; *How's it going?*

phone technical name for speech sound

phoneme minimal unit of sound that distinguishes meaning

phonemics study of the phonemic system of a language

phonetics description of how sounds are articulated

phonograph writing symbol that approximates the pronunciation of a sound in a word

phonology sound system of a language

phrase structure basic type of word arrangement in the construction of sentences

pictography use of pictures to represent things, ideas, actions, and so on

pidgin simplified language made up of elements of two or more languages

plosive another name for *occlusive*

poetic function type of speech pattern that aims to have an emotive effect; *roses are red, violets are blue*

point of articulation place in the mouth touched by the tongue (or other organs) where a sound is produced

pop language language spoken in the media and pop culture that has spread to society at large

poverty of the stimulus notion that children must already know a lot about language since they start talking simply by being exposed to partial and imperfect input

pragmatics general analysis of language use

prefix affix that is added before another morpheme; /il-/ in *illogical*

prosody set of tones and intonations used in language

protolanguage undocumented language that has been reconstructed

prototypical concept basic member of a *cat* is a prototypical member of the feline category

qualitative analysis research based on observation

quantitative analysis research based on statistical analysis

referent what a word refers to

referential function use of words to refer to something other than the words themselves

register style of language used in social situations

repair gambit for correcting a mistaken or inappropriate language form

restricted code code (usually dialectal) restricted to ingroup use

root morpheme morpheme with lexical meaning; *logic* in *logically*

segmental any vowel or consonant sound

segmentation decomposing a form or a phrase into its minimal elements; the word *illogically* can be segmented into /il-/, /logic/, /-al/, and /-ly/

semantics study of meaning in language

sentence minimal syntactic unit

sibilant a consonant that is produced as a hiss; *s* (/s/) in *sip* or the *z* (/z/) in *zip*

sign something that stands for something other than itself

slang　socially based variant of a language used by specific groups or produced by various popular media

sociolect　social dialect

sound symbolism　use of sounds to construct words in such a way that they resemble the sound properties of their referents or to bring out some sound-based perception of meaning; *crash* stands for the actual sound it refers to

source domain　concrete part of a conceptual metaphor; the *sweet* in *love is sweet*

specialized vocabulary　vocabulary used to describe specific things as part of a collectivity; color terms, sitting devices, and so on

speech　language as it is used vocally or in writing

speech act　specific use of language to imply an action

speech community　group of speakers of a language

speech network　group of speakers who relate to each other in interconnected ways

standard deviation　degree to which data cluster around the average

standard language　language that societies agree to use for formal purposes

standardization　process whereby a dialect or variant is turned into a standard language

stop　another name for *occlusive*

stress　degree of force used to pronounce a vowel

structuralism　type of analysis aiming to study language as a system of structures

style　distinctive form of language connected to some social system of meaning

subordinate concept　concept that provides detail; for example, *Siamese* details a type of *cat*

suffix　affix added to the end of a morpheme; /-ly/ in *logically*

supresegmental　feature used with a segment (vowel or consonant), such as tone or accent

syllabary　list of symbols representing syllables

syllable　minimal breath group in the pronunciation of words

synchronic analysis　study of language at a particular point in time, usually the present

synchronous communication　communication that occurs in real time

synecdoche　concept in which the part represents the whole; *head* in *head of the organization*

synonym　word that has the same (approximate) meaning as another word; *happy—content*

syntax　study of how phrases, clauses, sentences, and entire texts are organized

tag　word or phrase added to the end of a sentence to secure consent or approval; *You agree, don't you?*

target domain　topic of a conceptual metaphor; *love* in *love is sweet*

tenor topic of a metaphor; *professor* in *The professor is a sweetheart*

text any combination of sentences to produce a singular message

text message type of message created by some mobile device

topic what the metaphor is about; the *love* in *love is sweet*

toponym place name

t-test statistical test used to determine if the data have significance

tweet message on Twitter

twitterlect sociolect that emerges in some Twitter community

Universal Grammar set of rule-making principles present in the brain at birth that make up the language faculty

unmarked category default form in a class of forms

uvular sound produced in the area of the uvula (at the back of the throat); *ich* ("I") in German

variation process whereby forms vary according to geography, social class, individuals

vehicle concrete part of a metaphor; the *sweet* in *love is sweet*

velar sound produced with the back of the tongue close or in contact with the soft palate; *k* (/k/) in *kitchen*

vocabulary set of lexemes in a language

vocalization process by which a consonant is changed to a vowel

voiced sound produced by vibrating the vocal cords in the larynx; *z* (/z/) in *zip*

voiceless sound produced by keeping vocal cords taut in the larynx; *s* (/s/) in *sip*

voicing process whereby a voiceless consonant is voiced

vowel sound produced with no significant obstruction to the airstream

Whorfian Hypothesis theory that posits that a language predisposes its speakers to attend to certain aspects of reality as necessary

Zipf's Law claim that language forms are condensed, abbreviated, reduced, or eliminated to minimize the effort expended in producing and using them

Index

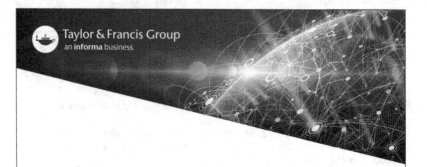

Printed in the United States
by Baker & Taylor Publisher Services